Documentation and Reimbursement for Long-Term Care

Ella James, BS, RHIT, CPHQ

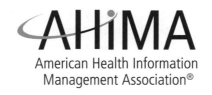

AHIMA
American Health Information
Management Association®

ISBN 1-58426-110-2
Product No. AB101804
IPC No. 1000-404

Michelle Dougherty, RHIA, Reviewer

American Health Information Management Association
233 North Michigan Avenue, Suite 2150
Chicago, Illinois 60601-5800

http://www.ahima.org

Contents

CD-ROM

About the Author

Ella James, BS, RHIT, CPHQ, is director of corporate health information management and health information security and the privacy officer at Hospital for Special Care in New Britain, Connecticut. The corporation, Center of Special Care, includes a 200-bed long-term acute hospital, a 280-bed skilled nursing facility, and specialty clinics in the community.

Ella is past president of the Connecticut Health Information Management Association and an American Health Information Management Association (AHIMA) Community of Practice (CoP) facilitator for long-term care. She also chairs the bylaws committee of AHIMA and is the coding task force coordinator for the National Association of Long Term Hospitals (NALTH).

Ella has presented programs on the Health Insurance Portability and Accountability Act (HIPAA) at the state, regional, and national levels, and has presented programs on long-term acute care coding for NALTH. An active member of the Connecticut Hospital Association Security Workgroup for HIPAA compliance, she also has served as a contributing author to *LTC Spectrum,* the former newsletter of the AHIMA long-term care section.

Ella is currently working toward her master's degree in healthcare administration at Saint Joseph's College in Maine.

Acknowledgments

The author and the AHIMA publications staff would like to extend their thanks to the following individuals for their time and help in making this publication a reality:

Jane Burster, RHIT, founder, Clinical Record Consultation, Tacoma, Washington, and part-time faculty, Tacoma Community College

Michelle Dougherty, RHIA, health information management practice manager, AHIMA, Chicago, Illinois

Deborah James, MBA, OTR/L, senior financial analyst, Health New England, Springfield, Massachusetts

Deborah Johnson, RHIT, founder, D. A. Johnson Consulting, Veradale, Washington

Charlotte Lefert, RHIA, long-term care consultant, Madison, Wisconsin

Carmilla "Kelli" Marsh, RHIA, vice president of support services, Westhaven Services, Perrysburg, Ohio

Barbara S. Michaelis, RHIA, health information management and long-term care consultant, Post Rock Solutions, Inc., Hays, Kansas

Sue Mitchell, RHIA, long-term care consultant, Omnicare Pharmacy of Perrysburg, Perrysburg, Ohio

Cheryl Olson, RHIA, health information director, Life Care Centers of America, Cleveland, Tennessee

Mary Turley, BS, RRT, clinical resource consultant, respiratory therapy, Hospital for Special Care, New Britain, Connecticut

And special thanks from Ella also goes to her husband, Tom, for his support, encouragement, and understanding, and to her mother.

Preface

Documentation and Reimbursement for Long-Term Care begins with a general discussion of health information management practices (chapter 1). Chapters 2 through 5 describe the admission process and discuss required consents, advance directives, and the face sheet before moving on to the supporting documentation for the comprehensive assessment process, discussed in chapter 6. The book outlines the importance of the resident assessment instrument (RAI), the minimum data set (MDS) for long-term care, and the resident assessment protocol (RAP) in chapter 7. Chapters 8 and 9 discuss care planning, narrative charting, and Medicare documentation.

Rehabilitative, physical, occupational, speech/language, and respiratory therapy are discussed in chapter 10. Physician documentation, physician orders, and the importance of medical oversight are discussed in chapters 11 and 12. Other documentation discussions included in the book are contained in medication and treatment records, flow sheets, laboratory and special reports, discharge documentation, and incident and accident reports.

The remaining chapters contain information on data quality, reimbursement, automation of health information, and confidentiality, privacy, and security of the resident's health record.

The book provides many forms and useful auditing tools and techniques to ensure proper documentation of resident care. It discusses the importance of documentation, the need for accurate assessment, and the connection among the resident assessment instrument, quality indicators, and quality measures. Integration of the assessment process with quality initiatives also is discussed.

Although documentation is the focus of the book, touching on each discipline's specific requirements, reimbursement is discussed in more detail in chapter 20. This chapter ties the accurate, concise, timely documentation practice into the reimbursement cycle, demonstrating why documentation is so important.

The appendices, located in the CD-ROM at the back of this book, provide detailed tools to ensure quality documentation practices, including a crosswalk of regulations and standards (appendix A), audit tools (appendix B), inappropriate abbreviation listings (appendix C), legal documentation standards (appendix D), a complete chart order policy (appendix E), and a sample long-term care record (appendix F).

This book covers the regulatory and accreditation requirements for documentation in detail, emphasizing the importance of establishing effective health record documentation policies and effective processes from the start. Complete, accurate documentation of all aspects of its residents' care provides the facility with a wealth of knowledge and information with which to run its business—the business of individualized healthcare for its residents' highest possible outcomes.

Introduction

According to the *State Operations Manual* published by the Centers for Medicare and Medicaid Services (2001, p. 1), a **skilled nursing facility** is "an institution (or a distinct part of an institution) which is primarily engaged in providing skilled nursing care and related services for residents who require medical or nursing care, or rehabilitation services for the rehabilitation of injured, disabled, or sick persons, and is not primarily for the care and treatment of mental diseases; has in effect a transfer agreement . . . with one or more hospitals having agreements in effect under §1866; and meets the requirements for a SNF described in subsections (b), (c), and (d) of this section."

A **nursing facility** is "an institution (or a distinct part of an institution) which is primarily engaged in providing skilled nursing care and related services for residents who require medical or nursing care, rehabilitation services for the rehabilitation of injured, disabled, or sick persons, or on a regular basis, health-related care and services to individuals who because of their mental or physical condition require care and services (above the level of room and board) which can be made available to them only through institutional facilities, and is not primarily for the care and treatment of mental diseases; has in effect a transfer agreement . . . with one or more hospitals having agreements in effect under §1866; and meets the requirements for a NF described in subsections (b), (c), and (d) of this section." The difference between the two definitions relates to level of skilled care individuals require.

Other long-term care facilities such as rehabilitation or assisted living may be defined by state-specific guidelines. CMS defines skilled nursing and skilled rehabilitation services as follows:

Skilled Services—Defined.—Skilled nursing and/or skilled rehabilitation services are those services, furnished pursuant to physician orders, that:

- Require the skills of qualified technical or professional health personnel such as registered nurses, licensed practical (vocational) nurses, physical therapists, occupational therapists, and speech pathologists or audiologists; and

- Must be provided directly by or under the general supervision of these skilled nursing or skilled rehabilitation personnel to assure the safety of the patient and to achieve the medically desired result (CMS 2002, p. 2-16.1).

The Omnibus Budget Reconciliation Act of 1987 brought sweeping changes to the nursing home industry and created a set of standards that facilities had to meet to ensure higher-quality resident care. The legislation required that facilities create policies that define resident rights to care and treatment. No longer can nursing home administrators allow poor-quality care, abuse, or harassment to occur within their facilities. The accreditation manual issued by the Joint Commission on Accreditation of Healthcare Organizations (JCAHO) has an entire chapter dedicated to resident rights that also addresses organizational ethics.

The resident's bill of rights gave residents the opportunity to choose their physician and have a voice in their treatment and care planning. Healthcare organizations may no longer simply allow residents to exercise their rights but must protect and promote such rights. Persons admitted to a healthcare facility continue to have the same civil and property rights they had before entering the facility. Residents need to understand their rights, and staff must thoroughly understand residents' rights as well in order to respect and honor them.

The goals of the Omnibus Budget Reconciliation Act of 1987 and the subsequent JCAHO standards were to ensure that residents receive high-quality care. These regulations and standards provide mechanisms to improve resident outcomes. They create safeguards and controls that ensure that residents maintain their dignity and receive the respect they deserve. In following the mandates of federal regulations and voluntary accreditation standards, however, long-term care facilities should not neglect any state or local laws that apply.

High-quality resident outcomes should be the paramount concern in all aspects of service in the long-term care industry. Documentation supports resident outcomes and constitutes proof that residents have attained or maintained the highest possible physical, mental, and psychosocial functioning through the assessment, reassessment, and care-planning process. Reimbursement should be a consequence of high-quality care and appropriate documentation practices, but not the focus of long-term care.

This book emphasizes the connection between documentation practices and resident outcomes. Documentation performed according to accepted standards and guidelines provides a clear indication that the residents' needs, preferences, and abilities have been taken into account and describes all the interventions, treatments, and services provided to help residents attain or maintain an optimal level of well-being.

Gathering detailed clinical information, developing a comprehensive assessment and reassessment, and conducting effective care planning are key processes in determining each resident's healthcare needs throughout his or her stay. The integrity of clinical data and comprehensive assessments trigger quality indicators (QIs). The new quality measures (QMs) are provided to the public for necessary decision-making capability on healthcare needs and placement. These are driven from documentation practices and data quality monitoring. The nursing home QMs are derived from the minimum data set (MDS) assessments documented at specific intervals in nursing homes and are required for all residents. The assessment data, when converted into QMs, provide the resident, resident's family, or responsible party with a source of information about how well nursing homes may be caring for their residents' healthcare needs. These QMs provide a mechanism for comparing one nursing home to another prior to resident placement.

The comprehensive assessment process is based on the resident assessment instrument (RAI), which comprises the minimum data set for long-term care and the resident assessment protocol (RAP). These tools constitute the foundation for the care-planning process in long-term care as required by federal regulations. The comprehensive assessment of the resident's needs and correlation of the assessment to the individualized care plan for the resident ensure high-quality outcomes for both resident and facility. Along with many supporting reports, this core information supports the facility's secondary outcome: reimbursement for the services provided to the patient. The provision of services focused on the documented healthcare needs of residents produces high-quality resident outcomes as well as sound financial results for the facility and stable, long-term care services for the community.

References

Centers for Medicare and Medicaid Services. 2002. Coverage of services. *Skilled Nursing Facility Manual.* Available at http://cms.hhs.gov/manuals/12_snf/sn201.asp#_1_17.

Centers for Medicare and Medicaid Services. 2001. *State Operations Manual.* Available at www.cms.gov.

Chapter 1

Health Record Management

The **health record** is the long-term care facility's record of services and programs provided to its residents. It supports reimbursement claims and provides information for quality and peer review. It also contains documentation showing that the care provided was medically necessary. As a formal record of care provided, it becomes the primary source of information to be used to defend the facility when disputes arise and lawsuits are filed. The resident's health record supports the following:

- Clinical significance

- Intensity of care

- Complexity of decision making

- Diagnostic and therapeutic procedures, treatments, and tests

- Resident's condition, either improvement or decline

- Diagnoses, including all coexisting diagnoses on admission and at discharge

- Length of stay

According to the **American Health Information Management Association's** (AHIMA's) definition of the term, a health record is a paper- or computer-based tool for collecting and storing information about the healthcare services provided by a healthcare facility to an individual patient. According to the AHIMA, health information management (HIM) is the management function responsible for ensuring the availability, accuracy, and protection of the clinical information required to deliver high-quality healthcare services and to make high-quality healthcare-related decisions (LaTour and Eichenwald 2002, p. 728).

Basic Documentation Guidelines

The same basic guidelines for creating and maintaining health record documentation apply to all healthcare settings (LaTour and Eichenwald 2002, p. 141):

1. All entries in the health record must be **authenticated,** or confirmed by signing, to identify the author (name and professional credentials), and dated.

2. No erasures or deletions should be made in the health record.

3. All entries in the paper health record should be in ink.

4. Blank spaces should not be left in progress/nursing notes. If there are blanks, they should be marked out with an X so that additional information cannot be inserted on the paper out of proper date sequence.

5. When a correction must be made in a paper health record, one line should be neatly drawn through the error, leaving the incorrect materials legible. The error then should be initialed and dated so that it is obvious that the mistake was corrected.

6. Original reports should always be maintained in the health record.

7. All blanks on forms should be completed, especially on consent forms.

8. When incomplete health records are filed, a statement should be attached to indicate that the health record is incomplete.

The following additional basic guidelines apply in long-term care settings:

1. The information recorded in the resident's record should relate to objective observations, never subjective opinions.

2. Documentation should be as specific and complete as possible.

3. Documentation should use only standard abbreviations approved by the facility.

4. Physician orders communicated by telephone should be clearly recorded, and every order should be related to a specific condition or diagnosis.

5. Every physician's visit should be noted in the resident's record.

6. Documentation should describe the resident's responses to medications and other treatments.

7. Care should be documented as soon as possible after it is provided.

It is important to remember that only care that has been properly documented can be considered to have been done.

Role of the Health Information Department

The health information department plays an important role in the management and oversight of the resident's health record as well as the maintenance of many important facility reports and functions to support its business practice. Health information personnel may be asked to oversee compilation of the resident roster (if applicable), the **master resident index,** census statistics, assignment of health record numbers, tracking of physician visits, initiation of the health record, compilation of documentation from referral facilities, and proper coding and indexing of admitting diagnoses. Some facilities may require that health record staff provide assistance with the **Minimum Data Set** (MDS) process. Health information staff also may input resident assessments and submit them as required.

Health information personnel are trained in the filing, archiving, and retrieving of resident information. They work to ensure the quality of clinical data and the data integrity of automated information management systems. In addition, they are trained in release of information (ROI) principles and practices and ensure that resident health information is confidential and well maintained.

Upon the resident's admission to the facility, health information staff may provide the initial health record with the required admission forms for clinical staff to complete. Health information staff also may be responsible for ensuring that state-specific requirements for referral documentation are present upon admission. If these reports are not present, health information staff may be responsible for obtaining them. It is the responsibility of the health information department to ensure that all the documents created during the resident's stay are appropriately managed, filed, indexed, and easily retrieved, as needed, to ensure that the resident's health record is complete. To assist a long-term care facility with maintaining complete health records, health information staff may also perform record audits upon admission, concurrently during a resident's stay, and upon discharge.

The **Joint Commission on Accreditation of Healthcare Organizations** (JCAHO) requires that "the organization can provide access to all relevant information from a patient's record when needed for use in resident care, treatment, and services" (JCAHO 2004, IM 6.607.9).

Health Record Requirements

State and federal agencies and accrediting organizations all require that each resident within the facility have a health record. The JCAHO requires that "the organization has a complete and accurate clinical record for every individual assessed or treated" (JCAHO 2004, IM.6.10).

Federal requirements further state that "the facility must maintain clinical records on each resident in accordance with accepted professional standards and practices that are complete" (CMS 2001, PP-197).

Federal requirements for the compliance initiative specify that policies and procedures must exist for the following areas:

- Creation of records

- Distribution of records

- Retention of records

- Destruction of records

- Complete, accurate, and timely documentation of all services

- Privacy and security

Moreover, the facility must maintain the following types of documents in addition to the resident's health record:

- Billing and claims records required for federal, state, and private healthcare services

- All corrective actions taken in response to surveys

- Records, audit information, and reports that support and clarify cost reports and other financial performance

- Record to illustrate facility integrity through compliance programs

- Record showing compliance efforts with applicable regulations

Record Numbering and Filing

Different types of record numbering and filing approaches are designed to file and reference records in different ways. The most common approaches used in long-term care are alphabetical and numeric. Each has its own advantages and reference needs, and each results in distinct patterns of arrangement and indexing. In long-term care facilities, a health record number is assigned to each resident upon admission. The individual health records of all the facility's residents are then filed according to facility policy.

The size of the health record number varies from facility to facility, but a six-digit number provides 999,999 different sets of unit numbers for a facility (000000 through 999999). Assignment of the health record number should occur only after the resident has actually been admitted to the facility. This ensures that record numbers remain chronologically sequenced in the files. Additionally, this method guarantees that the master resident index contains only actual admissions.

Alphabetical Filing Systems

Alphabetical filing systems are used widely in long-term care facilities because they are simple to understand and require no special supplies to accomplish the filing. However, alphabetical filing can be problematic because misfiled records are difficult to locate. In addition, when residents have the same last name, it can be difficult to locate the exact resident record required.

Unit Numbering System

In the **unit numbering system,** the same health record number is applied to the record for a resident each time he or she is admitted or readmitted to the facility. This system provides a mechanism for filing all the resident's records together as one set for easy access and retrieval, which becomes the composite record of all the resident's admissions.

When residents have multiple admissions, the health record number remains constant, but the visit or volume number tracks the unit record. Figure 1.1 shows an example of a record for a resident who was admitted to the same facility several times. In this example, the unit record of Jane Doe currently contains four visits to the organization and a total of eight volumes of clinical data. This unit record might increase if the resident were readmitted to the facility. It would not increase if the resident did not return. The unit record positions all of Jane Doe's records together; thus, the records for Jane Doe 01-01-01 are easily accessible and retrievable. Using the unit numbering system ensures that there would be no confusion even if several residents with the same name were treated in the facility.

Terminal-Digit Filing

In the **terminal-digit filing system** (also known as reverse-digit filing), the health record number is divided into smaller number sets, usually three groups of two numbers. This system speeds up retrieval and reduces filing time because files can be grouped according to the last two digits in the record number (00 to 99). For example, health record number 705500 would be hyphenated to produce health record number 70-55-00. The last two digits on the right (00)—the terminal digits of the number—are considered first when the record is being filed. The middle two digits (55) are considered second in the filing process, and the first two digits (70) are considered last. In this example, record 70-55-00 would be filed after 69-55-00 and before 71-55-00.

Figure 1.1.   Tracking of a health record number for multiple visits

			Health Record Number		
Resident Name	**Date of Admission**	**Date of Discharge**	**##-##-##**	**visit #**	**vol. #**
Jane Doe	12/01/2000	12/15/2000	01-01-01	visit 1	vol. 1
Jane Doe	01/17/2001	3/10/2001	01-01-01	visit 2	vol. 2 & 3
Jane Doe	04/15/2001	7/23/2001	01-01-01	visit 3	vol. 4 to 7
Jane Doe	09/21/2001	2/01/2002	01-01-01	visit 4	vol. 8

Terminal-digit filing ensures that each resident's files are located together, but it does require more space because areas in the files are left open for expansion. Terminal-digit filing methods are good for large systems with many records but require frequent shifting of files when large blocks of files are added or removed. Files would typically be purged to on-site or off-site storage on a predetermined basis to allow room for expansion of the health record files for the upcoming year.

The major advantage of terminal-digit filing is that the files form an equal growth pattern. (See figure 1.2.) This system was developed to overcome congestion in large filing systems when the most active records are being filed in consecutive order. When filing by terminal digit, all records that have the terminal digits or primary digits of 00 are filed together. To make terminal digits less complicated, facilities have adapted the process so that all 01-xx-00 are filed together, and when 02-xx-00 follows, they are filed behind the 01-xx-00 section in numerical order. This process requires less space to be reserved for future volumes.

In the preceding example, it is easy to see that space would be left for the numbers between 01-92-00 and 01-99-00, but excessive space is not required because the numbers follow in sequence by terminal digit only. As previously stated, the unit record of Jane Doe is easily filed as a unit record when the health record number is used for filing. Filing by health record number alleviates confusion among residents with the same first and last name. (See figure 1.3.) For example, in the alphabetical method of filing, the records for all persons named Jane Doe risk being interfiled. However, in the terminal-digit filing system, every resident named Jane Doe would be assigned a different health record number and thus avoid being filed together. Figure 1.3 demonstrates how each resident with the name Jane Doe is separated by a terminal digit. Terminal-digit filing provides an easy mechanism to keep residents with the same name not only separate, but also easily retrievable.

Figure 1.2.   Expansion space as seen in terminal-digit filing

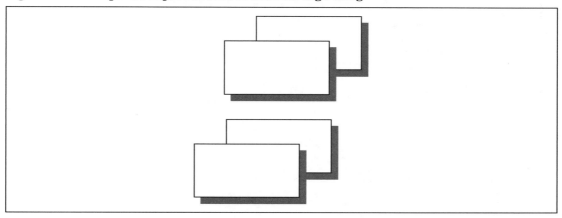

Figure 1.3.   Terminal-digit filing for residents with the same name

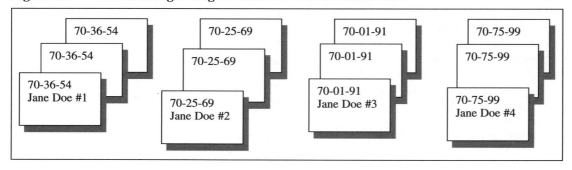

Figures 1.4 through 1.7 show file folders that have been converted or prepared for the terminal-digit filing system. Each terminal digit has its own color so that even misfiled charts can be easily located. Alphabetical filing makes it difficult to determine misfiled information.

The color scheme presented in figure 1.8 may not be indicative of the colors currently used in some facilities because color-coding depends on the vendor utilized for the actual purchase of the individual numbers. The figure simply indicates how each number may have a specified color assignment that makes it easy to determine misfiled health records.

Figure 1.4.   Resident binder prepared for terminal-digit filing

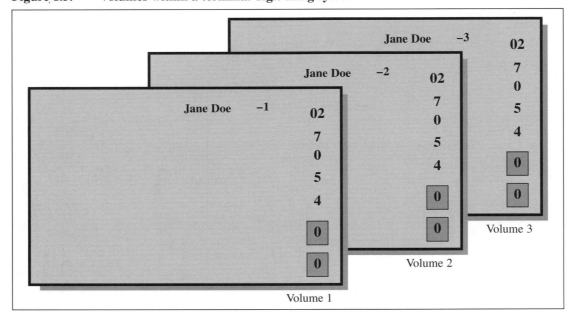

Figure 1.5.   Volumes within a terminal-digit filing system

It is inadvisable to use the resident's Social Security number as the health record number; rather, a predetermined set of numbers should be established for use as per facility policy. The problem with using the Social Security number is that some people may have more than one number and others may have no number at all. Another problem is that the Social Security number is a nine-digit number, which is too long to easily adapt to terminal-digit filing techniques.

In the long-term care setting, the size of health records can become unwieldy. Typically, more than one volume is needed to house the entire clinical record of a single resident. Moreover, the resident often has multiple admissions and discharges. Using terminal-digit filing in combination with a visit number and a volume number makes the sorting and filing of large volumes of resident records much easier.

Figure 1.6.   Placement of a terminal-digit file

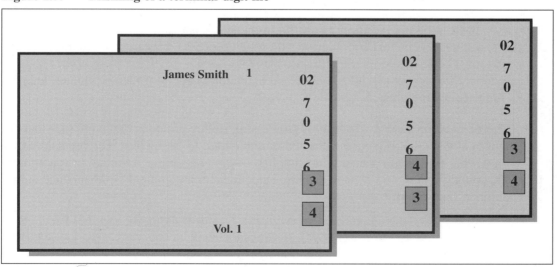

Figure 1.7.   Misfiling of a terminal-digit file

Figure 1.8.   Typical terminal-digit color schemes

0 = Green	2 = Black	4 = Purple	6 = Grey	8 = Blue
1 = Pink	3 = Yellow	5 = Red	7 = Brown	9 = Orange

Figure 1.5 shows the record of Jane Doe as an example. Her record, placed on the files in this order, makes it easy to determine that she has had three separate and distinct visits, but the health record number assignment has remained consistent. Terminal-digit filing provides a simple means to better track resident records. Should a visit require two or more volumes to house the entire stay, this would be indicated on the cover as volume 4, volume 5, and so on with visit 4 indicated after the resident's name.

Figure 1.6 shows that the file prepared in figure 1.4 for terminal-digit filing is placed on the shelf in the 00 section between 70-54-00 and 70-56-00. Figure 1.7 shows how use of the colored terminal digit makes it easy to see any misfiled information quickly and easily. The record with health record number 70-56-43 is out of sequence.

Health Information Department Policies and Procedures

Health information department policies and procedures provide guidance in ensuring that a consistent record-handling process is delivered. A **policy** is a governing principle that authorizes or limits actions. **Procedures** are steps taken to implement a policy. Written policies should have the following components:

- *Purpose statement:* The reason for the policy
- *Policy statement:* A specific description of what the policy of the facility is
- *Procedures:* The step-by-step instructions to carry out the policy
- *Responsibility:* The person responsible for overseeing the policy
- *References:* Any references used in the creation of the policy, as applicable
- *Approval:* The person or governing body that approves the policy
- *Date:* The date(s) the policy went into effect or was reviewed

Policies need to be reviewed on a specified schedule. State standards or regulations may drive this schedule. The facility should have a thorough process for writing and reviewing policies, which must be followed by the HIM department.

Long-term care facilities should develop and maintain health information policies and procedures in the following areas:

- The **admissions and readmissions processing policy** provides the guidelines that are required when the resident is admitted or readmitted to the facility. The procedure outlines what staff are expected to accomplish when a resident is admitted or readmitted. This policy also should contain specific guidelines for assignment of the medical record number. (See figure 1.9.)

- The **alias policy** is implemented when resident confidentiality is required by the resident, family, or responsible party. It outlines the steps needed to ensure that the individual's identity is protected while the person is a resident and that record-handling processes are in place to ensure confidentiality after the person has been discharged.

- The **analysis of discharged health records policy** outlines steps to be taken to process discharged resident records. It provides instruction on assembly and analysis expectations and time frames, and specifies what forms to flag for physician signature and other requirements of the department for processing discharged records.

Figure 1.9.   Sample admissions and readmissions processing policy

---

XYZ Organization

Procedure manual   Health Record Department

Admissions and Readmissions Processing

Purpose: To provide guidelines for medical record personnel when a resident is admitted or readmitted, ensuring continuity of resident care information, uniformity of the admitting process, and assignment of health record number for each resident

Policy: Health record personnel will adhere to guidelines established upon admission or readmission of residents.

Health record staff will ensure proper assignment of medical record number.

Health record staff will ensure integrity of demographic data.

Procedure: 1.   Health record staff will assign and verify health record number.

2.   Health record staff will verify demographic information online.

3.   Resident information will be entered into the computer:
3.1   Attending physician
3.2   Admitting and principal diagnosis
3.3   Secondary diagnoses

- The **census-reporting policy** outlines the process for census reporting and tracking. It should contain the list of individuals who would receive the census report if it is not computerized. Steps for confidential handling of the census also should be included.

- The **chart depletion policy** outlines the documents that can be removed, or depleted, from resident records over time. This practice also may be called thinning the health record. It is needed because residents in a long-term care facility have extended lengths of stay. This policy also defines the filing process for depleted documents and establishes a depletion schedule so that staff understand the expectations of the chart depletion function.

- The **chart order policy** defines the chart order within the facility. It provides a detailed listing of all documents and defines their order and section location within the health record. This policy requires updating each time a new form is approved for use in the resident health records.

- **Chart-tracking/requests policy** outlines the way in which charts are signed out of the permanent files and how requests for records are handled. This policy clearly defines the chart-tracking mechanism used, thus ensuring that the department can quickly locate a resident's record. The process may be a paper sign-out method, a computerized bar scan, or some other computerized method. The policy needs to state the process that is followed in the department to ensure that chart tracking is completed. This policy also spells out how requests for health records are handled and time frames for having records available for requesters.

- The **confidentiality policy** outlines the steps to take organizationwide to protect information about residents and the facility from unwanted disclosure. The facility should have an organizationwide confidentiality policy. In addition to, or in lieu of, this policy, many health record departments require each staff member to sign its own confidentiality statement. The policy outlines the expectations for maintaining confidentiality of resident's records. It may outline security mechanisms that have been established as well.

- The **correction, addendum, and appending health records policy** outlines how corrections, addenda, or appendages are made in the resident's health record. The policy needs to contain language from Health Information Portability and Accountability Act (HIPAA) regulations concerning the fact that residents may append their own records.

- The **damaged record recovery policy** outlines the steps the facility should take to recover paper and/or electronic records in the event of a disaster, whether fire, water, or other disaster. It is important to have guidelines in place to ensure proper handling of damaged records.

- The **downtime procedures for health records policy** outlines steps the department should take when computerized equipment fails or systems are down for long periods of time. If the facility is not computerized, the policy can outline steps to take in the event of a power or other type failure that would affect normal business operations.

- The **health record department access policy** outlines employee access to the health record department and the chart-tracking mechanism for signing out records. The policy on employee access provides a list of the categories of employees who may access health records, such as physicians, nurses, therapists, administration, and others. It expressly defines only those categories of staff that may access records. It also details how health record staff should respond to an unknown individual. The policy addresses requests to see identification in the form of an employer identification badge. Signing out of health records should refer to the chart-tracking policy for details on the chart-tracking process.

- The **faxing policy** outlines the steps to take for faxing individually identifiable health information and business records and should limit what information may be faxed.

- The **forms management policy** outlines the process for the creation of new forms. New forms design and detail should be outlined in the policy as well as the steps taken to have the form included in the resident's record. Moreover, the policy should specify that each new form requires a trial period before there is final approval to ensure that all data fields are included and that the form serves its full purpose.

- The **general health record documentation policy** outlines documentation practices within the facility. It should spell out the categories of persons who can document in the health record and sets time lines for documentation practices. This policy also defines a complete health record. The JCAHO's information management standard (JCAHO 2004, IM.6.10) offers the following that should be considered for the documentation policy:

  —List of authorized individuals who are allowed to make entries in the health record

  —Countersignature requirements

  —Guidance on dating and signing entries. Include the minimum documents listed in the Elements of Performance in the IM.6.10 standard

  —Guidance on timely entries

  —Definition of a complete record (organizations may choose to make this a separate policy)

- The **history and physical documentation requirements policy** specifies the detail required in the history and physical examination done by the physician or **physician**

extender. This policy typically is written by the HIM professional in conjunction with the medical director and is provided to each physician for reference material to use when the history and physical is documented.

- The **liability files policy** outlines procedures for limiting access to, and maintaining the security of, information related to liability cases.

- The **master resident index maintenance policy** outlines procedures on the maintenance of the master resident index and the steps to take to verify and cross-check all entries. This process is typically overseen by HIM professionals.

- An **MDS processing policy** is needed when health record personnel are included in the MDS data entry or submission of the MDS data. The policy should include a discussion of the roles and functions provided.

- The **health record committee policy** outlines the goals of the committee, the audit tools used, the number of audits required and specific time frames for completion of audits, and the results-reporting mechanisms.

- The **incomplete records policy** outlines how physicians are notified of records needing signatures. JCAHO standard IM.6.10 requires that "the organization define a complete record and the time frame within which the record must be completed after discharge, not to exceed 30 days" (JCAHO 2004, IM 6.10).

- The **off-site storage policy** details how and when records are processed for shipment off-site.

- A detailed **physician query process policy** is needed in facilities that sometimes request additional information from physicians as part of the coding and reimbursement process. A useful reference for developing a physician query process has been developed by the AHIMA (Prophet 2001).

- The **records purging policy** is used in conjunction with the off-site storage policy. When off-site storage is not utilized by facilities, the policy stands alone. It defines how and when records are purged from the main or permanent files.

- The **records disaster recovery policy** is required to establish how records should be handled in a disaster such as fire, smoke, or water damage. It should outline steps to take to recover both paper and electronic records.

- The **release of protected health information policy,** discussed in detail later in this chapter, outlines how residents and others may obtain copies of their health records. It should provide detailed procedures on handling each request for disclosure. It also may provide guidance for HIM staff to determine the validity of a request. It should clearly define the use of a compliant **authorization** and provide guidance to medical record staff on steps to take to ensure that proper disclosures are made.

- The **records removal policy** outlines how and when records may be removed from the health record department. It also outlines who may remove such records. This policy covers quality review, physician requests, requests to have the record brought to the resident stations or unit, administration review, and the like. A general statement in this policy should define when or whether records may leave the facility.

- The **records retention policy** specifies the length of time that health records are kept as required by law. Each state may have different criteria for retention. It is important to check your state regulations to determine health record retention expectations. Moreover, states may differ when defining record retention periods for hospitals, skilled nursing facilities, home care agencies, physician offices, and other healthcare agencies. Be sure that you have the correct retention periods when establishing this policy.

- The **resident's right to access** his or her health record encompasses the mechanisms in place to allow residents to review their own health information.

- The policy on **signing out of health records internally to other facility departments** establishes mechanisms to ensure that charts are tracked when taken out of the HIM department. This policy outlines how charts are signed out for use and which classes of employees can request resident health records (for example, quality or nursing departments, physicians, or administrator).

- The **subpoena policy** outlines the steps required to handle the subpoena processing for protected health information. This policy should provide details on how a subpoena is accepted, processed, and delivered.

- An **unapproved abbreviations policy,** which defines the abbreviations that are unacceptable for use in the health record, may become a facility requirement. The JCAHO has changed its focus on abbreviation listings and now requires organizations to establish such policies to identify the abbreviations that should never be used in healthcare documentation.

Organizations may have other policies and procedures for their health information department depending on the functions performed.

Release of Information

The resident's right to privacy is fundamental. The release of information (ROI) form authorizes the release of specific health information about the resident. (See figure 1.10.) The authorization form explains the federal and state regulation statutes concerning confidentiality and privacy of health information. (See chapter 3 for more discussion of authorizations.)

The purpose of the authorization is to protect the privacy and confidentiality of the resident's individually identifiable information. The facility uses the authorization as a security mechanism on the resident's behalf to ensure that only those individuals who need to know about their health conditions have access to confidential information.

The signed authorization to release information also protects the facility from disclosing information to unauthorized individuals. A well-defined process for the ROI function ensures that only authorized requests are honored.

Federal regulations (42 CFR, Part 2) prohibit healthcare facilities from making further disclosures without the specific written consent of the resident. Before releasing resident health information, the facility should have a signed and dated authorization.

In addition, HIPAA has very specific stipulations concerning the release of a resident's health record. (See chapter 22 for more details.)

However, the health records of patients being transferred from one facility to another constitute an exception to these rules. Federal regulations outlined in the Medicare *Conditions of Participation for Hospitals* (42 CFR 482.43) state that "the hospital must transfer or refer patients, along with necessary medical information, to appropriate facilities, agencies or

Figure 1.10.   Request for information

TO:

DATE:
RE:
Record #:
Tax ID #:

The enclosed information is sent in accordance with your request.

Further use of the information enclosed for other than the stated purpose is prohibited. Destruction of the information after the stated need has been fulfilled is required.

☐ Discharge Summary
☐ History and Physical
☐ Progress Notes_____
☐ Consultations_____
☐ Medications
☐ Physician's Orders
☐ Laboratory Reports
☐ The record on this patient is incomplete at this time but will be forwarded as soon as possible.
☐ X ray
☐ EKG/EEG
☐ EMG
☐ Therapies_____
☐ Nurse's Notes
☐ Social Work
☐ Above-named patient was not seen at _____.
                                                        (organization name)
☐ Other_____
☐ Information from _____ to _____
                          (date)   (date)
☐ Your request for records was received without a current signed authorization from the patient. Upon receipt of the authorization, we will be happy to comply with your request.
☐ Your payment of $_____ is being requested. Upon receipt of this payment, your request will be furnished.

☐ No charge
_____ Pages of health record at $_____ for each copy
_____ Total charge

Please make your check payable to: [insert organizational name]
Attention: Health Records Department

Sincerely,

[insert name and title of manager]

outpatient services, as needed, for follow-up or ancillary care." The requirements for states and long-term care facilities state that "the resident's right to refuse release of personal and clinical records does not apply when the resident is transferred to another health care institution or record release is required by law" (42 CFR 483.10). Further, "In cases of transfer of a resident with mental illness or mental retardation from a nursing facility to a hospital or to another nursing facility, the transferring nursing facility is responsible for ensuring that copies of the resident's most recent PASARR and resident assessment reports accompany the transferring resident" (42 CFR 483.106). The PASARR is the federally mandated Preadmission Screening and Annual Resident Review program designed to prevent inappropriate admission and retention of people with mental disabilities in nursing homes. (PASARR is discussed in greater detail in chapter 6.)

Process of Release of Information

Confidential information from health records is needed for a number of clinical and business purposes such as quality management and reimbursement. Disclosures of information are made in several formats, including direct use of paper-based or electronic information, verbal or e-mail communications, abstracts, and photocopied or faxed duplications. A valid authorization should be obtained for the ROI as defined by HIPAA rules and/or state regulations. However, federal requirements related to residents' rights state that "an oral request is sufficient to produce the current record for review" (CMS 2001, p. 5). In case of emergencies, where verbal release is required, documentation of the release should be made and the facility must follow specific HIPAA and state requirements.

Facilities should never ask residents to sign blank authorizations for release of information that are to be kept on file and used in the future when needed. Authorizations to release information must be obtained at the time they are needed. When the facility requires confidential information from other healthcare providers, the resident or his or her legal representative should be asked to sign an authorization form for the specific release. HIPAA regulations clearly define the required contents of the authorization form. They also provide examples of improper authorizations. In addition, authorizations must fulfill state requirements.

The ROI authorization process must be clearly defined and, when possible, centralized to ensure that the resident's fundamental right to privacy is upheld. The process should be outlined in HIM policy and procedures. The provisions of the HIPAA regulations have brought renewed attention to the ROI process. Centralization is important because it allows facilities to manage the process more effectively. Creation of a logging or tracking mechanism makes it possible to review volumes of requested information and monitor the timeliness of response. Auditing for quality improvement activity can be easily obtained from such tracking logs.

The ROI process also should include provisions for verifying the validity of authorizations before the information is released. Procedures should spell out the wording requirements of both requests and authorizations.

All ROI requests should be made in writing. Requests from attorneys for release of health information should be submitted on letterhead, and the specific information requested should be described in the request. Blanket requests for "the entire record" should be questioned to ensure that only the information required is released.

Some states have very specific laws governing the release of information related to treatment for acquired immune deficiency syndrome (AIDS), psychiatric illness, and drug and alcohol addiction that may supersede federal requirements. The facility may have an authorization for release of information and another for request of patient information. (See chapter 3.) The HIM department must stay current on legislation governing ROI, confidentiality, privacy, and security at both the state and federal levels. As regulations change, the authorization form and process must be reviewed and revised as necessary.

Release of Information Policies and Procedures

Long-term care facilities should have detailed policies and procedures on the release of confidential healthcare information. Policies should outline the content of the authorization form and valid signatures. ROI policies should include information on how much the facility charges for making copies of records and the process of making information requests and giving authorizations. Additionally, ROI policies and procedures should be based on both federal and state regulations.

A cover letter should be attached that details all the information that is released. The cover letter and the release form are placed together in the resident's health record. The cover letter becomes the *invoice* for the release of information. Items on the cover letter might include:

- Facility name

- Date of letter

- Resident name and health record number

- Address of the person/place to whom the information is released

It is always an excellent idea to mail the released information to an individual person (not a place or box number), and the address line should contain an "attention to" line. This practice ensures that the destination's mailroom can quickly forward the envelope to the individual to whom it is addressed. Providing this information decreases the chance that the record may be lost due to insufficient address and save recopy time and effort. The letter also might include:

- Facility's tax identification number

- Summary of check-off boxes indicating what was sent

- Cost of the copies (as defined by state laws in most instances)

- Signature of the person overseeing the ROI function

The facility should have a mechanism in place to track all requests for, and releases of, information. The information tracked may include:

- Date of request

- Date of release or disclosure

- Resident name

- Requester (name of the entity or person who received the protected health information and, if known, the address of such entity or person [DHHS 2002])

- Information requested (brief description of the protected health information disclosed [DHHS 2002])

- Statement of the purpose (brief statement of the purpose of the disclosure that reasonably informs the individual of the basis for the disclosure [DHHS 2002])

- Cost of release of information

- Payment received

- Comments if desired

The tracking mechanism may be an information-tracking system inherent in a health record software package or a simple spreadsheet that provides the data entered by date and sorted by month and year. The information system has predefined reporting capability, and the spreadsheet can be sorted by the criteria listed in its header for easy reporting and quality checking. A manual list also may be used to track requests for and release of information.

The ROI authorization is placed in the miscellaneous section of the resident's health record along with any applicable written requests for the record and the copy of the cover letter. They are filed in date order.

"Upon an oral or written request to access all records pertaining to himself or herself including current clinical records within 24 hours (excluding weekends and holidays); and after receipt of his or her records for inspection, to purchase at a cost not to exceed the community standard photocopies of the records or any portions of them upon request and two working days advance notice to the facility" (CMS 2001, p. 5). This requirement allows greater access than HIPAA and probably most state laws. Facilities must remember that this requirement applies only to the resident or his or her legal representative.

Quality Audits

To ensure proper ROI practice, a mechanism for checking validity of the authorization should be developed. Criteria to consider in developing the process are:

- Purpose of the request is completed.

- Specific records requested are defined.

- Authorization contains the correct signature.

- Authorization is signed and dated.

- Authorization is complete. (This is an important aspect under HIPAA regulations.)

- Authorization is still valid (or has it expired?).

Quality audits of the ROI function should be conducted. Figure 1.11 is a sample of an audit tool that can be utilized for departmental quality assurance.

Figure 1.11.   Audit tool for departmental quality assurance

Health Record Release of Information QA

Month:_____

Resident name (Last/ first initial)	Request is in writing from requestor Y/N	Signed authorization with request Y/N	Requested information	Information released (Progress notes, etc.)	Correct information released Y/N	Correct resident Y/N	Sent to a specific person Y/N	All pages stamped Y/N	%

Other Health Record Management Issues

Several other health record management issues affect documentation in long-term care facilities.

Legibility of Documentation

Health record information is used extensively throughout long-term care facilities and fulfills the following functions:

- Enhancing communication among physicians and the rest of the healthcare team

- Improving the care provided to residents

- Supporting adequate and appropriate quality-of-care measures

- Substantiating reimbursement claims

- Supporting research and education

- Protecting the legal interests of residents, clinicians, and facilities

When health record documentation is illegible or ambiguous, the record cannot support or protect the facility. Although the focus is currently on acute care hospitals, the legibility of clinical records is a problem in every healthcare setting. The legibility of health records should be monitored and reported through the organization's quality initiatives.

Legibility from a health record standpoint affects the coding and sequencing of diagnostic codes. The ability of the coding staff to read and interpret a physician's handwriting may jeopardize the organization's compliance efforts. Missing or simply misreading diagnoses can impact reimbursement for the facility. This says nothing of the possible errors from a clinical standpoint due to the inability to read what is documented. "Missing, incomplete, or illegible documentation can seriously impede resident care and the defense of a malpractice claim, even when the care was appropriate" (Harvard 2002).

Legibility may well remain problematic unless the facility determines that an electronic version of a health record can be pursued. In the interim, health record staff needs to develop a policy to query the physician about illegible diagnoses. The query process is an effective means to communicate with the physicians (Prophet 2001).

Chart Tracking

As previously discussed, facilities must be able to collect, store, and retrieve resident records in a timely and easy manner. Thus, chart tracking is an important function within the health record department. Any number of mechanisms can be used to ensure that chart tracking is completed. In electronic systems, chart-tracking screens allow staff to check charts out of the department. Records are easily generated to ensure that staff can identify where charts are located. However, most long-term facilities do not have the luxury of electronic systems.

In the noncomputerized environment, an outguide is placed in the file at the location of the pulled chart. It is easy to locate charts that are checked out by looking at the placement of the outguide. Outguides are available in colors to make them easier to view.

Depending on the style of outguide used, there are areas to indicate the resident's name, date of the pull, and who requested or removed the chart. A policy outlining the use of outguides helps to ensure proper processing of chart-tracking activity.

Physician Queries

The facility may determine that it needs a process for querying physicians when the documentation in a resident's health record needs clarification before a diagnosis can be coded. The **physician query process** is a communication tool and educational mechanism that provides a clearer picture of specific resident diagnoses when in question. It should be used at a minimum and be the exception rather than the rule.

The physician query process form should be included in the content of the health record. The process will have to be specific, and the facility must ensure that the process does not lead, direct, or probe the physician. There should be no yes or no questions on the forms, and the form must never indicate any financial impact of the responses. It cannot be designed so that the physician simply signs it. The following are components for the physician query form:

- Resident name

- Admission date

- Health record number

- Coding professional's name and contact information

- Specific open-ended questions relevant to health record documentation or clinical information

- Space for the physician's response

- Space for the physician's signature and date

The physician's response to the query must be contained in the health record and included on a progress note or as an addendum to a history and physical examination or the discharge summary. The AHIMA (Prophet 2001) practice brief on developing a physician query process describes the process in more detail.

Quality Management

The health record department should consider monitoring the quality of record management processes in the following areas:

- Accurate code assignment

- Admission and readmission process as it pertains to records management

- Chart tracking

- Confidentiality statements

- Correct documentation practices, including adherence to documentation requirements and standards

- Data integrity: Correct name, health record number, admission and discharge dates, and so on

- Master resident index

- Physician record completion

- Physician visit tracking

- Record assembly
- Referral information
- Release of information
- Timely policy review
- MDS completion, transmission, and RUG assignment

Health Information Managers

The HIM department should be overseen by an AHIMA-credentialed professional as either a direct supervisor or a consultant. The HIM professional is highly trained in specific records-handling processes as well as quality initiatives, correct coding principles, documentation practices, privacy and security, release of information, information systems, MDS processing, and chart content requirements. Long-term care facilities need to consider the value-added benefits that an AHIMA professional can bring to the organization.

Summary

Health information professionals play an important role in managing the resident's health record, which is the legal record for the facility. The HIM department must have specific policies and procedures in place that define its scope of practice and responsibility. Important issues include pertinent polices, the physician query process, and the need to include that information in the resident's health record.

In addition, the facility should have policies and procedures in place to determine how its residents can easily request or access their records. Moreover, it should have policies and procedures in place on how staff can access resident health information. There should be a thorough policy detailing the management of release of information, including subpoenas. All the facility's policies must take into consideration both federal and state-specific requirements.

Each resident must have a health record that indicates all of the care and services provided. This record must be maintained accurately, legibly, and in a timely manner. Documentation should be captured as close to the provision of care as possible.

Health information management—the safe keeping of the facility's legal record—must be managed efficiently and effectively. The HIM professional provides value to the organization through knowledgeable application of record management practices and functions that are required to meet federal, state, and accrediting agency regulations and standards.

References

Centers for Medicare and Medicaid Services. 2001 (October 31). Guidance to Surveyors—Long-Term Care Facilities, appendix PP in *State Operations Manual.* Available at www.cms.gov.

Department of Health and Human Services. 2002. *Federal Register,* August 14. Available at www.cms.hhs.gov.

Hughes, Gwen. 2002. Practice Brief: Required content for authorizations to disclose (updated). *Journal of the American Health Information Management Association.*

Hughes, Gwen, and Cheryl Smith. 2001. Practice Brief: Required content for authorizations to disclose. *Journal of the American Health Information Management Association* 72(10):72A–72D.

Joint Commission on Accreditation of Healthcare Organizations. 2004. *Comprehensive Accreditation Manual for Long-term Care.* Oakbrook Terrace, Ill.: JCAHO.

LaTour, Kathleen M., and Shirley Eichenwald. 2002. *Health Information Management: Concepts, Principles, and Practice.* Chicago: American Health Information Management Association.

Prophet, Sue. 2001. Practice Brief: Developing a physician query process. *Journal of the American Health Information Management Association* 72(9):88I–88M.

Risk Management Foundation of the Harvard Medical Institutions. 2002. *Risk Management Issues: Issues in Documentation.* Copyright ©1996–2002. Available at www.rmf.harvard.edu.

Chapter 2

Documentation of the Admission Process

Long-term care encompasses a wide range of nonacute healthcare services that include skilled nursing, rehabilitation, and subacute medical care. Most long-term care is provided in residential environments such as skilled nursing facilities and assisted living facilities. The purpose of every long-term care facility is to provide high-quality clinical care and services in the most appropriate healthcare setting. According to the **Centers for Medicare and Medicaid Services** (CMS), "Each resident must receive and the facility must provide the necessary care and services to attain or maintain the highest practicable physical, mental, and psychosocial well-being" (2001a, p. 83).

Fulfilling this goal begins with the process of admitting residents to the facility. Every long-term care facility must develop and maintain effective admission policies and procedures to ensure that residents receive the care and services they need during their stay. The policies and procedures should encompass the documentation that is required during the admission process and the important steps in the admission process. This documentation is the basis for initial assessments and the resident's placement in the proper program within the facility.

It is extremely important that the admission process flow well for every resident. The goal for the facility should be to make the process as simple and easy as possible for residents and their families. Actual admission to the facility should be fast, efficient, and seamless to ensure that residents are taken to their rooms as quickly as possible and made comfortable. The admission documentation must be captured accurately and completely to ensure that all the relative information is available for the physician, clinician, and allied health staff, as well as for financial services personnel, who require the data for proper care and service to the resident.

Long-Term Care Admission Process

The purpose of the admission process is to ensure that residents are placed in the healthcare setting most appropriate to their needs. The admission process also sets the stage for an open relationship among the facility's staff, the resident, and the resident's family or legal representative. It is key to developing effective communication throughout the resident's stay in the facility. The discussions that take place before and at the time of admission ensure that the resident and the resident's family or legal representative are knowledgeable enough to discuss any concerns surrounding the resident's placement in long-term care as well any issues that surface during the resident's stay.

Admission Policies and Procedures

Federal regulations described in the Medicare *Conditions of Participation* require that long-term care facilities establish and maintain effective admission policies and procedures. Specifically, federal regulations require that physician's orders describing the resident's immediate care requirements be provided to the facility at the time of admission. A **physician's certification** of the resident's need for long-term care services also is required when the resident is eligible for Medicare benefits. In addition, Medicare regulations stipulate that a health record must be established for every resident at the time of admission.

Similarly, the standards published for long-term care facilities by the Joint Commission on Accreditation of Healthcare Organizations (JCAHO) state that the long-term care facility should "accept for care, treatment, and services only those residents whose identified care, treatment, and services needs it can meet " (JCAHO 2004, PC.1.10, PC-10).

The **Commission on Accreditation of Rehabilitation Facilities** (CARF) examines "service design and delivery that focus on the needs of the persons served" and determines whether "accomplishment of predicted outcomes" (http://www.carf.org/) was achieved among other valuable quality components of rehabilitation or assisted living facilities. CARF standards focus on the goals and activities of the resident and the outcomes of care. Thus, CARF standards look at the needs of the resident, proper placement, and the outcomes of care.

State regulations and state Medicaid regulations also apply to long-term care facilities. Depending on state requirements, the admission process may start when potential residents are placed on the facility's waiting list, for which states may have specific requirements. All states require that residents of long-term care facilities remain under the care of a physician throughout their stay.

Every long-term care facility's admission policies should outline the steps to take to fulfill federal and state admission requirements as well as applicable accreditation standards. Procedures describing the storage and maintenance of admission applications and other paperwork also should be included in the facility's admission policies.

Identifying, defining, and flowcharting the process of admissions in the facility is a good way to ensure that the system in place runs smoothly for all departments involved. Quality design of the admission process includes the following components:

- Resident comfort
- Proper placement
- Proper staffing levels
- Identification and completion of required documentation
- Institution of the resident record
- Needed supplies, pharmaceuticals, and equipment
- Needed services and interventions
- Notification for clinical and nonclinical services
- Room preparation
- Decreased duplication of effort
- Quality data gathering
- Accurate master resident index

- Sound census verification

- Compliance with federal, state, and accreditation requirements

Steps in the Preadmission Process

The admission process begins long before the actual arrival of the resident at the long-term care facility. However, preadmission processes vary among facilities, although preadmission planning is always central to the appropriate placement of residents. The most important element of preadmission planning is the preadmission assessment. A preadmission assessment of the resident's needs ensures that he or she will receive appropriate care. It also helps the facility to identify each resident's clinical needs. This information makes it possible for the facility to adjust staffing and resources before a new resident is admitted for care.

Many departments are involved in preadmission planning and the admission process. Figure 2.1 provides a checklist that outlines critical points in the admission process. Describing the process in a flowchart can help facilities understand the process and ensure communication among participating departments. Figure 2.2 offers a simple flowchart showing the important steps in the admission process.

Documentation of the Admission Process

A number of documents need to be completed before a resident can be admitted to a long-term care facility. Requirements depend on the regulations of the state in which the facility operates. In addition to the documentation of preadmission and admission assessments, some or all of the following forms, records, and consents may be created and maintained in the resident's health record:

- Completed application (kept in the admitting office)

- Consent to treat

- Consent to photograph (per facility policy)

- Physician certification for Medicare

- Interagency transfer form (from the referring facility) (See figure 2.3.)

- Acknowledgments

Figure 2.1.   Admission checklist

1.	Preadmission assessments are completed.
2.	Resident who meets admission criteria as indicated in facility policies is admitted.
3.	Resident is placed at appropriate level of care, and the station/unit/room assignment is determined.
4.	Resident receives an orientation to the facility that includes an explanation of his or her rights.
5.	Resident and appropriate staff discuss the importance of advance directives.
6.	A health record is established and assigned a permanent identification number in accordance with the facility's record-handling policies and procedures.
7.	Staff is notified of the admission.
8.	An admission assessment is completed.
9.	The care-planning process is initiated.
10.	Immediate care services are provided according to the order of the resident's physician.

Figure 2.2.   Admission process

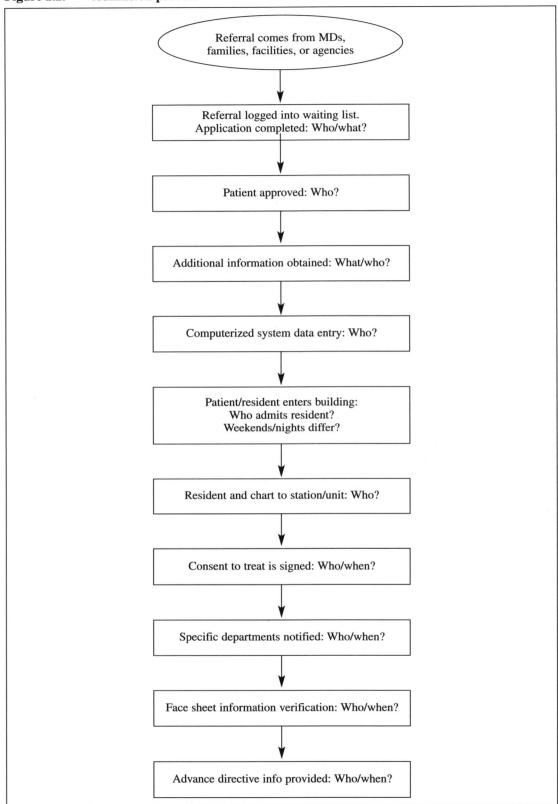

Figure 2.3.   Interagency patient referral report (W-10)

Interagency Patient Referral Report (W-10)

Identifying Data

Patient's Name (Last, First, Middle)   Sex   Birth Date   Admission Date   Discharge Date

Patient's Home Address   Home Phone No.   Marital Status   Religion
(No. and Street, Town or City, State, Zip Code)

Responsible Person or Agency (Name and Address)   Relationship   Telephone No.

Referred by (Name and Address of Facility or Agency)   Contact Person or Unit   Telephone No.

Referred to (Name and Address of Facility or Agency)   Contact Person or Unit   Telephone No.

Follow-up by (Name and Address of Physician or Clinic)   Telephone No.   Date of Next Appointment
1. _____
2. _____

Medical Record No.	Medicare No.	Social Security No.	Dept. of Inc. Maint. No.	Other

Orders and Patient Care Information

Pertinent History/Diagnosis/Reason for Transfer _____

Behavior Status Issues: ☐ Yes ☐ No   Describe _____

Restraints: _____

Vital Signs: _____   Diet: _____

Cognitive Status: Alert: ☐ Yes ☐ No   Oriented: ☐ Yes ☐ No

Personal Needs

    Bathing: _____   Feeding: _____   Sight: _____

    Dressing: _____   Admin of meds: _____   PPD: _____

    Transfer: _____   Ambulation: _____   Lab/X rays _____

    Toileting: _____   Speech: _____

Responsible party notified? _____

Prosthetic(s) sent with client: (X if applicable)

    Dentures: _____   Hearing aid: _____   Cane/walker: _____

    Glasses: _____   Ostomy appliance: _____   Other: _____

Height: _____   Weight: _____

Bladder Control: _____   Bowel Control: _____   Last BM: _____

Skin Condition: _____   Decubitus present ☐ Yes ☐ No

Other Skin Problems(s) Location/Description _____

Advance Directives ☐ Yes ☐ No (If appropriate, attach copies)

Code Status: _____   Organ Donor: _____

Medications (Drug, Strength, Mode)	Frequency	Last Given	Medications (Drug, Strength, Mode)	Frequency	Last Given
1.			2.		
3.			4.		
5.			6.		
7.			8.		

Allergies: Diagnosis Given: _____   Prognosis: _____

    Explained to: ☐ Patient ☐ Family   Explained to: ☐ Patient ☐ Family

Therapeutic Goals: _____

Patient Serv Start Date: _____   Services Requested:

      ___ Nursing   ___ Occ. Therapy   ___ Speech therapy

      ___ Physical therapy   ___ H.H. aids   ___ Other

Is treatment for condition for which patient was hospitalized   Patient essentially homebound:

(if NO, explain) ☐ Yes ☐ No   ☐ Yes ☐ No

Hereby certify that the above services should be provided by

Acute Hosp.   Chronic   SNF   ICF   Home Health Agy.   Rehab. Center

Signature _____   Date Signed _____

- Mental illness and mental retardation form (state specific)

- Face sheet for the health record

- Acknowledgment of the Notice of Privacy Practices

- The resident bill of rights (depending upon facility policy)

- The admission agreement (depending upon facility policy)

The remainder of this chapter discusses admission criteria, the application form and admission agreement, the release of information (ROI) agreement, acknowledgments, and the statement of resident's rights. Consents, assessments, face sheets, and other types of documentation are discussed in detail in subsequent chapters.

Preadmission Screening

Long-term care preadmission screening is a requirement of both state and federal agencies. It identifies appropriate and cost-effective services for persons applying for placement in a long-term care facility.

Preadmission screening also is required for mentally ill and mentally retarded individuals as outlined by the CMS in the *State Operations Manual* (2001b, p. 82.7). This preadmission screening is captured in the mental illness/mental retardation assessment. (The Preadmission Screening Assessment and Annual Resident Review [PASARR] is discussed in chapter 6.)

Preadmission screening entails the collection and review of resident-specific clinical information. This information is used to place the resident in the appropriate delivery setting and at the appropriate care level and to document the necessity of clinical interventions.

State licensing bodies and/or accreditation organizations establish the required time frames for conducting a preadmission screening. Every long-term care facility must have a predefined process. It is important to check all regulations to ensure that the facility is compliant with the most stringent regulation.

Admission Assessments

The JCAHO stipulates that the nursing assessment must be completed as specified in writing by the organization. The following time frames are minimum JCAHO standards requirements:

- MDS assessment with 14 days

- Subacute initial assessments are started with 24 hours prior to admission and completed within 72 hours after admission

The physician history and physical must be completed as specified by state regulations. The JCAHO does set requirements for completion of the history and physical or medical assessment. "This time frame must not exceed 24 hours before admission or within 72 hours after admission" (JCAHO 2004, PC.2.120). A history and physical received from the attending physician or licensed independent practitioner that has been completed within 30 days prior to admission may be used as long as "a summary of the resident's condition and course of care during the interim period, and the summary also includes the resident's current physical/ psychosocial status" (JCAHO 2004, PC.2.120). Residents in subacute care units must undergo a medical examination within forty-eight hours of admission. JCAHO requirements for history and physicals are located in the Provision of Care, Treatment, and Services (PC) chapter of the JCAHO *Accreditation Manual.* Physician history and physical requirements are discussed further in this book in chapter 12, Documentation of Physician Services. The JCAHO also requires that oral examinations be performed no more than ninety days prior to admission or no later than fourteen days after admission.

The **resident assessment instrument** (RAI) must be completed according to specified time frames. The completion schedule for residents who are eligible for Medicare benefits is slightly different from the schedule for other residents. (See the bulleted list below and chapter 7 for more detail on the RAI process.)

The facility must not condition the admission of the resident for any reason. Under federal regulations, the facility cannot ask residents or applicants to waive their rights to Medicare or Medicaid benefits. State laws may supersede some federal regulations. However, it is extremely important to check all applicable state laws to ensure that the facility is following the most stringent application requirements, whether federal or state.

During the RAI process, several assessments may need to be completed, including any or all of the following:

- Physician history and physical

- Nursing assessment

- Wound and skin assessment

- Fall assessment

- Bowel and bladder assessment

- Pain assessment

- Basic mental/cognitive examination

- Restraint assessment (only if applicable)

- Minimum Data Set assessment

- Nutritional assessment

- Therapy assessments, as required

- Therapeutic recreation assessment

- Pastoral care assessment

Application for Admission

The application for admission is an assessment tool used by the facility to determine the care needs of each patient applying for admission. It is used to ensure that the individual is properly placed. Every applicant must meet the facility's eligibility requirements before he or she can be placed on its waiting list.

Application Process

Many states do not require an application process, but in those that do require one, specific state requirements should drive the content of applications and other screening assessments.

The first step in the application process is to perform a thorough assessment of the applicant's needs. The application gathers information on the applicant's financial situation, preadmission clinical assessment, level of care determination, and care-planning requirements. It includes details about the applicant's medical condition, requirements for assistance with daily activities, information about the client's lifestyle, and facility choices. Eligibility for placement is based on criteria set by the organization. When the assessment has been completed, applications for placement are processed. The facility then reviews the application to determine whether it is able to meet the applicant's needs. Finally, the applicant goes on the waiting list for the facility and the type of services required.

An application to a long-term care facility simply indicates an individual's desire to be admitted to the facility. States may specifically regulate how applications and waiting lists are maintained. Additionally, they may specify that applicants must be admitted in the order that they applied and were placed on the waiting list.

The application process ensures that there is no discrimination in the admitting process and that the facility abides by both federal and state requirements related to admissions to long-term care facilities. In most instances, the regulations based on state Medicaid laws supersede the federal regulations. Because each state regulates its Medicaid program differently, each state has created different admission regulations.

State requirements for admissions to long-term care facilities may be very stringent. The processing and maintenance of applications, waiting lists, and other necessary paperwork also may need to fulfill very strict requirements. Additionally, time frames for responding to requests for an application may be very specific. The state may even define the content of the application and the wording for specific areas of the application.

Applicants or their legal representatives need to complete written applications as fully as possible to allow the long-term care facility to complete a good assessment of each applicant's needs. The application documents and waiting lists must be maintained according to relevant regulations to ensure that sound processes are in place and the information is readily available to state licensing agencies. The applications should be stored in the admitting office.

Content of Applications

The content of the application may include any or all of the following elements:

- Prospective resident information
  - Name, address, and telephone number
  - Date of birth
  - Marital status
  - Sex
  - Birthplace
  - Education
  - Religion
  - Citizenship status
- Power of attorney or conservator's name
- Individual responsible for paying the bill

—Name, address, and telephone number

—Relationship to resident

- Emergency contact: Name, address, and telephone number
- Primary physician, address, and telephone number
- Clinical data, mental status, ambulation, activities of daily living (ADL) needs
- General medical information
- Hospitalizations
- Prior nursing home placement
- Financial information
- Social Security number
- Medicare identification number
- Other insurance coverage
- Monthly income
- Transfer of assets
- Veteran status
- Signature and date of resident or resident's family member or responsible party
- Signature of guarantor and date
- State-required notices

Admission Agreement

The **admission agreement** is a legal contract. The long-term care facility requires prospective residents or their legal representatives to sign an admission agreement. The agreement specifies the facility's responsibilities and fees for providing healthcare and other services. It explains the daily rate, noncovered services, deposit and refund practices, and other policies and operating procedures.

Each resident or his or her legal representative signs an admission agreement that includes proposed charges, process for notification of changes in costs, right to appeal involuntary discharge, and discharge criteria. The state reviews the facility's admission agreements as part of the licensure process.

The admission agreement is part of the package provided to the resident upon admission to the facility. The Nursing Home Reform Act (discussed later in this chapter) mandated improvements in the quality of care provided in nursing homes. The admission agreement may contain state-specific requirements derived from the federal legislation.

The resident or his or her legal representative must be able to easily understand the contents of the admission agreement. The statement should clearly state what services are included in the basic daily rate and list the charges for items and services that are not included. Admission agreements should be kept according to facility policy. Some facilities may choose to place the admission agreement in the resident's record. However, because of the sensitive data such documents may contain, many facilities file them in the admitting office or other appropriate office for security and confidentiality reasons.

Content of Admission Agreements

State regulations may require specific components within the admission agreement. Following is a list of such components:

- Daily rates

- Billing procedures

- Charges for rates not covered

- Pharmacy charges

- Bed hold policy and rate

- Residents' rights and responsibilities

- Notice of right to apply for Medicare or Medicaid and right to appeal

- General policies of eviction conditions and notification procedures, visitation, banking hours, church services, and so on

- Resident transfers and discharges

- Policy on resident account funds

- Advance directives

- Storage space for personal items

- Theft and loss policies

- Procedure for filing complaints or grievances

- Availability of special telecommunication devices for residents who are deaf or hard of hearing or who have other disabling conditions

- Beauty parlor services

- Authority of the licensing agency to inspect the facility and to review records

- Provisions for terminating the agreement

Acknowledgments

The **acknowledgment** is a form that provides a mechanism for the resident to acknowledge receipt of important information. Depending on the facility, more than one acknowledgment may be required. Common acknowledgments of information provided during the admission process include acknowledgments of important information and of privacy notice.

One acknowledgment documents the receipt of the Important Message from Medicare. (See figure 2.4.) In some instances, the facility may require that the resident sign for the receipt of the following types of information:

- Resident bill of rights

- Leave of absence policy

- Bed hold policy

- Complaint and lost valuable policy

- Resident responsibilities

- Summary of charges and room rates

- Nondiscrimination policy

- Spousal assets assessment notification

- Notice of participation in Title 18 and 19 programs

- Copy of the resident handbook

- Personal funds policy

- Notices regarding Medicaid

- Privacy Act notification

- Other state-required notifications

- Other pertinent facility policies

This list may be included in one acknowledgment form as appropriate with a signature line and date required to prove receipt of the information.

HIPAA requires that every patient or resident of a healthcare facility receive a notice of privacy practice in the facility. The acknowledgment form for the notice need not be a separate form unless specified by state law. The acknowledgment can be included on the general consent to treat form as two check-off boxes indicating the following options:

- I acknowledge that I received the notice of privacy practice.

- The facility offered the notice of privacy practice, but the resident did not take the information.

Figure 2.4.   Acknowledgment form

[insert organization's name and address]

ACKNOWLEDGE OF RECEIPT

Resident/Patient Name:_____

Health Record Number:_____

Acknowledge of Receipt: My signature only acknowledges my receipt of the Important Message from Medicare provided by [insert name of organization] on _____ and does not waive any of my rights to request a review of or make me liable for any payment.

_____
Signature of beneficiary or person
acting on behalf of the beneficiary

If you have any questions, you may contact [insert name or department to be contacted].

The resident or his or her family or legal representative signs the general consent to indicate that treatment may begin and that the acknowledgment of privacy notice was obtained.

The notice of privacy practice need only be provided to the resident once. By including the acknowledgment on the general consent, the facility actually provides the resident with the information at each admission. This system is important because the notice of privacy practice may change over time.

Acknowledgment Process

Practices on acknowledgments vary by facility, need, and policy. The process ensures that the information was provided to the resident and provides documentation that the information was given.

The federal and state-specific regulations provide guidance on the type and content of acknowledgment forms that each facility must have. Facility policy may mandate the use of other acknowledgments.

All acknowledgments may be filed in either the admission section or the miscellaneous section of the resident's health record in date order and by type of acknowledgment.

Resident's Bill of Rights

In a 1986 study initiated by Congress, the Institute of Medicine (IOM) showed that residents of nursing homes often experienced abuse and neglect and commonly received inadequate care. The IOM's report proposed extensive reforms to improve the quality of life for residents of nursing homes.

The proposed reforms became law in 1987 with passage of the **Nursing Home Reform Act,** part of the **Omnibus Budget Reconciliation Act of 1987.** The basic purpose of the Nursing Home Reform Act is to guarantee the quality of nursing home care and to ensure that the care residents receive helps them to achieve or maintain the "highest practicable" level of physical, mental, and psychosocial well-being. Specifically, the act requires that nursing homes and other long-term care facilities provide certain basic services to every resident and to establish a resident's bill of rights. The legislation created a minimum set of standards for residents' rights and care. According to Medicare rules, every "resident has a right to a dignified existence, self-determination, and communication with and access to persons and services inside and outside the facility. A facility must protect and promote the rights of each resident" (CMS 2001a, p. 2).

The Nursing Home Reform Act allows residents to exercise their rights and gives them autonomy in healthcare decision making. It allows all residents to have a "choice, to the maximum extent possible" concerning their way of life, specifically, "how they wish to live their everyday lives and receive care" (CMS 2001a, p. 2). Of course, the facility's policies and rules also must be taken into consideration.

Policies on the Resident's Bill of Rights

The legislation of a resident's bill of rights changed the legal requirements for nursing homes and other long-term care facilities. Under federal regulations, all nursing homes must have written policies that describe the rights of residents. These polices help define and clarify the resident's bill of rights and the responsibilities of the facility. Long-term care facilities must give all new residents a list of their rights under the regulations in a format that each resident can understand. For example, when a resident does not understand English or is hearing impaired, the facility must provide an interpreter who can explain the resident's rights. Moreover, facilities are required by law to provide a written copy of the resident's bill of rights to any resident who requests it.

Many states also have regulations that mirror the federal requirements and require policies that address resident rights. Every long-term care facility must abide by the federal, state, and local regulations governing a resident's rights to qualify for Medicare and Medicaid reimbursement.

Rights information should be made easily available to residents and families. Posting these rights in lounges, lobbies, and other common areas for residents and families helps residents keep their rights in mind.

Evidence that residents have received their rights may be checked by regulatory agencies and accreditation organizations. Thus, the form that acknowledges receipt of the resident's rights should be kept in the resident's health record. It can be placed with admission paperwork. Regulatory agencies and accreditation organizations also may ask residents specific questions regarding their rights.

The federal government outlines several rights that the resident retains upon admission to a long-term care facility. These rights include:

- The ability to exercise rights

- The need to be informed about rights and responsibilities

- The ability to have personal funds managed

- The ability to choose a physician or treatment and to participate in decisions and care planning

- The right to privacy and confidentiality of healthcare information

- The ability to voice grievances and to respond to any grievances

- The ability to review survey results

- The ability to work or not work

- The ability to have confidential mail service

- The ability to have visitors

- The ability to have telephone privacy

- The ability to keep personal possessions to the extent allowed by space and safety

- The ability to share a room with a spouse when requested

- The ability to self-administer medications when determined safe

- The ability to refuse a transfer within the facility

- The ability to be restraint free

- The ability to choose activities, programs, and healthcare options consistent with interests, assessments, and care plans

The JCAHO recognizes that "residents deserve care, treatment, and services that safeguards their personal dignity and respects their cultural, psychosocial, and spiritual values"

(JCAHO 2004, RI-1). The JCAHO resident's rights standards are published in the JCAHO *Comprehensive Accreditation Manual* in the chapter titled "Ethics, Rights and Responsibilities." The organization must have mechanisms in place to ensure that residents experience the respect they deserve. Additionally, mechanisms must be in place to address ethical issues in healthcare. The accreditation standards for resident's rights contain the following provisions:

- The long-term care organization must inform residents of their rights before or upon admission.

- The organization must resolve conflicts over care decisions with residents.

- The organization must support residents in achieving independent expression, choice, and decision making, as allowed by law.

- The organization must respect the resident's values, beliefs, cultural and spiritual preferences, and lifelong patterns of living.

Each long-term care facility must ensure that residents retain the rights provided in figure 2.5.

Figure 2.5.   Resident rights

- Personal freedom and dignity
- Impartial access to treatment or accommodations
- Confidentiality of information
- Privacy, safety, and security
- Freedom to exercise citizenship privileges
- Unlimited contact with visitors and others
- Appropriate assessment and management of pain
- Freedom from chemical or physical restraint
- Freedom from mental, physical, sexual, and verbal abuse as well as neglect and exploitation
- Freedom to perform or refuse to perform tasks in or for the organization
- Freedom to participate in, or refuse to participate in, social groups and community activities
- Freedom to keep and use personal clothing and possessions
- Ability to preserve one's dignity and contribute to a positive self-image
- Freedom to manage or delegate management of personal financial affairs
- Access to transportation services when appropriate within the care plan
- Effective communication from caregivers
- Freedom to engage in a complaint process
- Resident council
- Freedom to give informed consent
- Freedom to decide on withholding resuscitative services and providing, forgoing, or withdrawing life-sustaining treatment
- Healthcare decision making at the end of his or her life
- Freedom to select medical, dental, and other licensed independent healthcare practitioners
- Freedom to communicate with his or her medical, dental, and other licensed independent healthcare practitioners
- Freedom to refuse care or treatment to the extent permitted by law
- Ability to involve his or her family in making care or treatment decisions
- Freedom to formulate advance directives
- Freedom to participate in or to not participate in research, investigations, or clinical trials

State Long-Term Care Ombudsman Program

The long-term care ombudsman program was created in the mid-1970s to advocate the rights and needs of long-term care residents. The program operates in all fifty states, and each state has an Office of the State Long-Term Care Ombudsman to guide these efforts. The ombudsman has the following responsibilities:

- To receive, investigate, and resolve complaints from residents
- To pay regular visits to long-term care facilities
- To address instances of poor practice
- To maximize community awareness and involvement
- To influence public policy
- To ensure effective program administration

The state ombudsman is empowered to review the health records of residents with permission of the resident or his or her legal representative as allowed by federal and state laws. According to Medicare regulations, "The facility must provide immediate access to any representative of the Secretary of the Department of Health and Human Services, the State, the resident's individual physician, the State long-term care ombudsman, or the agencies responsible for the protection and advocacy of developmentally disabled or mentally ill individuals" (CMS 2001a, p. 27). Such representatives are not subject to visiting hour limitations.

Each long-term care facility must post information on the ombudsman program in a prominent place so that all residents or their family members have immediate access to the information.

Summary

When an individual seeks admission to a long-term care facility, he or she must go through a process during which documentation is gathered that will be used to determine the most appropriate program to fit his or her care needs. This admission process establishes communication between the resident and his or her family or representative and the facility's staff. A preadmission screening is used to obtain information so that the facility can best determine the potential resident's appropriate care level and capture all anticipated care needs and interventions.

Another tool used by the facility to determine a potential resident's level of care is the application for admission. Every applicant must meet the facility's eligibility requirements before he or she can be placed on the waiting list. The admission process also involves completing an admission application and signing an admission agreement, which is a legal document specifying the facility's responsibilities and fees. The resident also signs an acknowledgment, acknowledging receipt of important information.

In addition, facilities must inform potential residents of their rights under the Nursing Home Reform Act, which was designed to guarantee the quality of nursing home care and to ensure that residents are able to receive care that helps them to achieve or maintain optimal well-being. Residents also must be informed about the state long-term care ombudsman program, a program created in the mid-1970s to advocate for the rights of long-term care residents.

The admission process is prescribed by the facility's admission policies and procedures. Although policies and procedures may vary somewhat from one facility to another, most are determined in large part by federal and state regulations, including federal and state Medicare regulations in the case of Medicare residents.

References

Centers for Medicare and Medicaid Services. 2001a (October 31). Guidance to Surveyors—Long-Term Care Facilities, appendix PP in *State Operations Manual*. Available at http://www.cms.gov/manuals/pub07pdf/AP-P-PP.pdf.

Centers for Medicare and Medicaid Services. 2001b (October). Requirements for States and Long Term Care Facilities. Code of Federal Regulations, Title 42, Volume 3. Available at http://frwebgate.access.gpo.gov/cgi-bin/get-cfr.cgi.

Centers for Medicare and Medicaid Services. 2003 (January). Conditions of Participation for Hospitals. Code of Federal Regulations. Title 42, Volume 3. Available at http://frwebgate.access.gpo.gov/cgi-bin/get-cfr.cgi?TITLE=42&PART=482&SUBPART=C&TYPE=TEXT.

Department of Health and Human Services. Health Insurance Portability and Accountability Act of 1996. Administrative Simplification. Available at http://aspe.os.dhhs.gov/admnsimp.

Joint Commission on Accreditation of Healthcare Organizations. 2004. *Comprehensive Accreditation Manual for Long-term Care*. Oakbrook Terrace, Ill.: JCAHO.

Rehabilitation Accreditation Commission (CARF). www.carf.org.

Chapter 3

Consents and Authorizations

Several different kinds of consent and authorization forms are used in long-term care organizations. **Consents** provide a means for residents to convey to healthcare providers their implied or expressed permission to administer care or treatment or other medical procedures. In contrast, **authorizations** document the resident's formal, written permission to use or disclose his or her protected health information for purposes other than treatment, payment, or healthcare operations.

Policies and Procedures

Every long-term care facility should have a comprehensive policy that outlines how authorizations and consents are to be requested and documented. Formal procedures ensure that the facility is aware of all of the consents and authorizations in use and that residents fully understand every document they are asked to sign.

The policy should list each type of consent and authorization and describe its use as well as the parties responsible for explaining the documents to residents and requesting their signatures. The policy should provide specific information on the admission agreement, acknowledgment of receipt of Medicare benefits, and an outline of the facility's procedure for witnessing signatures.

Different Consent Forms

General and specific consents to treatment are the most common forms of consents. A **general consent to treatment** (figure 3.1) or **general consent** covers ongoing medical and nursing care or treatment and usually includes the resident's agreement to pay for the services provided by the facility, to assign insurance benefits to the facility, and to allow the facility to obtain or release health records for payment purposes. More **specific consents to treatment** explain the potential risks and benefits of a particular treatment or procedure and constitute the resident's permission to the healthcare provider to perform the treatment or procedure. Examples of specific consents include those to receive blood or blood products and to undergo a diagnostic test. It should be noted that HIV testing requires the specific consent of the resident. Consent for HIV testing cannot be inferred from a general consent to treatment.

Other consents commonly documented by long-term facilities include consent to photograph (figure 3.2) and consent to restrain.

Resident's Rights and Informed Consent

The purpose of obtaining consents is to provide adequate information to the residents to allow them to make the best decisions about their care and disclosure of health information. The consent goes hand-in-hand with resident rights. The consent is a mechanism for the resident to exercise his or her rights and allows the resident to have autonomy in decision making and the care provided. It enhances the fact that all residents have a "choice, to the maximum extent possible," concerning their way of life, specifically, "how they wish to live their everyday lives and receive care" (CMS 2001, p. 2).

Figure 3.1.   **General consent to treatment**

(Please have legal counsel review before use)

XYZ Organization
Anytown USA 00000

GENERAL CONSENT

Consent to Treat: I consent to (name of the organization) to provide and perform such medical/surgical care, treatments, interventions, tests, procedures, drugs, and other services and supplies as are considered necessary or beneficial for my health and well-being. I acknowledge that no representations, warranties, or guarantees as to the results or cures have been made to me or relied upon by me.

Release of Medical Records: I authorize (name of the organization) to release information from my medical record to my insurance carrier(s), or third-party payers, including the Medicare program or its intermediaries or carriers, or to the professional review organizations for processing of claims for medical benefits or government agency for the processing of claims for medical benefits. I have the right to revoke this authorization in writing at any time except to the extent that action has been taken in reliance on it. Revocation of this consent will be signed and addressed to the manager of medical records.

Assignment of Benefits: I assign any benefits that I or the insured may have or may be entitled to (name of the organization) toward payment of my charges unless I pay my account in full each month. I request that my insurance company(s) honor my assignment of insurance benefits applicable to the services and pay all assigned insurance benefits directly to (name of the organization), on my behalf.

If I am eligible for, I request Medicare benefits. I also appoint (name of the organization) as my agent to act on my behalf to collect claims for my charges. I also understand that my insurance benefits are subject to verification by (name of the organization) and that I am responsible for any charges not covered by this assignment.

Financial Arrangements: I understand all accounts are the full responsibility of the resident and/or the resident's responsible party/guarantor. If I am or become a Medicaid resident, I will pay all applied income monthly without billing from the facility. In the case of default payment, I promise to pay any legal interest on the balance due, together with any collection costs and reasonable attorney fees incurred to effect collection of this account or future outstanding accounts.

I certify that I have read and do understand the above general consent statements and that I am indeed authorized to sign this form and agree to all of the terms contained within.

_____   _____
Resident's Signature   Date

_____   _____
Responsible Party   Date

Figure 3.2. **Observation and photographic consent**

(Please have legal counsel review before use)

XYZ Organization
Anytown USA 00000

OBSERVATION AND PHOTOGRAPHIC CONSENT

Resident Name: _____ Health Record Number: _____

I, the undersigned, give full permission to (name of organization) to take photographs, videotape, or other photographic images of _____
(resident's name)

and to use or disclose such photographic image(s) for the following purposes:
☐ treatment ☐ training of personnel ☐ education
☐ advertising ☐ written publication(s) ☐ fund-raising
☐ public relations ☐ television/Web site ☐ research
☐ Other:_____
(please specify)

NOTES: _____

_____
(Please give any specific details of intended use.)

The photographic image(s) to be taken, used, or disclosed may include:

Full-face photograph, videotapes for treatment or other reason(s), television pictures, digital images, other (specify below)_____

I understand that this consent form is valid and enforceable for a period of _____ days.

If the purpose of this consent/authorization is for photographic images for journalistic and/or media purposes, I also authorize a representative of the news media involved to observe any procedures or treatments required for the photographs and allow the media to discuss them with my physician/healthcare provider.

Videotapes/photographic images that are not taken solely for treatment purposes are not considered part of the medical record and are destroyed at the convenience of the hospital/facility.

I expressly waive any right to control copying, reproduction, or distribution of any pictures taken in accordance with this consent form/authorization, and I expressly waive any right to any compensation whatsoever for any use of such photographic images.

I understand that this authorization is only for the specific, stated purpose and may be revoked by me at any time upon written request to the medical record manger, except to the extent that action has been taken in reliance on this authorization.

I understand that if the person or the entity that receives the photographic images and any related protected health information is not a healthcare provider or health plan covered by the federal privacy regulations, the information described above may be redisclosed and no longer protected by those regulations.

I understand that I may refuse to sign this authorization and that my refusal to sign will not affect my ability to obtain treatment, payment for my care, or my eligibility for benefits. I may inspect any photographic images released under this authorization.

I certify that I am over eighteen (18) years of age and have the legal right and authority to sign this consent form for myself. I understand the meaning of this consent form, and I hereby release (name of the organization) from any claim or liability whatsoever in connection with the taking or use of photographic images and related observation.

_____ _____
Signature of Resident/Patient/Legal Guardian or Representative   Date

Relationship to the patient, if applicable: _____

_____ _____
Witness: (If resident/patient is unable to sign/write)   Date

Both federal and accreditation standards require that patients provide their **informed consent** before undergoing medical procedures or treatment. The Joint Commission on Accreditation of Healthcare Organizations' (JCAHO's) closed health record audit asks for evidence of informed consent in the resident's health record. State-specific guidelines also may be applicable to informed consent as well as to other required consents. It is important to check all state regulations with respect to all consents.

The person who will perform the medical procedure should obtain the informed consent. In the case of the consent to treat, the facility in which the resident would reside will obtain the consent. However, in the case of the resident being sent to an acute care facility for surgery, the physician performing the surgery would be required to obtain the informed consent. Some states and case laws may permit the actual obtaining of the resident signature on the consent form to be delegated to others. However, this requires that the physician performing the surgical procedure will have first discussed the procedure with the resident.

The resident must be capable of providing a consent. If he or she is not legally or mentally capable of understanding the reason for the consent, the guardian, legal representative, or next of kin as defined by state law may act on the resident's behalf. The responsible party must be given all the information about the medical and surgical procedures before signing any consent. The medical and surgical procedure must be discussed with the resident in terms that he or she can understand for any type of consent. In cases where the resident may need interpreter services because of language barriers or hearing impairment, these services must be provided to the resident.

The resident must be free from coercion or undue influence when providing consent. He or she has the right to refuse any treatment and the right to refuse to provide consent for medical and surgical procedures.

General Requirements

Each consent form contains specific information that is needed for the particular consent required. Federal and state governments and regulatory agencies as well as the facility's own policies mandate what information should be included on each specific type of consent.

The quality concern with any consent is the necessity to have it completely filled out. All areas on the form that contain a check box, initials, or other required information should be filled in. If particular areas are not applicable or if the resident does not consent to a specific part or section of a consent form, this should be so indicated.

All consent forms become part of the resident's health record as evidence that consent was obtained. Each specific form has a designated location within the health record. (See the sample chart order policy in appendix E for placement of specific consents.)

Types of Consent to Treatment

In long-term care facilities, residents are asked to give their general consent to undergo treatment at the time of admission. The general consent gives the facility's staff permission to perform routine medical and nursing services for the resident. More specific consents to treatment are required before more invasive procedures can be performed, such as surgical procedures.

Long-term care facilities also may need to develop consent forms for other activities that occur in the institution. State regulations may require specific consent forms that are not listed in figure 3.1. Always check with state regulations and accrediting body agency rules to ensure that the facility has the proper consents outlined in the consent policy.

General Consent to Treatment

As mentioned earlier, a general consent to treatment or general consent is the consent signed upon admission to the facility that allows the clinical staff to provide care and treatment for the resident; thus, it must be signed before any treatment is initiated. The general consent certifies that the resident or resident's responsible party has agreed to the medical care that is available at the facility. "The general consent form records the [resident's] consent to routine services, general diagnostic procedures, medical treatment, and everyday routine touching of the [resident]" (Pozgar 1996, p. 399). Written consent provides visible proof of the resident's wishes for services. The general consent does not, however, override formulated advance directives. (See chapter 4 for information on advance directives.)

The general consent to treatment provides a record of the resident's permission to receive medical care at the facility. It is interesting to note that failure to have a consent to treatment signed could result in a claim of battery.

> Battery is an intentional touching of another's person, in a socially impermissible manner, without the person's consent. . . . [T]he principle of law concerning battery and the requirement of consent to medical and surgical procedures is critically important. . . . Procedures ranging from bathing to surgery involve some touching of a [resident]. Therefore, medical and surgical procedures must be authorized by the [resident]. If they are not authorized, the person performing the procedure could be subject to an action for battery (Pozgar 1996, pp. 59–60).

The process for signing the consent to treatment must be well established in the long-term care facility. This process protects the resident's rights to decision making and provides a mechanism for the facility to show that all residents are provided opportunities to consent to treatment and care interventions.

Permission to obtain or release health records in the general consent form pertains only to the information that may be needed for reimbursement purposes. The general consent form does not constitute carte blanche permission to release all health records. States may have specific rules and regulations that pertain to the release of information, and these regulations and rules must be considered when developing the general consent form.

The general consent to treatment usually includes statements covering permission to provide treatment, agreement to pay for services, assignment of benefits, and permission to obtain or release health records for payment purposes. It not only allows treatment but also covers other general categories of information that may be needed to ensure that the bill can be paid. State regulations may have specific requirements for the content of the consent to treatment or general consent form.

Like other health record forms, the general consent to treatment must include the name of the facility. The form also must contain a general statement of the resident's consent to undergo treatment. By signing the form, the resident agrees to undergo diagnostic, laboratory, and other general medical procedures or examinations not included under informed consent. The consent section also explains that there are no guarantees or promises as to the results of care to be performed. Also included is a statement that the resident consents to further testing deemed appropriate by the facility's infection control nurse. A disclaimer should be added to indicate that the form does not cover HIV/AIDS testing.

In addition, the general consent to treatment should include a statement of agreement to pay for the care provided; that is, the resident agrees to pay for the care the facility provides. When the resident is covered under the Medicaid payment system, the agreement states that the resident agrees to pay all applied income. The resident also agrees that should the account become delinquent, the payment will also include the cost of collection and legal fees.

Further, the general consent contains a statement of assignment of benefits whereby the resident agrees to assign insurance payment benefits to the facility. In this section, residents who are eligible to receive Medicare benefits agree to request Medicare benefits and to allow the facility to act as the agent to collect claims. The resident also agrees that insurance benefits are subject to verification and agrees to pay all charges not covered by insurance plans. The resident may choose to pay personally for any treatment so that information concerning diagnoses would not be released to the insurance plan.

Permission to release health records for purposes of providing treatment also is covered in the general consent to treatment. By signing the form, the resident agrees to permit the facility to release any health record information to the resident's insurance carrier; other healthcare agencies; or any utilization, managed care, and/or quality review organizations affiliated with the insurance carrier. This section of the form should have a clause stating that the consent may be revoked except to the extent that action has already been taken.

The section of the form that pertains to obtaining health records allows the facility to obtain any information from other sources related to the resident's treatment plan.

Another section of the form provides check-off boxes that indicate whether the resident received a copy of the facility's privacy practices notice.

Finally, the form must be signed and dated by the resident or the resident's legal representative. The representative's relationship to the resident and the witness's dated signature also should be included, if required.

It should be noted that states may have defined requirements for the content of the general consent. The consent form may differ depending upon facility policy as well.

Informed Consent to Treatment

An informed consent to treatment should be granted for specific procedures or treatments. The exact procedure to be performed must be sufficiently explained. Extenuating circumstances that could occur during the procedure also should be explained so that the resident understands that the procedure could be more extensive than originally planned. The resident must be given the opportunity to ask questions and receive answers about the procedure from the person explaining the procedure. He or she must understand the risks, benefits, the nature and purpose, reasonable alternatives, and risks of refusing the proposed procedure before the resident or responsible party authorizes the consent.

The resident should also understand that, as a result of unforeseen circumstances during the course of the procedure, additional operative or medical procedures might be necessary. The consent should allow a section for the resident to authorize the healthcare provider to modify the proposed procedure or to perform any additional procedures that are required or desirable in the exercise of his or her professional judgment. There should be a statement on the consent form that indicates that there are no guarantees of the outcome of the procedure.

The resident's signature indicates that he or she has had sufficient opportunity to discuss the condition and the treatment and that all questions have been answered satisfactorily. A statement that the resident has adequate knowledge upon which to base an informed consent to the proposed treatment should be included. The facility should consider telephone consent policy and include that option on the form. The form should be signed and dated by the person explaining the procedure to the patient and include witnesses, as appropriate. The forms must be signed and dated by the resident or authorized representative (along with an indication of the relationship to the resident).

The following items should be considered when developing an informed consent, depending on state regulations. The person performing the procedure is the person who provides the information to the resident unless stipulated differently in state regulations and requirements. The following must be discussed and explained to the resident's satisfaction:

- The procedure(s)/treatment(s)

- The benefits of the procedure(s)/treatment(s)

- The reasonably foreseeable risk involved in the procedure(s)/treatment(s)

- The reasonably foreseeable risks of not having the procedure(s)/treatment(s)

- The reasonable alternatives for care or treatment

- The potential use of blood and/or blood products

- The benefits and reasonable foreseeable risks of anesthesia or intravenous conscience sedation

Other Types of Consents

The resident's consent is also required in other healthcare contexts. For example, the facility must request the resident's permission before taking photographs or videotaping the resident. The use of restraints to protect the resident from injury also may be necessary in long-term care facilities, and a special consent form applies to the use of restraints.

Consent to Photograph

There are several reasons that a long-term care facility might wish to photograph the residents. Each purpose may need its own consent form. Typical reasons for photographing residents include:

- A consent to photograph for purposes of observation and recording of treatment provides permission from the resident to have pictures or videotapes made to demonstrate to other clinical staff members how treatment should be performed. The photograph might show positioning of the resident in a bed, recliner, or wheelchair, or be used for other identified reasons. It is a mechanism for communicating to staff what treatment options are best for the resident.

- Consent to photograph also may be used to document wounds and the their healing process. Such photographs also may be used to support skin assessments and help identify areas of concern such as location and size of decubitus ulcers, bruises, and other skin conditions. The photographs typically do not help to identify the patient but, rather, to identify skin condition locations and size. Thus, some facilities may not require a consent for photography to be completed for this particular documentation.

- Consents to observe, photograph, or videotape patients for educational purposes provide educational opportunities for staff to learn new types of treatment options. They are not used to help provide care to the resident but, rather, to educate staff on specific techniques or procedures.

- Consents to photograph may also be used for identification purposes. The photo is usually placed in the resident's health record or medication administration record (MAR) to help identify the resident when medications and treatments are provided.

- A consent to photograph residents during leisure activities permits the activity department to photograph residents at functions or parties. It allows the facility the opportunity to take snapshots of residents in leisure activities for posters or displays that can be hung in public areas within the facility. If photos will be used for publicity purposes, on a Web site, or in a facility newsletter sent to families and associates, a separate consent should also be signed.

- A consent to videotape/photograph upon an attorney's request provides authorization for the attorney to videotape or photograph the resident for legal reasons or litigation.

Consent to Restrain

The **consent to restrain** is used in those few instances when the resident must be restrained to ensure quality of life. "The resident has the right to be free from any physical or chemical restraints imposed for purposes of discipline or convenience, and not required to treat the resident's medical symptoms" (CMS 2001, p. 44). Restraints should be used only when the resident's medical symptoms indicate a need to protect the resident as defined in the federal regulations. A consent to restrain does not advocate restraining residents. In fact, facilities look for the least restrictive device to attain the highest level of functioning for the resident.

Two types of restraints are used in long-term care and other healthcare facilities: physical restraints and chemical restraints. According to the CMS, **physical restraints** include any manual or mechanical device, material, or equipment attached or adjacent to a resident's body, which the individual cannot easily remove. Physical restraints restrict the resident's freedom of movement and prevent the resident's normal access to his or her body. Chemical restraints include any drug that is used for purposes of discipline or convenience and is not required to treat the resident's medical symptoms (CMS 2001, p. 44).

The resident or the resident's legal representative must be told in language that can be understood why the restrictive device is required. The consent to restrain is not signed until the resident or resident's legal representative has been clearly informed. The restrictive device cannot be applied until the resident and/or responsible party has authorized the device.

Except in emergencies, the resident or resident's legal representative must be informed of the reason for the restraint, including the risks and benefits of its use. A physician order must be obtained as specified by state law when the restraint is to continue for the resident. The order must contain the type of restraint, frequency, and duration, and specify the indication for use.

Facility clinical staff must monitor the use of the restraint to "promote the highest practicable level of physical, mental, and psychosocial well-being of the resident" (CMS 2001, p. 83). Moreover, there must be ongoing assessments of the need for the device. Residents who are restrained must be checked periodically, and the restraint must be released according to regulations. The physical restraint RAP should be used to assess the relevance of the restraint.

State law may govern the use of restrictive devices, and thus the content of the form may differ from state to state. The consent to restrain may contain the following information:

- Explanation of the reason for the restrictive device, including "how the use of restraints would treat the resident's medical symptoms and assist the resident in attaining or maintaining his/her highest practicable level of physical or psychological well-being" (CMS 2001, p. 46)

- The benefits of the restrictive device

- The reasonably foreseeable risk involved in using the restrictive device

- The reasonably foreseeable risks of *not* applying the restrictive device
- The reasonable alternatives for the restrictive device

Devices that may be considered a restraint, depending on how they are used, include:

- Leg restraints
- Arm restraints
- Hand mitts
- Soft ties or vests
- Lap cushions
- Lap trays the resident cannot remove easily
- Recliner chairs
- Ambulation devices such as merry walkers
- Wheelchair brakes
- Bed rails
- Height of the bed from the floor
- Use of restrictive mattresses
- Mechanisms to keep residents in a confined area, such as beds against walls, black floor mats, chairs behind counters, and such

Facility practices that constitute a restraint include:

- Side rails that restrict the resident to bed
- Tucking in bed linens or using Velcro to restrict a resident's movement
- Restrictive devices used in combination with a chair to prevent the resident from rising
- Chairs that prevent the resident from rising
- Placement of furniture too close to objects preventing the resident from rising

"Side rails sometimes restrain residents. The use of side rails as restraints is prohibited unless they are necessary to treat a resident's medical symptoms" (CMS 2001, p. 45). Documentation of the need for the side rail should be contained in the resident's health record.

The facility must have a detailed restraint policy for the organization. The goal of the facility is to promote an environment that is as restraint free as possible. Prior to a restrictive device being applied, a restraint use assessment must be completed and filed in the health record. (See chapter 6 for the restraint use assessment criteria.) Restrictive devices for the resident are only used based on a thorough assessment finding. Nonrestrictive alternatives are explored and utilized prior to the request for consent for restraint. Those residents who require restrictive devices must have ongoing evaluation and reassessments on a periodic basis. The resident has the right to refuse restrictive devices.

The JCAHO standards pertaining to restraints are located in the resident rights (RI) and treatment of residents (PC) chapters of the accreditation manual. These standards mirror the federal regulations for restraints.

The restraint consent is filed in the resident's health record.

Miscellaneous Consents

Additional consents that may be used in the long-term care setting include:

- *Consent to test for HIV:* An infection control–specific consent to test for HIV/AIDS virus in the event that sure testing is deemed necessary

- *Consent to receive influenza immunization:* An informed consent permitting the facility to administer to the resident an annual influenza vaccination (this form must contain the same content criteria as previously discussed for informed consent) (See figure 3.3.)

- *Consent for autopsy:* A consent that allows an autopsy to be performed on the resident

Documentation of Consents in the Health Record

Every type of consent should have the facility name on the form. The consent would clearly outline to what the resident is consenting. The form should be in language that is easily understood. Each form should have signature lines and date lines and contain witness signature and date areas, if needed. Each should have an expiration date included in the body of the consent. Each consent form should be signed as close to the activity occurring as possible, but never after the activity has taken place.

The general and informed consents to treatment should be filed in the resident's health record. Other consents also may be placed in the health record. When the consent expires, it

Figure 3.3.   Information consent for influenza immunization

XYZ organization
AnyTown USA 00000

Influenza Immunization Informed Consent

Please check the appropriate choice and sign in the space provided below:

- ☐ I give XYZ facility permission to administer an influenza vaccination to me annually, in the fall.

- ☐ I do not give XYZ facility permission to administer an influenza vaccination to me annually, in the fall.

I have been instructed that as a result of this vaccination, I may experience some side effects such as the following:

- slight discomfort
- soreness of the administration site
- redness of the administration site
- slight fever
- muscle aches

_____   _____
Signature of Resident   Date

_____   _____
Signature of Conservator/Responsible Party   Date

_____   _____
Signature of Witness   Date

should be moved to the overflow files within the health record department for filing with the entire record upon discharge. Consents should be placed in the resident's health record in alphabetical order, by date, so that each type of consent form is placed together. (See the chart order, admission, and discharge policy in appendix E.)

Authorization to Release Information

A resident's confidential information should not be divulged without his or her expressed authorization or the permission of his or her legal representative. The release of health record information provides a mechanism for the resident to authorize disclosure of his or her protected health information. (See figure 3.4.)

The Health Insurance Portability and Accountability Act (HIPAA) of 1996 mandates use of an authorization to release health records at the federal level. This legislation is the minimum required for the release to occur. State-specific regulations may be more stringent and would preempt the HIPAA requirements.

"Those who come into possession of the most intimate personal information about [residents] have both a legal and ethical duty not to reveal confidential communications. . . . All health care professionals who have access to medical records have a legal, ethical, and moral obligation to protect the confidentiality of the information in the records" (Pozgar 1996, p. 378). The release of information is not required when reporting vital statistics, diagnoses, or other required reporting to government agencies.

The release of information ensures that the resident's protected health information is disclosed as provided by federal, state, and accrediting bodies. (See chapter 2 for the description of the process for release of information.)

General Requirements

The federal and state rules and regulations dictate the general requirements of the release of information (ROI) authorization. Because state laws differ from state to state, individual states will have different requirements on the ROI form.

The authorization to release health record information should be completed at the time of the request for the release. The authorization may be good for specified periods of time as outlined in the actual release form. If the authorization for ROI has expired, the resident or his or her legal representative must sign a new one. An authorization for release of health records must be completed for each person or entity to whom the resident wants the information sent.

When developing the authorization, it is important that facilities use federal (HIPAA) requirements as well as appropriate state requirements. The authorization to release information should contain the following elements, but may have additional components depending on state specifications:

- Resident's name

- Health record number

- Date of birth

- Name of the person or facility that will release the information

- Statement on the authorization of release

Figure 3.4.   Sample authorization to release information

[ORGANIZATION NAME]

AUTHORIZATION

**RELEASE OF RESIDENT/PATIENT INFORMATION
INCLUDING HIV/AIDS-RELATED INFORMATION**

Resident/Patient Name:_____   Date of Birth: _____

I authorize [insert ORGANIZATION NAME] to release the following information from my health record relating to the diagnosis and treatment for medical, psychiatric, drug, or alcohol abuse**, if applicable, to the party named below. In addition, I authorize [insert ORGANIZATION NAME] to release information from my health record relating to confidential HIV/AIDS*** related information, if applicable, to the party named below.

Information to be released to:

_____
(Name)

_____
(Address)

_____
(City, State, Zip Code)

For the purpose of: _____
                    (continuity of care, medical review, benefit review, etc)

This information covers the period of care from _____ to _____
_____Discharge summary   _____Physician orders   _____Nurse's notes
_____History and physical   _____Laboratory   _____Therapies
_____Progress notes   _____X ray/EKG/EEG   _____Other_____
_____Consultations   _____Social work   _____

I understand that with respect to psychiatric information, refusal to grant consent to release of information will not jeopardize the resident/patient's right to obtain present or future treatment except where disclosure is necessary for treatment.

I understand that this consent is only for the specific, stated purpose and may be revoked by me at any time upon written request communicated to the Nursing Home, except to the extent that the Nursing Home has already acted in reliance upon the consent. If not previously revoked, this consent shall expire on the earlier of _____ or six (6) months form the date I have signed it.

*The confidentiality of your health and psychiatric records is required under [insert CITATION of STATE STATUES]. This material shall not be transmitted to anyone without written consent or other authorization as provided in the aforementioned statues.

**In the event that information released is protected by the HHS Confidentiality of Alcohol and Drug Abuse Resident/Patient Records regulations:

This information has been disclosed to you from records protected by federal confidentiality rules (42 CFR Part 2). The federal rules prohibit you from making any further disclosure of this information unless further disclosure is expressly permitted by the written consent of the person to whom is pertains or as otherwise permitted by 42 CFR Part 2. A general authorization for the release of medical or other information is NOT sufficient for this purpose. The federal rules restrict any use of the information to criminally investigate or prosecute any alcohol or drug abuse resident/patient.

*** In the event that information released constitutes confidential HIV/AIDS related information protected under [insert CITATION of STATE STATUES]:

This information has been disclosed to you from records whose confidentiality is protected by state law. State law prohibits you from _____.

***I understand that "confidential HIV-related information" [insert CITATION of STATE STATUES].

Signature of Resident/Patient/Legal Guardian: _____

Relationship: _____   Date: _____

Witness: _____   Date: _____
(If resident/patient is unable to sign/write)

- Name and address of the person to whom release is granted

- Purpose of the release of information

- Types of information to be released and dates of service for which the information was created

- Protections for information related to AIDS or HIV status

- Protections for psychology/psychiatry documentation

- Expiration date of the authorization to release

- Revocation clause

- Federal or state statutes

- Statement on redisclosure

- Statement that treatment cannot be conditioned on refusal to sign the authorization

- Statement to identify whom the resident or resident's family may contact with questions on disclosure activities (privacy officer or facility-specified individual)

- Signature of resident, legal representative, or other authorized party

- Date the authorization was signed

- Witnesses, as appropriate

Documentation in the Health Record

Refer to chapter 2 for the placement of the authorization to release health records or see appendix E for the chart order policy.

Miscellaneous Authorizations

Other authorizations that may be necessary under specific circumstances include:

- *Authorization for communication of information:* An authorization that designates with whom the resident prefers to share his or her health information (the form may indicate that the resident prefers not to share information with anyone).

- *Authorization to participate in a resident fund:* An authorization that allows the facility to manage the resident's fund account in accordance with federal and state law.

- *Authorization to forward mail:* An authorization that empowers the facility to forward any business or personal mail to an individual, a department within the facility, or another option.

- *Authorization to release information to the media:* An authorization that allows the facility to release information about the resident to the news media. Such an authorization must be completed prior to any release of information to the media or press. (The facility must establish a policy and procedure to manage the release of information to the media.)

Requests for Information

From time to time, the facility may need to obtain protected health information from other facilities when a resident is admitted or discharged. The authorization to request information is specifically designed for such times. (See figure 3.5.)

Facilities should have policies and procedures for managing a request for information. The resident or resident's responsible party signs the request for information specifying what protected health information is required. Usually, the form is then sent to the health record department for processing and tracking of the request.

The request for information form is similar to the release of information form. Again, state laws may define requirements for the request for information.

The timeliness of the request for information is similar to the release of information. The request for information is filed in the miscellaneous section of the resident's health record.

The content of the request for information may include the following information:

- Organization's name
- Facility/practice name and address from where the information is being requested
- Resident's full name and date of birth
- Dates of treatment
- Information requested
- Reason for the request
- Expiration date of the authorization to release
- Revocation clause
- Federal or state statues
- Signature of resident or authorized responsible party
- Date the authorized was signed

State laws and facility requirements, as outlined under policies that have been developed as a result of HIPAA, should be checked for additional specifications concerning requests for information.

Summary

Many consent forms may be present in the long-term care facility driven by federal, state, and regulatory agencies. The consent documents the permission of the resident to provide a service or function. Certain consents may be detailed in format; others provide information for a specific function within the facility and have less detail on the form.

Consents are important documents for the resident. They protect his or her rights that are inherent in the constitution of the United States. Facilities must get permission from residents for specific procedures or services to occur within the organization. The policies and procedures that govern these consents must be clearly written and followed by all facility staff to ensure that the resident's rights are protected.

Figure 3.5.   Sample authorization to request information

[ORGANIZATION NAME]

AUTHORIZATION

**REQUEST OF RESIDENT/PATIENT INFORMATION
INCLUDING HIV/AIDS-RELATED INFORMATION**

I, the undersigned, hereby request: _____
                                                                    (Facility/Practice name)

_____
(Address)

_____
(Address)

_____
(City, State, Zip Code)

to release the following information from my health record, relating to the diagnosis and treatment for medical, psychiatric, drug, or alcohol abuse**, if applicable, to [insert ORGANIZATION NAME]. I also request the above facility to release confidential HIV/AIDS*** related information, if applicable, to [insert ORGANIZATION NAME], to be used for the purpose of continuing care, evaluation, and further treatment.

I understand that this permission can be revoked by me at any time upon written request (not retroactively) and that this consent will automatically expire in 90 days from the date of issue.

I understand that with respect to psychiatric information, my refusal to grant consent to release of information will not jeopardize my right to obtain present or future treatment except where disclosure is necessary for treatment.

Patient Identifying Information

Resident/Patient Name: _____   Date of Birth: _____

Dates of Treatment: _____ to _____

Information/reports requested:
_____Discharge summary   _____Physician orders   _____Nurse's notes
_____History and physical   _____Laboratory   _____Therapies
_____Progress notes   _____X ray/EKG/EEG   _____Other_____
_____Consultations   _____Social work   _____

*The confidentiality of your health and psychiatric records is required under [insert CITATION of STATE STATUES]. This material shall not be transmitted to anyone without written consent or other authorization as provided in the aforementioned statutes.

**In the event that information released is protected by the HHS Confidentiality of Alcohol and Drug Abuse Resident/Patient Records regulations:

This information has been disclosed to you from records protected by federal confidentiality rules (42 CFR Part 2). The federal rules prohibit you from making any further disclosure of this information unless further disclosure is expressly permitted by the written consent of the person to whom it pertains or as otherwise permitted by 42 CFR Part 2. A general authorization for the release of medical or other information is NOT sufficient for this purpose. The federal rules restrict any use of the information to criminally investigate or prosecute any alcohol or drug abuse resident/patient.

*** In the event that information released constitutes confidential HIV/AIDS [insert CITATION of STATE STATUES].

This information has been disclosed to you from records whose confidentiality is protected by state law. [insert CITATION of STATE STATUES].

***I understand that "confidential HIV-related information" [insert CITATION of STATE STATUES].

Signature of Resident/Patient/Legal Guardian: _____

Relationship: _____   Date: _____

Witness: _____   Date: _____
(If resident/patient is unable to sign/write)

Authorizations provide a mechanism for the resident to grant permission for disclosures of protected health information. Authorizations should be based on both federal and state requirements and contain all the elements mandated by HIPAA. Authorizations should be used for both release of information and request for information disclosures.

References

American Health Information Management Association. 2002. Practice Brief: Required content for authorizations to disclose. Available at www.ahima.org.

Centers for Medicare and Medicaid Services. 2001 (October 31). Guidance to Surveyors—Long-Term Care Facilities, appendix PP in *State Operations Manual*. Available at www.cms.gov.

Health Insurance Portability and Accountability Act of 1996. Available at http://aspe.os.dhhs.gov/admnsimp.

Pozgar, George D. 1996. *Legal Aspects of Healthcare Administration*. 6th ed. Gaithersburg, Md.: Aspen.

Chapter 4

Advance Directives

Advance directives are documents that give individual residents a way to state in advance the kinds of treatment they would or would not want if they were ever to become mentally or physically unable to make their own healthcare decisions or communicate their wishes. Through advance directives, residents also are able to authorize another person to make those decisions for them in the event they became incapacitated.

Types of Advance Directives

According to the Joint Commission on Accreditation of Healthcare Organizations (JCAHO), advance directives include do-not-hospitalize orders, **do-not-resuscitate (DNR) orders,** and organ donation processes (JCAHO 2004, RI.2.80).

Although state legal requirements vary, the two most widely accepted advance directives are the living will and the **durable power of attorney for healthcare** (DPAHC). A **living will** is a directive that allows an individual to describe in writing the type of healthcare that he or she would or would not wish to receive. A DPAHC is a directive that allows an individual to appoint a proxy, or agent, to make healthcare decisions in the event that he or she is no longer able to make or express his or her own decisions. It also may describe the type of healthcare the individual would or would not wish to receive. (See figure 4.1 for a sample advance directive.)

Patient's Right to Self-Determination

Federal regulations mandated by the **Patient Self-Determination Act** (PSDA) require hospitals, skilled nursing facilities, hospices, home health agencies, and health maintenance organizations (HMOs) that provide services to Medicare and Medicaid beneficiaries to provide their patients with information about advance directives. Regulations also require these healthcare providers to explain each patient's legal right to make decisions about his or her own medical care.

The PSDA became effective on December 1, 1991. Specifically, the act stipulates the following requirements:

- Healthcare facilities must provide written information on the following subjects to all patients and residents upon admission to the facility:

    —The patient's rights under the law to make healthcare decisions, including the right to accept or refuse treatment and the right to complete advance directives as permitted by applicable state laws

—The facility's written policies concerning the execution of those rights

- Healthcare facilities must document the fact that the resident has an advance directive in the health record.

- Healthcare facilities must not place conditions on the care they provide to an individual nor may they discriminate against an individual on the basis of the existence of an advance directive.

- Healthcare facilities must take steps to ensure compliance with advance directives.

- Healthcare facilities must provide education for staff and the community on issues concerning advance directives.

The PSDA also requires states to develop their own regulations concerning advance directives. Each state is required to develop a written description of the legal requirements for advance directives and provide that information to all healthcare providers within the state. Because the requirements of states may differ significantly, it is crucial that healthcare providers understand

Figure 4.1.   Sample advance directive

Resident Name: _____

Attending Physician: _____ Telephone No.: _____

Please indicate your decisions below by circling choices A through E.

A.   **Full code:** Residents are given total medical support including cardiopulmonary resuscitation (CPR) if required. In the absence of an order identifying another category, total support is always provided.

B.   **No CPR:** Indicates we will do all but CPR. Residents will remain candidates for aggressive medical treatment and transfer to a hospital for treatment of acute medical problems. Survival remains a goal, and every indicated therapeutic approach is utilized except to the point of cardiac arrest. If cardiac arrest occurs, CPR is not provided and the resident is permitted to die.

C.   **Comfort measures only/No CPR:** Indicates we will attempt to relieve pain and suffering, meeting the physical, emotional, and spiritual needs of the resident. Underlying diseases will not be treated aggressively, and hospitalization will only be ordered if the physician deems it necessary to provide comfort. Artificial methods of nutrition, hydration, and respiration will not be initiated.

D.   **No artificial nutrition support:** If I am unable to take adequate nutrition or fluids by mouth, I do not wish the placement of feeding tubes (nasogastric or gastrostomy).

E.   **I do not wish to make a decision** at this time and understand a full code will be performed.

F.   **Specific requests or additional comments:**

_____

_____

_____

_____   _____
Resident's Signature   Date

_____   _____
Responsible Party/Relationship   Date

I have been in communication with the resident or responsible party and am satisfied that he or she understands the risks and benefits of his or her decision.

_____   _____
Physician's Signature   Date

and abide by their state requirements for advance directives. Some states recognize only one form of advance directive; other states recognize several. In certain states, more than one form of advance directive is required to ensure that specific treatments are selected or avoided. Each state law is different, and no single form of advance directive is accepted in all fifty states.

The PSDA requires that facilities provide information about advance directives, but it is important to remember that completing an advance directive is a voluntary act of the resident. The law does not require that an advance directive be completed; rather, it requires only that information be given to the resident about such options.

Policies and Procedures

Every long-term care facility should develop an advance directive policy that describes what procedures the facility will follow to honor advance directives and durable powers of attorney for healthcare. Policies should cover the specific requirements involved in complying with every type of advance directive. For example, some states may require that the resident's attending physician determine the resident's capacity to make healthcare decisions. In such cases, the facility would need a process for making such determinations in a timely way because most long-term care facilities do not have an attending physician on staff.

Policy also should stipulate that advance directives be documented in the residents' health records. (See figure 4.2.) There is no requirement in the PSDA or state law on the extent of the provider's responsibility to get an actual copy of the advance directive. The facility should encourage the resident or resident's legal representative to provide a copy of the advance directive to the institution. But, ultimately, it is the responsibility of the resident or resident's legal representative to provide that copy for the health record and inform the facility of the resident's healthcare choices.

Facilities need to consider the following points in developing policies to ensure proper compliance with the PSDA:

- Requirements for a valid advance directive under state law

- Methods for witnessing advance directives and other legal documents

- Answers to the most commonly asked questions concerning advance directives

- The principal resource on advance directives for guidance of staff and residents

The JCAHO's requirements are stipulated under standards RI.2.70 and RI.2.2.8025. These standards provide for the resident's right to refuse care or treatment as allowed by law and allow the formulation of advance directives. The JCAHO expects long-term care facilities to institute policies and procedures to manage the advance directive process in a number of areas, including:

- Informing residents of their rights

- Determining and documenting organ donation status

- Honoring the resident's wishes concerning organ donation

- Reviewing advance directives

- Honoring advance directives

- Involving the family in decisions related to advance directives

Figure 4.2.   **Sample advance directives checklist**

XYZ Corporation   Patient Name: _____
100 Anywhere St.
Any Town, ZO 00000   Health Record Number: _____

ADVANCE DIRECTIVES CHECKLIST

Advance Directives

1. _____ Have you been given information regarding advance directives, which includes a summary of the hospital policy to implement advance directives? (Fill in yes or no.)

2. Have you executed an advance directive? Please indicate what types of advance directives you have executed. (Fill in yes or no.)

     _____ Living will

     _____ Healthcare agent

     _____ Durable power of attorney for healthcare

     _____ Conservator

     _____ Designation of individual to appoint as conservator

     _____ Other: _____

3. _____ Has an original or copy of any current advance directive document been provided for placement in the medical record? (Fill in yes or no).

     3.1 _____ If a current advance directive document exists but is not available on admission, has it been requested so that a copy can be placed in the patient's chart? (Fill in yes or no.)

4. I hereby release, on behalf of myself/the patient and my/the patient's heirs and assigns, the Hospital for Special Care and its agents, servants, and employees (Hospital), from all liability, of whatsoever nature, in connection with or resulting from my failure to inform the Hospital of the existence of an advance directive and/or to supply the Hospital with a copy of such document.

                            _____
                            Patient or Legal Representative

                            _____
                            Witness

Documentation in the Health Record

Advance directives should be placed in a dedicated section of the resident's health record. All other pertinent documentation such as powers of attorney, living wills, conservator papers, and so on should be filed in the advanced directive section as well.

Summary

The first advance directives were developed in response to the Patient Self-Determination Act of 1991. This law requires healthcare facilities that treat Medicare and Medicaid residents to have mechanisms in place to provide written information about advance directives to each resident admitted. Advance directives are legal documents that allow residents to identify in advance the kinds of treatment they want or do not want in the event they become incapacitated. Advance directives also may designate a responsible person who would be allowed to make healthcare or financial decisions on behalf of the resident. The facility must have policies and procedures in place for the advance directive process, and the resident's health record must show evidence that the information was provided.

Federal law necessitates the advance directive obligation for facilities, but each state has been mandated to provide specific requirements for the advance directive process. The state requirements may differ widely from state to state. It is crucial that each facility define its policies and procedures not only around the federal regulations, but also any state-specific mandates. Finally, the facility must incorporate necessary accrediting body requirements into policies and procedures.

References

Joint Commission on Accreditation of Healthcare Organizations. 2004. *Comprehensive Accreditation Manual for Long-term Care.* Oakbrook Terrace, Ill.: JCAHO.

Monagle, John F., and David C. Thomasma. *Health Care Ethics, Critical Issues for the 21st Century.* 2nd ed. Boston: Jones & Bartlett Publishers, 1998.

Chapter 5

Face Sheet

The **face sheet** is usually the first page of the resident's health record. (See figure 5.1.) It contains the resident identification, demographics, original date of admission, insurance coverage or payment source, referral information, hospital stay dates, physician information, and discharge information. It also contains the names of the responsible party, emergency contacts, and additional contacts, and the diagnoses of the resident. Facilities with appropriate capabilities may computerize the face sheet. Many times, support staff types the information on the sheet. The face sheet also may be called the patient summary sheet, the patient identification sheet, or the intake sheet.

Face Sheet Information

The purpose of the face sheet is to provide sufficient information to completely identify the resident. It provides clinical staff and allied health professionals with information concerning next of kin or emergency contacts. The form provides a mechanism to house all the necessary identification and demographic information concerning the patient in one accessible location. Typically, it also provides a list of the diagnoses known at the time of admission or that affect the resident's stay.

Facility policies should define the mechanisms used to document all diagnoses. Placing the entire list of diagnoses on the face sheet may be cumbersome because many data are contained on the form. Using the face sheet for the entire listing of diagnoses may not always be effective if there are no mechanisms for updating diagnoses codes on a regular basis. In more recent years, facilities have reexamined the need for placement of all diagnoses on the resident face sheet. Diagnosis tracking sheets (such as a problem or diagnosis list) have been developed to ensure that all current, relevant diagnoses are captured in the resident's health record and that resolved diagnoses are removed on at least an annual basis. (See figure 5.2.) This process eliminates the need to capture all diagnoses on the face sheet and simply allows the required diagnoses for therapy to be placed there.

The information entered on the face sheet that is obtained prior to admission should be verified when the resident has been admitted to the facility. Policies and procedures should be developed to outline the process for verification of face sheet information. These policies and procedures should consider the following criteria:

- Process for review of the face sheet

- Personnel responsible for, and timeliness of, the review

Figure 5.1.   Sample face sheet

XYZ Organization Anytown, XX 00000		**Face Sheet**	

Original Adm. #/Date	Room #	Current Adm. #/Date
Original Pay Source		Current Pay Source
Referred By		Current Status
Medicare Full/Copay Days		Hospital Stay Dates

Resident Information	**Resident Preferences**

Resident Information

Resident Address
City/State/ZIP
County
Phone

SSN   Sex
Date of Birth/Age   Marital Status
Place of Birth   Military Service
Religion   U.S. Citizen
Language   Race

1. American Indian/   3. Black (not of   5. White
   Alaskan Native   Hispanic origin)
2. Asian/Pacific Islander   4. Hispanic

Medicaid #   Date
Authorization #   Date
Medicare (A) #   Date
Medicare (B) #   Date
Advanced Directives

Resident Preferences

Physician Address
Alternate Address
Dentist
Podiatrist
Eye Doctor
Psychiatrist
Mortuary
Church
Pharmacy
Hospital
Ambulance

Insurance
Phone
Certificate #
Name

Responsible Party

Name
Address
Phone
Relationship

Emergency Contact

Name
Address
Phone
Relationship

Additional Contact Information

Name
Address
Phone
Relationship

Diagnoses

Allergies

Additional Contact Information

Name
Address
Phone
Relationship

Diagnoses

Comments

Discharge Summary

Cause of Death or Final Diagnosis ———————   Condition on Discharge ———————

Physician Signature ———————   Date ———————

Mortician Signature ———————   Date and Time ——— Date of Death ———

Figure 5.2.   Diagnosis tracking sheet

MEDICAL RECORD DIAGNOSIS TRACKING SHEET			

NAME: _____   ADMIT DATE: _____

FROM: _____   MED. REC. #_____

MD: _____   ROOM #: _____

[__] – NEW ADMISSION   [_____] – NF1   [_____] – PRIVATE   [_____] – PENDING

[__] – RE-ADMISSION   [_____] – NF2   [_____] – SEMI-PRIVATE   [_____] – VA

[__] – LEVEL CHANGE   [_____] – SNF   [_____] – TITLE IX   [_____] – CWR

[__] – RETURN FORM   [_____] – PRIVATE INS.   [_____] – 4 BED
         MEDICAL LOA   [_____] – MEDICARE
                                               CIRCLE ALT STATUS

DIAGNOSIS

ADMISSION		ADDENDUM DIAGNOSES	
Diagnosis	**Code**	**Diagnosis**	**Code**

- Personnel responsible for, and timeliness of, the data correction

- Process and time frames for placement of the face sheet in the health record when it has been corrected

- Process and time frames for updating face sheets regularly

The federal regulation specifies, "The facility must maintain clinical records on each resident in accordance with accepted professional standards and practices that are complete. . . . [T]he clinical record must contain sufficient information to identify the resident" (CMS 2001).

For those facilities that are accredited by the Joint Commission on Accreditation of Healthcare Organizations, "The organization has a complete and accurate clinical record for every individual assessed or treated" (JCAHO 2004, IM.6.10).

The face sheet is generated when the resident is admitted to the long-term care facility. It may be computer generated or typed as outlined in facility policy.

For the long-term care resident, the information gathered during the preadmission and admission processes helps identify continuity of care issues as well. Information on hospital stay dates clearly defines whether prerequisites for Medicare eligibility are met. The typical information placed on the face sheet includes:

- Full name of the resident

- Resident's health record number

- Resident's address

- Date of birth

- Pay source(s)

- Medicare days used

- Room number

- Hospital stay dates

- Social Security number

- Religion

- Sex

- Marital status

- Military service

- Citizenship

- Race

- Insurance/Medicare numbers

- Authorization number

- Presence of an advance directive

- Responsible party name, address, phone number, and relationship

- Emergency contact(s) name, address, phone number, and relationship

- Other contact(s), name, address, phone number, and relationship
- Resident preferences

    —Physician's address and telephone number

    —Dentist

    —Podiatrist

    —Eye doctor

    —Psychiatrist

    —Mortuary

    —Church

    —Pharmacy

    —Hospital

    —Ambulance service

- Diagnoses
- Allergies
- Comments section
- Discharge summary

    —Cause of death or final diagnosis

    —Physician signature and date

    —Mortician's signature with date and time signed and date of death

    —Condition at discharge

- Other information to fulfill state requirements

The JCAHO requires that the following information be contained in the health record:

- Resident's name
- Address
- Date of birth
- Religion
- Marital status
- Social Security number
- Gender
- Name of any legal representatives

Each section of the face sheet should be completed to ensure quality of documentation. If any section is not applicable, it should be so noted. When information contained on the face sheet cannot be obtained, the reason should be noted. Accurate data capture is paramount. Creating a process to ensure that the data are accurately entered makes the clinical staff's job easier should situations arise when family members need to be contacted or emergencies occur. Accurate insurance information and authorization numbers ensure that proper billing processes can be completed as well.

Documentation in the Health Record

The face sheet should be placed in the resident's health record on the day of admission. Even when information still requires verification, it is essential that a face sheet be placed in the record on the day of admission. This is to assist clinical staff in the event an emergency arises. When the face sheet data are verified, the updated face sheet should replace the original face sheet so that the health record reflects the most accurate information. Although a face sheet is not required to be in a patient's health record, the information is imperative to keeping accurate records for each patient.

Updates to the Face Sheet

When the face sheet has been verified and placed in the health record, the information should be updated as appropriate. "The facility must record and periodically update the address and phone number of the resident's legal representative or interested family member" (CMS 2001, p. 13). Social services can be instrumental in providing updated information on the resident's face sheet. Health information management (HIM) services also can be instrumental in updating electronic versions of the face sheet and filing them in the appropriate record. The facility should have a clearly defined process in place to ensure that the information is kept as up-to-date as possible.

Summary

Although a face sheet is not required by federal law to be kept in the resident's health record, its inclusion does provide easy access to the resident's demographic data. The face sheet provides a centralized location to reference these valuable data in addition to the resident's demographic data. By consistently placing the face sheet at the front of the resident's health record, the staff has the resident information within easy reach in the event of emergencies.

References

American Health Information Management Association. 2001. Long-Term Care Health Information Practice and Documentation Guidelines. Available at www.ahima.org.

Centers for Medicare and Medicaid Services. 2001 (October 31). Guidance to Surveyors—Long-Term Care Facilities, appendix PP in *State Operations Manual*. Available at www.cms.gov.

Glondys, Barbara A. 1999. *Documentation Requirements for the Acute Care Patient Record*. Chicago: American Health Information Management Association.

Joint Commission on Accreditation of Healthcare Organizations. 2004. *Comprehensive Accreditation Manual for Long-term Care*. Oakbrook Terrace, Ill.: JCAHO.

Chapter 6

Documentation of Assessments

Federal, state, and accreditation organizations drive the assessment and documentation process in long-term care. In an effort to capture the supporting documentation of the resident assessment instrument (RAI), which includes the **Minimum Data Set** (MDS), a federally mandated resident assessment that must be done for every resident in a nursing home, facilities have developed several types of assessments. These assessments establish mechanisms for gathering appropriate and necessary information about each resident. (For further information on the MDS, see chapter 7.)

The assessment process is an ongoing evaluation of the resident's needs, functional abilities, and requirements, and is used to identify and provide for appropriate interventions and services. The entire assessment process is fundamental to the care-planning requirements. Without continued assessments and reassessments, care planning becomes stagnant and the resident suffers adverse outcomes due to outdated treatments and interventions and ill-defined care needs.

The MDS is a primary document in the resident's health record, but unless the interdisciplinary team takes the initiative to complete further in-depth assessments and reassessments, the MDS may be inadequate to demonstrate all the required interventions and treatments the resident needs to maintain mental and functional well-being. With the supporting documents of the many assessments discussed in this chapter, the resident will be assured of high-quality outcomes and the facility will experience better outcomes as well.

According to the Joint Commission on Accreditation of Healthcare Organizations (JCAHO), **assessment** is "the process established by an organization for obtaining appropriate and necessary information about each individual seeking entry into a health care setting or service. The information is used to match an individual's need with the appropriate setting, care level, and intervention" (JCAHO 2004, GL-3).

Documentation of the assessments conducted in the long-term care setting is driven by federal and state regulations and accreditation standards. Medicare prospective payment system (PPS) requirements also affect clinical documentation efforts. Because state laws in this area differ widely, this chapter deals only with the minimum documentation required by federal regulations and JCAHO standards. It is imperative that facilities incorporate the requirements of state regulations and the other accreditation agencies into their assessment and documentation policies. It also is extremely important that facilities keep abreast of legislative changes at both the federal and state levels.

General Requirements for the Assessment Process in Long-Term Care

As discussed in chapter 1, facilities must keep health records on every resident they treat. The records must be complete, accurately documented, and systemically organized. Documentation gathered through the resident assessment process must provide a clear, accurate picture of the resident's health status. The crux of the documentation in the health record supports the resident's care plan and treatment program throughout his or her stay. Assessment is not a one-time process but, rather, an ongoing evaluation of the resident's health, needs, and condition. Reassessments are required at regular intervals throughout the resident's stay. In addition, facilities may need to screen residents to identify possible cases of abuse, neglect, or exploitation. Policy should address the process for collecting, retaining, and safeguarding material pertinent to the examination of the alleged abuse, neglect, or exploitation and define systems for notifying and releasing information to the proper authorities. Assessments in the area of abuse require consent from the resident or his or her legal representative unless otherwise provided by law. This chapter includes several types of commonly required assessments.

Several JCAHO requirements address the assessment of each resident. First, the facility must have a process for assessing and reassessing residents, and reassessments must be conducted at regular intervals. Moreover, assessments must be overseen by a registered nurse. In addition, initial nursing assessments must be completed as established by law or facility policy, but no later than fourteen days after admission. Initial assessments also must specifically address the status, needs, and potential of each resident and include the following information on his or her medical, physical, functional, psychosocial, and nutritional status:

- Relevant past medical history and medical status

- Diagnoses

- Medications

- Allergies

- Treatments

- Results of diagnostic or laboratory studies

- Prognosis

- Limitations

- Precautions

- Neuropsychiatric status: Mental, affective, cognitive, sleeping patterns or memory, recall ability, decision-making ability, and behavior

- Communication status: Hearing, speech, language, voice, and modes of expression

- Rehabilitation status: Previous and current functional status, ADLs, mobility, balance, strength, bowel and bladder function, sensory capacity and impairments, vision, ability to swallow, orientation, and rehabilitation potential

- Psychosocial status: Level of functioning, cultural and ethnic factors, current emotional status, social skills, family circumstances, family relationships, current living situation, relevant past history, past roles, and response to current status

- Spiritual status: Including spiritual orientation and the dying individual's esteem

- Physical status: Musculoskeletal, cardiorespiratory, gastrointestinal and integumentary, and foot care

- Level of activity: Use of free time; personal preferences, preadmission hobbies, interests, and lifestyle; past and current activities; and ability to participate

- Nutritional and hydration status: Potential nutritional risk and deficiencies; cultural, religious, or ethnic food preferences; special dietary requirements; and nutrient-intake routines

- Dental status and oral health: Condition of the oral cavity, teeth, and tooth-supporting structures; natural teeth or dentures; functioning with or without natural teeth or dentures

- Level of pain: Including its origin, location, severity, alleviating and exacerbating factors, and current treatment and response to treatment

- Response to stress caused by present situation, illness, and treatment

- Educational needs: Needs, preferences, abilities, and readiness to learn to include family members

The initial assessment also should determine the resident's need for further assessment and periodic reassessments at regularly scheduled times or at change in health status. The scope and intensity of any further assessments are addressed by screening criteria and based on the resident's diagnosis, treatment environment, desire for treatment, response to previous treatment, and discharge needs.

Preadmission Assessment

The preadmission assessment occurs prior to admission and acceptance to the long-term care facility. It provides a mechanism for determining whether the resident requires skilled nursing care in an institutional setting. Included in the preadmission assessment is the **Preadmission Screening Assessment and Annual Resident Review** (PASARR) for mental illness and mental retardation, which also must be completed prior to admission to the facility.

The purpose of the preadmission assessment is to provide a clear, detailed picture of the resident's level of care needs. It gives insight into the services and programs required by the resident and allows both the prospective resident and the facility to determine whether these needs can be met in the facility setting.

An integral part of the preadmission process, the preadmission assessment provides valuable data on the resident's current condition, supplies information for the application, and provides for the proper placement of the resident in the healthcare setting. The preadmission assessment process ensures that the facility can provide the appropriate care and services for each resident admitted. The preadmission assessment also provides valuable insight into the resident's appropriate placement in terms of unit and room assignment, and roommate. It is often used to estimate the reimbursement rate, when applicable, and to project the resident's acuity.

The preadmission assessment data can be used to help formulate the resident's interim care plan and helps establish what other assessments will have to be completed upon admission to the facility. This information also facilitates the initial MDS assessment process. It is through the preadmission assessment that the facility can determine what diagnostic tests the prospective resident has already had so that further testing on admission is kept to a minimum.

General Requirements

There are no requirements for a preadmission assessment at the federal level. States, however, may have specific criteria that must be followed. The preadmission assessment should include enough information to determine the needs and health status of the resident. This in turn allows the facility to prepare any special equipment or supplies the resident may require.

If the preadmission assessment is used to plan the interim care plan and the initial MDS, the information should be filed in the health record.

As mentioned earlier, the goal of the preadmission assessment is to place the potential resident into the correct care setting with the proper services and programs. The quality of the assessment ensures that the resident receives the best care setting and allows the facility to develop a thorough and comprehensive care plan for the resident. This in turn ensures that the resident receives the correct services and programs, which enhances his or her quality of life.

The preadmission assessment data may be included on the application form for the facility. In some facilities, the potential resident health information may be captured on a worksheet that queries the resident's data or on a preadmission form that captures the following data elements:

- Demographic information

- Next of kin and responsible party information

- Referring institution and physician

- Insurance coverage

- Allergies

- Medications

- Pain

- Fall risk

- Current episode or illness, health status, complications, procedures, and treatment needs

- Diagnoses, including infections and active problems

- Medical, psychosocial, and surgical histories

- Hospital stays

- Level of care required

- Advance directives

- Pertinent laboratory results and X-ray findings

- Nutrition

- Mental status, management, or behavior problems

- Wandering and/or elopement risk

- Functional status, mobility, and activity of daily living

- Communication

- Leisure interests

- Family and social history

- Discharge planning

- Special needs

- Other data required for the face sheet

- Recommendations

- Comments

- Signature and date

Documentation in the Health Record

The preadmission assessment should be done as close to the admission of the resident as possible to ensure that the facility receives the most current health information. The resident may apply to the facility in advance of admission, but the preadmission information should be gathered just prior to admission as the resident's health status may fluctuate over time. Using outdated health information from an application will not provide the resident with the best opportunity for placement in the correct care setting.

The preadmission assessment form should be placed in the admission section of the health record. If the nursing staff takes a verbal report from the referring facility on the day of admission, the information should be captured for communication to other clinical staff to help them understand the resident's current status and needs. This form may be placed as the first progress note or the first nursing note, depending on the facility's documentation practices.

Preadmission Screening Assessment and Annual Resident Review

The Preadmission Screening Assessment and Annual Resident Review (PASARR) is both a federal- and state-mandated requirement that provides a mechanism for screening mental illness and mental retardation (MI/MR). The PASARR for MI/MR is required under the Omnibus Budget Reconciliation Act of 1987 (OBRA). "The Omnibus Budget Reconciliation Act of 1987 (OBRA 87) sets forth three sections that address preadmission screening and annual resident review (PASARR) requirements:

- With respect to new admissions occurring on or after January 1, 1989, §1919(b)(3)(F) prohibits a nursing facility (NF) from admitting any new resident who has mental illness (MI) or mental retardation (MR) (or a related condition), unless the State mental health or State mental retardation authority has determined that, because of his/her physical and mental condition, the prospective resident requires the level of services provided by a NF. In addition, where it is determined that admission to the NF is appropriate, a determination must be made as to whether active treatment is required.

- With respect to all current residents who have MR or MI and who were admitted prior to January 1, 1989, §1919(e)(7)(B) requires the State mental health or the State mental retardation authority to have reviewed and determined by April 1, 1990:

    —Whether or not the resident, because of his/her physical and mental condition, requires the level of services provided by a NF or requires the level of services of an inpatient psychiatric hospital (for individuals under age 21) or of an institution for mental diseases (IMD) providing medical assistance to individuals 65 years or older in the case of residents with MI or the level of services of an ICF/MR in the case of residents with MR. In the case of residents with MI, the statute further specifies that the determination made by the State mental health authority must be based on an evaluation performed by an independent person or entity; and—Regardless of the outcome of the NF level of care determination, whether or not the resident requires active treatment for his/her MI or MR" (CMS 2002).

The PASARR has two levels of screening assessment. A physician or hospital discharge planner, the appropriate social services department, or a family member can request the PASARR level I process where persons with mental illness, mental retardation, and/or related conditions are evaluated. It determines whether the individual should be "referred to a state mental health or mental retardation authority for Level II screening." If the level I assessment indicates a need for the level II evaluation, the individual is referred for further review. Level II assessments identify specialized services needed by these individuals and help determine the most appropriate placement. All persons applying for admission into or residing in a Medicare- and Medicaid-certified nursing facility are subject to PASARR requirements.

The preadmission MI/MR level I contains demographic and insurance information for the resident as well as section A, Identification of Serious Mental Illness, which indicates whether the resident has any of the following symptoms: depression, delusions, paranoia, or hallucinations. Section A also indicates the resident's current psychiatric diagnosis as specified in the *Diagnostic and Statistical Manual of Mental Disorders, Fourth Edition, Text Revision (DSM-IV-TR)*:

- Schizophrenia
- Mood disorder (major depression or bipolar disorder)
- Delusional, borderline G, axis II thought disorder
- Psychotic disorders
- Other psychiatric disorder
- Personality adjustment
- Anxiety disorder

Section B of level II indicates possible mental retardation and other developmental disabilities, including:

- Cerebral palsy
- Epilepsy
- Autism
- Traumatic brain injury (TBI) onset prior to age 22
- Other developmental disorders

Section C indicates a diagnosis of dementia (only if yes is indicated in section A) and section D, the need for further evaluation (only if yes is indicated in either section A or B).

All individuals must undergo a level I screening. A level II screening should be completed when appropriate. Residents who have a significant change in mental health or mental retardation needs must be rescreened at level I as a status change.

The PASARR ensures that prospective residents admitted to or residing in a Medicare- and Medicaid-certified nursing facility receive the additional specialized services in the most appropriate setting. Those individuals who have severe mental illness would be placed in settings that are more appropriate for their care needs.

General Requirements

The MI/MR prescreening assessments must take into consideration cultural background, language, ethic origin, and means of communication. The PASARR assessment must involve the person being evaluated, his or her legal representative (if applicable), and his or her family, if available and if he or she agrees to family involvement. The PASARR is mandated by the federal government but driven by individual state regulations.

The PASARR is a written document that must be coordinated with the routine MDS assessment (CMS 2001a, PP-156–159). It must identify the name and professional title of the evaluator and the date of the evaluation. Additionally, it must contain a summary of medical and social history. If nursing facility services are recommended, it identifies the specific services needed to meet the person's needs. If no services are recommended, it identifies mental retardation or mental health services that are of lower intensity than nursing facility services. Information gathered by the screening must support the conclusions.

The results of the PASARR must be explained to the evaluated person and, when appropriate, to his or her legal representative. The evaluated person must receive a copy of the evaluation, as does the state authority per established guidelines. The report must be sent to the nursing facility, the attending physician, and the discharging hospital, when applicable.

The evaluation may be discontinued if the person being evaluated does not have MI/MR or has a primary diagnosis of dementia or a secondary diagnosis of dementia without a primary diagnosis of serious mental illness or is not diagnosed with mental retardation or related disorder.

The state survey process conducts periodic audits for compliance of OBRA regulations. Therefore, noncompliance of performance of the PASARR may subject facilities to administrative action.

Documentation in the Health Record

The PASARR must be permanently filed in the admission section of the resident's health record for care-planning activities. Copies of the PASARR form must be sent with the resident if he or she is transferred to another facility. The level I screens are valid until there is a significant change in the resident's status affecting mental health or mental retardation treatment requirements.

Physician certification may be required for sections C and D as defined by state requirements. The long-term care facility may be required to sign when review of the level I evaluation has occurred at the facility.

Admission Assessment

According to federal Medicare and Medicaid regulations, the long-term care "facility must conduct initially and periodically a comprehensive, accurate, standardized reproducible assessment of each resident's functional capacity" (CMS 2001a, p. 68). The admission assessment for this discussion is the initial nursing assessment, which must be done within specified time frames of the resident's admission to the facility. The federal government requires that the resident assessment instrument (RAI) be completed by the facility with defined time frames but goes no further in requiring an admission assessment. (See chapter 7 for further requirements of the RAI.)

The purpose of the admission assessment is to provide a detailed baseline assessment of the resident's health status and functioning ability. It is used in conjunction with the preadmission assessment to determine the resident's care needs and interim care plan.

The admission assessment is a detailed nursing evaluation of the resident's health status at the time of admission. It includes a full review of the resident's current condition. An important piece of the resident's overall healthcare needs planning, the admission assessment begins with the resident's initial stay and provides the basis for the ongoing assessment, evaluation, and planning for the episode of care. It helps the healthcare team identify pertinent nursing diagnoses and further develops and defines the nursing care plan and nursing interventions required for the resident. Further, it provides a basic assessment that triggers more in-depth assessments for pain, skin, gastrointestinal and genitourinary functions, and such. Each completed assessment identifies care-planning needs and enhances both the care-planning process and the MDS assessment process.

General Requirements

The federal government has no requirements for an admission assessment. State-specific guidelines may require specific areas for the assessment, or the standards may be more general and simply state that health history, mental and social status evaluations of problems, and rehabilitation potential must be completed within specified time frames by all disciplines involved in the resident's care.

JCAHO standards require a **registered nurse** to coordinate the resident's admission assessment. The standards further stipulate that the assessment must be completed as required by facility policy or state law.

Admission assessment requirements differ by state but may include initial assessments of resident health status and function. The initial assessment form should contain areas to identify the resident and resident care functioning status and problems. The assessment is a detail-oriented form requiring specific assessment criteria such as:

- Skin status

- **Activities of daily living** (ADL) status

- Rehabilitative needs

- Psychosocial status

- Mental status

- Cognitive status

- Neurological communication

- Mobility

- Comfort

- Activity

- Safety

- Gastrointestinal/genitourinary status

- Sexuality

- Cardiac status

- Respiratory status

- Patient family education

- Discharge planning

Other facilities may take a systems approach to the admission assessment and cover the following broad areas:

- Endocrine system

- Nervous system

- Circulatory system

- Respiratory system

- Digestive system

- Genitourinary system

- Integumentary system

- Musculoskeletal system

The content of the admission assessment may include the following components:

- Date and time of admission

- Resident demographics

- Arrival information, ambulance, accompanied by, and so on

- Name of referring physician

- Reason for admission

- Name of the responsible party notified with the date and time

- Allergies

- Vital signs: Temperature, pulse (regular or irregular), respirations, and blood pressure (lying, sitting, or standing)

- Communication

- Language spoken and interpreter needed

- Cognition

- Functional status: Independent, one-person assist, two-person assist

  —Bed mobility

  —Ambulation

  —Transfer

- —Toileting

- —Feeding

- —Dressing

- —Grooming

- —Bathing

- Assistive devices

- Sensory

- Hearing

- Vision

- Oral assessment

- Sleep patterns

- Skin

- Condition of feet

- Nutrition

- Bowel habits

- Bladder

- Safety

- Mood

- Behavior

- Personal habits

- Motivation for rehabilitation

- History of:

  - —Chest pain

  - —Shortness of breath

  - —Depression

  - —Anxiety

  - —Psychiatric

- Pain

- Discharge planning

- Nurse's signature and date (if not a registered nurse)

- Registered nurse's signature and date

The admission assessment as well as ongoing nursing assessments and evaluations should be completed in their entirety. If an area is not applicable, it should be so noted. The quality of the assessment is important to the ongoing assurance that the resident's needs are met and the care plan accurately reflects the resident's health status and health issues.

Documentation in the Health Record

Time frames for completion of the admission assessment may be mandated by state requirements. The JCAHO requires that initial assessments be completed for residents within fourteen days after admission. Subacute units must have the initial admission assessments started within twenty-four hours and completed within forty-eight hours of admission for all disciplines that are required as indicated by the reason for admission.

The admission assessment is often placed in the nursing section of the health record. Subsequent nursing assessments are filed in date order after the initial assessment.

Skin Assessment

A skin assessment should be conducted as part of the admission assessment process to determine whether the resident is at risk for developing skin conditions. After admission, formal and informal skin assessments should be conducted as part of ongoing nursing care. "Based on the comprehensive assessment of a resident, the facility must ensure that a resident who enters the facility without pressure sores does not develop pressure sores unless the individual's clinical condition demonstrates that they were unavoidable" (CMS 2001a, p. 93). Bed- and chair-bound residents and/or residents with impaired ability to reposition should be assessed for risk factors that increase the possibility for developing pressure ulcers. These risk factors include immobility, incontinence, nutritional factors (such as inadequate dietary intake and impaired nutritional status), and altered level of consciousness. Individuals should be assessed upon admission to the facility.

The entire healthcare team is responsible for assessing a resident's skin on a day-to-day and shift-to-shift basis. These assessments establish whether any risk factors are present that might contribute to the development of skin ulceration or skin breakdown. Residents who are found to have risk factors for developing skin breakdown should have a care plan in place to ensure that the skin remains intact.

Validated risk assessment tools, such as the Braden Scale or the Norton Scale, can be utilized to assess residents for the risk of developing a pressure ulcer. Facilities should use only validated assessment tools when conducting skin assessments. Skin assessments should be completed periodically, and all skin assessments should be documented.

Many long-term care facilities use the MDS and **resident assessment protocols** (RAPs) to help identify areas of concern for skin issues and supplement these assessment tools with the Braden Scale evaluating pressure sore risk.

Upon admission to a long-term care facility, the resident's medical history will specify that he or she may be at risk for pressure ulcer development. From information gleaned through the nursing assessment and physician history and physical, a referral to the registered dietitian may be needed for this higher-risk resident.

The initial nursing assessment helps determine if a care plan for skin is required. If it is determined that the resident is at risk for developing skin problems, a more thorough skin assessment should be completed and the care plan for skin integrity initiated.

A skin assessment usually contains a drawing to help nursing staff identify areas of the body where skin condition may be a problem. (See figure 6.1.) The assessment identifies the number of potential skin problems and the location of each. The nurse then marks the drawing to indicate where each skin problem exists.

Figure 6.1.   Skin assessment graphics

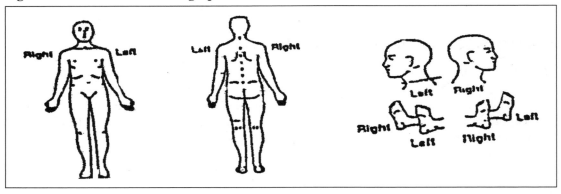

If the skin condition is a pressure sore, the nurse documents the stage of the pressure ulcer (I, II, III, IV). The appearance of each skin problem is noted, as is the size (in centimeters) of the area in question. The nurse also notes any drainage and/or odor associated with the skin problem. Color of the skin is noted as pink or red. Drainage is noted as serosanguineous or purulent, and odor is noted as none, mild, or foul.

The following are other areas that may be assessed:

- Occurrence or resolution of ulcers in the past ninety days

- Skin sensation

- General skin condition

    —Good

    —Fair

    —Dry

    —Dry and fragile

    —Surgical incision

    —Abscesses

- Diagnosis

- Treatments

- Weight loss

- Laboratory data

- Clinical signs and symptoms

Skin Condition as a Quality Indicator

Skin condition is considered a **quality indicator** (QI) for long-term care residents. In fact, it is identified as a sentinel health event QI. Just one occurrence of a **sentinel health event** QI is sufficient to justify a review by accreditation surveyors.

QIs derived from the MDS assessments in long-term care are intended to reflect the quality of the care delivered or the resident care outcomes that are a result of the care delivered by the facility and its clinical staff. The long-term care facility can then use the results of the QIs to enhance internal quality performance. Certain QIs have been identified as sentinel health events and are discussed further in chapter 7.

QIs look at either prevalence of the condition and/or incidence of the condition reported when completing the MDS assessment. The facility should develop mechanisms to reduce the prevalence or incidence of quality problems measured by the QIs.

QIs are used in conjunction with resident assessment protocols (RAPs), which are components of the resident assessment instrument (RAI). "Use of the QIs and QI reports in the survey process offers an additional source of information from which surveyors or supervisory staff may make planning decisions about the survey of a facility and from which a facility staff can plan their internal quality improvement initiatives" (University of Wisconsin 1999).

QI 24 is the prevalence of stages 1 though 4 pressure ulcers. Therefore, the initiative of assessing skin and providing skin care is extremely important for the facility. It is imperative that the facility have a sound skin assessment process that is grounded on the concepts of quality improvement. This QI looks at all residents who have been assessed with a pressure ulcer against all residents included in the most recent assessment.

The purpose of the QI reports is to provide a mechanism for the facility to identify possible areas of concern on which to focus quality improvement activities. Clinical indicators that could be associated with pressure ulcers include:

- New fractures

- Bladder/bowel incontinence

- Indwelling catheters

- Weight loss

- Dehydration sentinel health event

- Bedfast resident, chair-/wheelchair-bound, or decreased/lost mobility and ambulation

- Falls

- Use of nine or more medications

- Decline in late-loss ADLs

- Psychotropic drug use

- Daily physical restraints

Fecal impaction is the third sentinel health event QI and can easily be linked to nutrition, which is linked to dehydration and pressure ulcers.

The facility can begin to see the importance of the QI process in its assessment and care-planning activities. When skin problems are identified, they may be linked to another health problem. It is imperative that the treatment team complete the skin assessment accurately and thoroughly and plan care based on the assessment to ensure high-quality resident care.

Documentation in the Health Record

The skin assessment should be completed as soon as a problem is identified so that care planning and interventions can be quickly established to help restore skin integrity. The skin assessment is kept in a designated section of the health record and filed with other assessments in chronological or reverse chronological order.

Fall Assessment

According to the **Centers for Disease Control**'s Web site, every year one of every three Americans 65 years old or older suffers a serious fall. Falls are the leading cause of death from injury among people in this age range. About 9,600 people over the age of 65 died from fall-related injuries in 1998. Of all these deaths, more than 60 percent involved people who were 75 years old or older. Fall-related death rates are higher among men than women and differ by race. White men have the highest death rate, followed by white women, black men, and black women (www.cdc.gov).

Fall assessments represent a multidisciplinary clinical assessment of residents who are at risk for falling. Federal regulations require that "each resident receives adequate supervision and assistance devices to prevent accidents" (CMS 2001a, PP-105). The intent from the federal regulations is to ensure that facilities identify each resident who may be at risk for accidents and/or falls. The facility then must effectively plan for the care needs of these residents and execute programs to prevent accidents from occurring. "An 'accident is an unexpected, unintended event that can cause a resident bodily injury'" (CMS 2001a, PP-105).

The purpose of the fall assessment is to provide treatment and interventions and to address medical and safety issues that pertain to accidents that may cause falls. The facility must identify any resident with the potential of falls and provide adequate care plans that reflect appropriate activities to prevent them. The initial nursing admission assessments contain information on fall risk. Should the resident have a potential for falls as indicated in the admission assessment, a more detailed assessment should be completed.

The RAI includes a fall risk assessment for the MDS and RAPs triggers. The MDS addresses accidents with the purpose of identifying the resident's risk of future falls. Falls represent a QI for facilities. The fall assessment is important in the long-term care setting because the resident's condition can deteriorate based on inherent factors of health.

General Requirements

The CMS mandates the reporting of all fall incidents due to the possibility for serious injury from a fall. The cause of the accident must be investigated and action taken to prevent further falls. A fall recorded on the MDS will trigger a RAP that further assesses the resident's fall potential.

Inherent factors that might cause falls include:

- Age-related changes

- Slowed reaction time

- Sensory changes (reduced hearing, diminished tactile sense)

- Gait changes (decreased step height, decreased ankle movement, shuffling)

- Postural instability (decreased range of neck motion, increased body sway)

- Acute and chronic disease

- Acute exacerbation of disease (congestive heart failure, arrhythmia, syncope)

- Impaired vision (cataracts, macular degeneration, glaucoma)

- Lower extremity dysfunction (arthritis, muscular weakness, foot disorders, joint pain and stiffness)

- Cognitive impairment (dementia, depression, denial of mobility limitations)
- Orthostatic hypotension
- Hypotension, delirium, ataxia, dizziness
- Adverse effects of medication (diuretics, sedatives)
- Bladder dysfunction (frequency, urgency, nocturia, incontinence)

External factors that may cause falls include:

- Hazardous environmental conditions and obstacles
- Bed side rails interfering with safe bed exits
- Poor lighting
- Slippery floor surfaces (wet or polished floors)
- Bedroom and hallway clutter
- Low-seated chairs
- Low-seated toilets lacking sufficient grab bar support
- Improper use of ambulation and transfer devices
- Inappropriate size of device
- Faulty equipment
- Unlocked wheelchair brakes
- Worn tips on walkers, canes
- Nonworking wheelchair brakes
- Improper footwear

The fall assessment may take into consideration the following:

- Disease-related risk factors
- Medications
- Exercise
- Ambulation devices
- Assistance required, transfers needed
- Toileting schedules
- Supervision for confused and/or at-risk individuals
- Skilled occupational and physical therapy
- Weight bearing when transferring
- Hazardous conditions
- Mobility tasks

- Safety checks on bed wheel brakes, bed side rails, assistive ambulation devices, position of furnishings, clutter in hallways, and wheelchair brakes

- Proper footwear

- Long robes or nightgowns

- Hip-protecting aids

- Wheelchairs, canes, and walkers work properly

- Handrails

- Items within reach

- Lighting, without glare

- Hazards

The assessment conducted after a resident has fallen may be a checklist that contains some of the following data elements:

- Type of fall

- Consequences of the fall

- Resident's blood pressure and pulse

- Presence of swelling

- Presence of bruising

- Pain

- History of falling

- Immediate environment

- Quality of lighting in the area where the fall occurred

- Spills or obstacles on the floor

- Equipment check such as walkers, wheelchairs, canes, and such

- Type of footwear

- Witnesses

- Recommendations

- Comments

- Signature and date

Falls as a Quality Indicator

QI 2 is the prevalence of falls for long-term care residents. It compares all residents in the reporting cycle to all residents who have fallen in the past thirty days. A QI to reduce falls and prevent accidents helps facilities to achieve better resident care and demonstrate high-quality standards.

Clinical indicators that could be associated with falls include:

- New fractures

- Bowel and bladder incontinence

- Indwelling catheters

- Skin issues

- Use of nine or more medications

- Weight loss

- Dehydration

- Decline in late-loss ADLs

- Psychotropic drug use

- Daily physical restraints

There also may be a connection between a fall, a new fracture, and possible skin problems. The assessment process can help facilities to establish comprehensive care planning and enhance the **quality improvement** initiatives by tracking and correlating resident outcome data over time.

Documentation in the Health Record

The initial fall assessment should be completed upon admission and can be incorporated into the admission assessment process. Those individuals with potential for risk factors of falls should be monitored more frequently. The MDS monitors the resident falls from the time of admission. Assessments are submitted to the state at fourteen days, quarterly, and annually.

The fall assessment should be placed in a designated section of the health record in alphabetical, chronological, or reverse chronological order.

Bowel and Bladder Assessment

"A resident who is incontinent of bladder receives appropriate treatment and services to prevent urinary tract infections and to restore as much normal bladder function as possible" (CMS 2001a, PP-97). The MDS bowel and bladder assessment triggers RAPs for urinary incontinence, ADL functioning, and rehabilitation potential as well as cognitive loss and dementia. The facility must be fully aware of residents with bowel and bladder incontinence as well as those residents who may have indwelling catheters. The bowel and bladder assessment must take into consideration all of these aspects of care.

The purpose of the bowel and bladder assessment is to evaluate the resident for any bowel and bladder issues and to provide insight into existing problems. The assessment provides vital information to determine actions that might restore normal bladder and bowel function to the resident.

The bowel and bladder assessment identifies bowel and bladder problems and provides the clinical staff information for care planning and treatment of identified problems. It examines bowel and bladder issues in more detail, looking at specific reversible causes of urinary incontinence and bowel problems. In addition, it records any actions taken to restore the resident to normal functioning and looks at diagnostic reasons for urinary and bowel problems.

General Requirements

Clinical staff must look at the following when considering bowel and bladder assessments:

- Cause of incontinence

- Adequate hydration

- Urinary tract infections (UTIs)

- Bacterial colonization versus acute infection

- Risk factors of poor fluid intake, previous UTIs

- Assessments, care planning, and treatment to prevent UTIs in those with a history

- Infection control procedures

- Care received to restore or improve functioning (pelvic floor exercises, habit training, adequate hydration)

- Periodic evaluation

- Possibility that incontinence cannot be improved or maintained

- Evidence of prevention of incontinent-related complications to ensure resident dignity

- RAPS used

The MDS will trigger RAPs for urinary incontinence, ADL functional/rehabilitation potential, and cognitive loss/dementia. These RAPs are then used to provide an in-depth care plan for the resident concerning bowel or bladder problems. Facilities also may have specific urinary incontinence and bowel assessments and observation sheets as well as specific nursing reports to discuss treatment and care plan options and results.

The bowel and bladder assessment may contain the following elements:

- Resident's name

- Date

- Incontinence monitoring

- Reversible causes of urinary incontinence

    —Infection

    —Restraints

    —Medications

    —Fecal impaction

    —Inadequate fluid/fiber intake

    —Continuing medical conditions: Congestive heart failure, UTI, diabetes, multiple sclerosis, late effects of spinal cord injury, stroke, other conditions/causes

- Actions taken to address reversible causes

    —Urine C&S

—Fluid intake increased

—Dietary fiber increased

—Activity and ambulation increased

—Bowel regime initiated or changed

—Bedside commode, bedpan, urinal available

—Therapy consults (PT/OT) for mobility and transfers

—Restraint reduction

—MD consultation for improved function, treatment of medical condition, review of medications

—Toileting schedule

—Other (with explanations)

- Referable causes identified, including but not limited to:

—Marked prostate enlargement

—Possible cancer

—Pelvic prolapse

—Post void residual greater than 200 cc

—Hesitancy, straining, or interrupted urinary stream

—Hematuria

—Uncertain diagnosis

- Treatment plan

- Signature of the nurse

- Assessment completion date

Bowel and Bladder Conditions as Quality Indicators

Five quality indicators are tied into the bowel and bladder assessment structure. QI 8 is the prevalence of bladder or bowel incontinence. QI 9 is the prevalence of occasional or frequent bladder or bowel incontinence without toileting plan. QI 10 is the prevalence of indwelling catheters. QI 11 is the prevalence of fecal impaction, which is a sentinel health event QI. QI 12 is the prevalence of UTIs.

Clinical indicators that could be associated with bowel and bladder problems include:

- Use of nine or more medications

- Falls

- Weight loss

- Dehydration

- Bedfast residents

- Decline in late-loss ADLS

- Psychotropic drug use

- Daily physical restraints

- Pressure sores

Facilities should be aware of the connection between the QIs and the importance of assessing the resident for bowel and bladder function. The clinical staff at the facility needs to work closely with the quality arm of the organization to ensure that the resident has accurate and thorough assessments and care planning.

Documentation in the Health Record

The bowel and bladder initial assessment is often completed at the time of admission through the admission assessment process. Any identified areas of concern such as incontinence, UTIs, or others should be assessed as soon as indicated.

The documentation of the assessment should be placed in a designated section of the resident's health record in alphabetical chronological or reverse chronological order.

Physical Restraint Assessment

The purpose of the physical restraint assessment is to ensure that a restraint is necessary and that the least restrictive device required to treat the resident's medical symptoms is used.

" 'Physical Restraints' are defined as any manual method or physical or mechanical device, material, or equipment attached or adjacent to the resident's body that the individual cannot remove easily which restricts freedom or movement or normal access to one's body" (CMS 2001a, PP-44).

The glossary in JCAHO's *Comprehensive Accreditation Manual for Long-term Care* offers this definition: "Physical restraint: Any method of physically restricting a person's freedom of movement, physical activity, or normal access to his or her body" (JACHO 2004, GL-19).

The facility should strive to be restraint free but, in specific circumstances to maintain or improve the resident's medical condition, a least-restrictive restraining device may be required. The assessment ensures that this goal is met organizationwide. "The intent of this requirement is for each person to attain and maintain his/her highest practicable well-being in an environment that prohibits the use of restraints for discipline or convenience and limits restraint use to circumstances in which the resident has medical symptoms that warrant the use of restraints" (CMS 2001a, PP-44). It is important for the facility to keep this requirement in mind. The facility must always seek the "least-restrictive" device when implementing a restraint. The restraint assessment should be utilized to ensure that facility practice is according to regulation. It should be noted that a restraint may *never* be applied for the convenience of anyone, including the family.

General Requirements

The federal requirements are specific in discussing the resident's medical symptoms. These symptoms should not be considered alone but, rather, in the framework of the resident's overall condition, status, and surroundings. The assessment must use objective findings and not simply subjective symptoms. The facility must document the specific medical symptoms that required the restrictive device as well as how the restrictive device would be used to treat, protect, and assist the resident to attain or maintain the "highest level of physical and psychological well-being."

The following safety devices are considered physical restraints depending on how they are used:

- Leg restraints

- Arm restraints

- Hand mitts

- Soft ties or vests

- Lap cushions

- Lap trays the resident cannot remove easily

- Recliner chairs

- Bed rails

- Height of the bed from the floor

- Use of restrictive mattresses

- Mechanisms to keep residents in a confined area such as beds against walls, black floor mats, chairs behind counters, and such

The following facility practices constitute restraints:

- Side rails that restrict the resident to bed

- Tucking in bed linens or using Velcro to restrict a resident's movement

- Restrictive devices used in combination with a chair to prevent the resident from rising

- Chairs that prevent the resident from rising

- Placement of furniture too close to objects preventing the resident from rising

"Side rails sometimes restrain residents. The use of side rails as restraints is prohibited unless they are necessary to treat a resident's medical symptoms" (CMS 2001a, PP-45). Documentation of the need for the side rail should be contained in the resident's health record.

The resident's health record must contain documentation of the medical symptoms that support the use of restrictive devices. It also must contain the initial assessment, ongoing assessments, and care plans specific to the medical symptoms and use of the restrictive device.

CMS requires that a physician order for the restraint be written in the resident's health record, but this order is not sufficient to justify the use of a restrictive device. CMS also expects that facilities will work toward reducing the overall use of restrictive devices throughout the facility.

The assessment for the restrictive device must include the following review of resident information:

- Bed mobility

    —Will the device allow or assist the resident to move side to side?

    —Mobility: Is the resident immobile? Is assistance required to change position?

- Ability to transfer

  —Between positions

  —To and from bed/chair

  —Stand and toilet: Will the device add risk to the transfer process?

- Other approaches tried that were not effective

- Recommendations

- Signature and date

Documentation in the Health Record

There must be a physician order for the restrictive device. The physician order must be renewed as specified by state requirements. The resident's health record must contain the description of the medical symptoms that reflect the necessity for use of the restrictive device. There must be documented assessments and ongoing assessments as well as the document care plan pertaining to the restrictive device.

Interventions to consider for care planning include:

- Restorative care to improve abilities to stand, transfer, and walk

- Rehabilitation screening and/or treatment

- Devices to improve mobility in bed

- Lower beds (use of mats)

- Monitoring device that notifies when the resident rises

- Staff checks and routine toileting schedule

- Visual and verbal reminders

- Exercise and restorative programs

Use of Restraints as a Quality Indicator

QI 22 is the prevalence of daily physical restraints. This indicator includes trunk, limb, bed, or chair restraints used on a daily basis. Of the eleven clinical links among the MDS QI criteria, physical restraint falls into nine of these categories. QI categories for daily physical restraints include:

- Accident

- Behavior/emotional patterns

- Cognitive patterns

- Elimination and incontinence

- Nutrition

- Physical functioning

- Psychotropic drug use

- Quality of life and skin care

Restrictive devices can affect the resident's clinical outcomes adversely as demonstrated by the number of categories that the physical restraint QI is reflected within. Facilities must complete each physical restraint assessment accurately and thoroughly to ensure that the resident indeed receives the least-restrictive device while ensuring the highest quality of life. A methodology for ongoing assessments also must be established to ensure that the resident is continually examined and as restraint free as possible. The goal for the facility must be to remain as restraint free as possible.

Documentation in the Health Record

The physical restraint assessment should be completed when medical symptoms indicate the need to assess the resident for treatment options. The initial physical restraint assessment should provide for the use of the least-restrictive methods first, and subsequent assessments may uncover the need to provide the resident with a restrictive device.

The physical restraint assessment and nursing flow sheets and ongoing assessment may be placed in a designated section of the health record for ease in documentation and tracking of compliance with the assessments. Some facilities may require that these documents be placed in other sections of the health record. Ultimately, placement is driven by facility policy.

Psychotropic Medication Assessment

Antipsychotic medications are drugs that are used in the management of psychotic conditions, bipolar disorders, or major depression with psychotic features. "Residents who have not used antipsychotic drugs are not given these drugs unless antipsychotic drug therapy is necessary to treat a specific condition as diagnosed and documented in the clinical record" (CMS 2001a, PP-125–126). Those residents who do use antipsychotic drugs should have the doses gradually reduced and behavioral plan interventions, unless inadvisable clinically, so that these drugs can be discontinued.

The psychotropic medication assessment is used to evaluate those residents who are taking antipsychotic medications and to determine whether the dosage of the medication can be reduced as appropriate to clinical indications.

Psychotropic medication includes antipsychotic and hypnotic medications. The assessment evaluates the resident based on clinical indication and behavioral symptoms. Antipsychotic medications are used only when the clinical indication substantiates their use.

General Requirements

Antipsychotic drugs should be used only when the health record contains documentation that the resident has one or more of the following conditions:

- Schizophrenia

- Schizo-affective disorder

- Delusional disorder

- Psychotic mood disorder

- Acute psychotic episodes

- Brief reactive psychosis
- Schizophreniform disorder
- Atypical psychosis
- Tourett's disease
- Huntington's disease
- Organic mental syndromes related to:

    —Behavioral symptoms that are temporary or permanent

    —Interventions required

    —Events in the resident's life contributing to the behavioral symptoms

    —Environmental causes such as heat, noise, overcrowding

    —Medical causes such as pain, constipation, fever, infection

    —Behavioral symptoms that are persistent

    —Behavioral symptoms that are preventable

    —Behavioral symptoms that cause danger to resident or others

    —Behavioral symptoms that cause continual screaming, yelling, pacing, and decreased functional capacity

- Behavioral symptoms that cause psychotic symptoms
- Short-term (seven days) treatment of hiccups, nausea, vomiting, or itching

Antipsychotics should not be used when the following symptoms are the only indications of a behavioral disorder:

- Wandering
- Poor self-care
- Restlessness
- Impaired memory
- Anxiety
- Depression
- Insomnia
- Unsociability
- Indifference
- Fidgeting
- Nervousness
- Uncooperativeness
- Agitated behaviors that are not a danger to self or others

When these drugs are ordered, a monitoring assessment must be completed, signed, and dated. Any side effects of the medication must be monitored as well. The goal of the antipsychotic medication assessment is to determine whether the medication dosage can be reduced or eliminated based on clinical findings. Any reduction or justification of the antipsychotic dosage must be documented in the resident's health record. The effectiveness of the antipsychotic medication is monitored, and justification for the drug is documented on a regular basis. The physician must order the antipsychotic medication.

The facility should have policies and procedures outlining guidelines for clinical staff in the assessment and documentation of the antipsychotic medication use. Some assessments that may be required include:

- Antipsychotic use monitoring form

- **Antipsychotic Dyskinesia Identification System** (Condensed User Scale) or Discus monitoring form: This is one of several standardized forms for assessing and documenting abnormal movements (of face, eyes, mouth/tongue, or body) that may occur in the course of treatment with some psychotropic medications. Another similar form, the **Abnormal Involuntary Movement Scale** (AIMS), may be used in facilities as an alternative to the Discus form.

- Antipsychotic treatment form

- Antipsychotic medication dose guidelines

The content of the antipsychotic medication assessment may include the use of the antipsychotic use monitoring form, which includes the following elements:

- Resident's name and health record number

- Diagnosis

- Antipsychotic medications used and dosage

- Indication

- Medication start date

- Date of behavior management plan, if applicable

- Behaviors monitored are desired target behaviors

    —Short term

    —Long term

- Date of review

- Possible adverse reactions

- Positive changes

- Negative changes

- Recommendations

- Signature and date of review

The antipsychotic Discus monitoring form includes the following elements:

- Resident's name and health record number
- Antipsychotic medications used and dose
- Exam type
- Assessment
  —Face

  —Eyes

  —Oral

  —Lingual

  —Head/neck/trunk

  —Upper limbs

  —Lower limbs

  —Side effects

  —Lethargy

  —Parkinsonian effects

  —Hypotension

  —Hypertension

  —Slurred speech

  —Mental status changes

  —Urinary retention

  —Evaluation

  —Conclusion

  —Comments

  —Signature of rater and date

The antipsychotic treatment form (completed by the ordering physician when an antipsychotic medication is prescribed for regular use) includes the following elements:

- Primary diagnosis
- Indication for antipsychotic
- Antipsychotic used
- Dosages
- Duration
- Expected benefits of treatment
  —Short-term goals

  —Long-term goals

- Alternative measures considered

- Psychiatry evaluation and date

- Psychology evaluation and date

- Prescribing physician's signature and date

- Reviewed and approved by (resident or resident's legal representative) and date

Prevalence of Antipsychotic Use as a Quality Indicator

QI 19 is the prevalence of antipsychotic use in the absence of psychotic or related conditions. The QI looks at residents who receive antipsychotic medications on the most recent MDS assessment. Of the eleven clinical links among the MDS QI criteria, antipsychotic medications use falls into nine of the following categories:

- Accidents

- Behavioral and emotional patterns

- Clinical management use of nine or more medications

- Cognitive patterns incidence of cognitive impairment

- Elimination and incontinence

- Nutrition and eating

- Physical functioning

- Psychotropic drug use

- Quality of life

The facility should monitor those residents who are identified as taking antipsychotic medications for all of the clinical categories for potential areas of concern. When assessing the resident on antipsychotic medication use, the assessment should look at these clinical areas as well.

Documentation in the Health Record

The assessment should be completed on those residents who are taking antipsychotic mediations when they are admitted to the facility. When the assessment is completed upon admission to the facility, the resident must be monitored on an ongoing basis and reevaluated periodically for antipsychotic medication use. The antipsychotic assessment is placed in the nursing section of the health record and filed in alphabetical, chronological order.

Behavioral and Mood Problems Assessment

The long-term care facility must ensure the following:

- "A resident who displays mental or psychosocial adjustment difficulty, receives appropriate treatment and services to correct the assessed problem" (CMS 2001a, PP-100).

- "A resident whose assessment did not reveal a mental or psychosocial adjustment difficulty does not display a pattern of decreased social interaction and/or increased withdrawn, angry, or depressive behaviors, unless the resident's clinical conditions demonstrate that such a pattern is unavoidable" (CMS 2001a, PP-102).

The purpose of the behavioral and mood problem assessment is to determine whether the resident (1) has behavioral or mood problems and (2) is adjusting to the facility environment.

The behavioral and mood problem assessment helps clinical staff recognize behavioral and mood issues that are present in identified residents. It assists the clinical staff in planning care and interventions for identified problems in an effort to help the resident overcome behavioral issues or decrease mood occurrences.

Some residents have a difficult time adjusting to the long-term care environment or to functional impairment and the inability to participate in daily activities. Clinical staff, through the assessment process, can identify signs and symptoms of behaviorial and mood issues.

A general pain assessment tool can be used to identify some behavioral and mood problems and assist clinical staff to more clearly understand behavior and mood changes. The following lists the hierarchical value of the essential measures of pain intensity:

1. Self-reporting

2. Pathologic conditions or procedures

3. Behaviors such as facial expressions, body movements, crying

4. Reports of pain from parent, family, or others close to patient

5. Physiologic measures

Problems in mental and psychosocial adjustment can be indicated by the following:

- Impaired verbal communication

- Social isolation

- Sleep pattern disturbance

- Spiritual distress

- Inability to control behavior

- Unordinary response to any stressor

- Wandering

Facilities can incorporate the following interventions into care planning:

- Self-governance

- Well-organized orientation programs

- Community involvement for resident

- Cultural heritage considerations

- Former lifestyle

- Religious practices

- Contact with family and friends

- Psychiatry/psychology interventions and counseling

General Requirements

Facilities must be prepared to provide treatment such as crisis intervention, psychotherapy sessions, drug therapy, and rehabilitation services and programs.

A functional assessment includes the following three means to complete the assessment:

- Information gathering (interviews, document review, and rating scales)
- Direct observation of the resident
- Functional analysis

The form content may:

- Identify behaviors, including behaviors that occur together
- Assist in identifying events, times, and situations that predict behavior issues
- Assist in determining any results that allow the resident to continue the behavior, such as extra attention or others
- Describe particular behaviors and particular types of circumstances in which the behavior happens
- Describe observed situations that support assessment
- Forecast conditions in which the difficult behavior is likely to happen

A typical pain assessment for behavioral or mood problems will provide a rating scale to help identify the intensity of the pain and help clarify a behavioral or mood issue. (See figure 6.2.)

Documentation in the Health Record

If there are documented behavioral or mood issues, assessments that have been completed should demonstrate that there is consideration for the resident's deviation from usual and customary routines. Activities and programs that the resident is involved in should be documented to demonstrate that the facility is seeking to achieve the usual and customary routine for each resident. Treatment and care plans must be reviewed and rewritten, if necessary, for behavior or mood issues. Psychological or psychiatric evaluations should be on file for those residents who have required such services. Additionally, the facility should use the RAPs to assist in assessing behavior and mood problems.

Figure 6.2.   Sample pain-rating scale

No pain	Slight pain	Significant pain	Severe pain	Excruciating pain
0 1 2 3		4 5 6	7 8	9 10
(0–3) No pain, slight pain at rest		(4–5) Intermittent pain at rest	(6–8) Frequent, significant pain at rest	(9–10) Continuous severe pain at rest
Slight pain with movement		Significant pain with movement	Severe pain with movement	Excruciating pain with movement

Behavioral and Mood Problems as Quality Indicators

Three QIs have an effect on behavioral and mood indicators:

QI 3 Prevalence of behavioral symptoms affecting others
QI 4 Prevalence of symptoms of depression
QI 5 Prevalence of depression with no antidepressant therapy

These three QIs provide the facility with information on behavioral and mood problems. The clinical links among the MDS QI criteria for behavioral and mood include:

- Clinical management, use of nine or more medications

- Cognitive patterns

- Incidence of cognitive impairment

- Infection control

- UTIs

- Psychotropic drug use

- Quality of life

Identification of behavioral and mood issues may be contained in several documents within the health record, including the pain assessment, the MDS, and antipsychotic assessments. Some facilities may determine that a specific section for such information should be created within the health record or filed in the nursing section of the resident's health record.

Self-Administration Assessment

The purpose of the self-administration assessment is to ensure that the resident is indeed capable of self-administering his or her own medications. "An individual may self-administer drugs if the interdisciplinary team . . . has determined that this practice is safe" (CMS 2001a, PP-30).

The regulation to allow residents the ability to self-administer their own medications is a part of the resident's right to a *dignified existence.* It is the responsibility of the interdisciplinary team to determine that it is safe for the resident to self-administer medications before he or she may execute that right.

General Requirements

The interdisciplinary team is required to assess the resident to determine whether it is safe for him or her to self-administer medications. This same team also must decide who will be accountable for storage and documentation of the drug administration. This is either the resident or the nursing staff. The determination of the interdisciplinary team should be noted and placed in the resident's health record.

The determination must be reevaluated periodically to ensure that the resident is still safe to self-administer medications. Facilities should check individual state laws for specific requirements for self-administration of medications.

Medication errors that occur when the resident is allowed to self-administer medications are not counted in the facility's medication error rate. However, should errors occur, the facility should reconsider the resident's safety in the self-administration of drugs.

The content of the notation should include:

- Determination that the resident can self-administer medications

- The type of drugs, dosage, and times that the resident may self-administer

- Specific notation that the resident self-administers medications

- Levels of administration that may be identified, such as:

  —Meds at the bedside or kept in resident's room and resident is responsible

  —Medications given to the resident such as at meal times, and resident takes the medications during the meal but is not observed by staff members

Documentation in the Health Record

Documentation of the medication must be kept. JCAHO requires that every medication be documented. The determination to allow the resident to self-administer medication should be made "at least by the time the care plan is completed within seven days of the comprehensive assessment" (CMS 2001a, PP-30).

Documentation of the determination to allow the resident to self-administer medications may be kept in the medication section of the record. Some facilities may choose to keep this documentation at the front of the record until such time as the right is no longer granted due to safety issues. It then may be purged to the overflow files to avoid confusion on self-administration of the medications.

Nutritional Assessment

The purpose of the nutritional assessment is to guarantee that all residents have adequate nutritional status and assessments that evaluate the resident's clinical condition and identify any nutritional problems. "The facility must ensure that a resident maintains acceptable parameters of nutrition status" (CMS 2001a, PP-106). The facility includes in these parameters body weight, protein levels (unless clinically contraindicated), and a therapeutic diet when the resident develops a nutritional problem. The registered dietitian is responsible for completing an initial nutritional assessment for the resident.

The nutrition an individual receives is important to his or her well-being. Appropriate interventions must be implemented to ensure that each resident has adequate nutrition and nutritional assessments. The facility must incorporate mechanisms to monitor dehydration, weight loss and gain, and general physical wasting and malnutrition. The facility should monitor weight loss according to established parameters on all residents.

Risk factors for nutritional decline include:

- Drug regimes

- Poor oral status

- Depression or dementia

- Altered diet
- No access to favored foods
- Pace of eating
- Cancer

Clinical indications of poor nutrition include:

- Refusal to eat
- Chronic disease
- Increased need for more calories to compensate for wound-healing requirements
- Radiation or chemotherapy
- Kidney disease
- Gastrointestinal disorders

General Requirements

The nutritional assessment should address:

- Resident's nutritional status
- Resident's clinical condition
- Drug regimen
- Abnormal laboratory values (although not required)
- Appropriate intervention for nutritional problems
- Risk factors of malnutrition
- Review of the RAP for nutritional status
- Causation of decline
- Potential for decline
- Lack of improvement for those residents identified with risk factors
- Periodic evaluation of care plan goals
- Documentation of further intervention should goals not be met

The following information is used to complete the nutritional assessment:

- Activities of daily living
- Bowel and bladder
- Diagnoses including, but not limited to:
  —Cerebral vascular disease
  —Chronic obstructive pulmonary disease

—Chronic or end-stage renal disease

—Diabetes mellitus

—Dehydration

—Hip fracture and other fractures

—Immunosuppression diseases

—Liver disease and/or heart disease

—Malnutrition

—Peripheral vascular disease

—Pressure ulcers

—Sepsis

—Spinal cord injury

—Weight loss

—Multiple sclerosis

- Fluid intake and urine output
- Height, weight, and body mass index
- Laboratory values with dates (within thirty days of testing) including albumin, HgB, Hct
- Medical history, including risk factors
- Medications
- Nutrition history
- Oral assessment
- Resident's input
- Skin condition

Nutritional Status as a Quality Indicator

The following three QIs have an effect on nutritional assessment:

QI 13 Prevalence of weight loss
QI 14 Prevalence of tube feeding
QI 15 Prevalence of dehydration, a sentinel event

These indicators provide the facility with information on nutritional issues. But of the eleven clinical links, all eleven take into account at least one risk factor of nutrition. (See figure 6.3.)

Facilities need to examine the correlation between the risk factors and nutritional status of each resident. Nutrition is a key component of a resident's outlook on quality of life, and facilities should be prepared to provide appropriate interventions and assessments whenever necessary to improve the nutrition of their residents.

Figure 6.3.   Clinical links among MDS QI criteria for nutrition

• Accidents	for weight loss and dehydration
• Behavior and emotional patterns	for weight loss and dehydration
• Clinical management (use of nine or more medications)	for weight loss and dehydration
• Cognitive patterns	for weight loss and dehydration
• Elimination and incontinence	for dehydration
• Infection control	for dehydration
• Physical functioning	for weight loss and dehydration
• Psychotropic drug use	for weight loss and dehydration
• Quality of life	for weight loss and dehydration
• Skin care	for weight loss and dehydration
• Nutrition and eating	is its own category

Documentation in the Health Record

The nutritional assessment should be completed upon admission to the facility according to state requirements and accrediting agency requirements. The initial nutritional assessment may be placed in the nutritional section of the resident's health record. Subsequent assessments should be placed in date order and archived as needed from the nutritional section of the resident's health record.

Activities, Recreation, and Leisure Assessment

The purpose of the resident activity, recreation, and leisure assessment is to provide a program that meets the needs of the resident. The assessment evaluates the resident's needs, preferences, and abilities and takes into consideration resident desires for recreational activities. "The facility must provide for an ongoing program of activities designed to meet . . . the interests and the physical, mental, and psychosocial well-being of each resident" (CMS 2001a, PP-58). The activity program established for the resident must be in harmony with the comprehensive assessment, the resident's care plan, and his or her interests and preferences. The completed plan should promote physical, cognitive, and emotional health. The program should provide the resident with added enthusiasm or comfort depending on his or her identified needs.

The therapeutic recreation assessment performs an important role in ensuring that the resident is placed into appropriate programs that meet his or her needs and desires. The interventions provided through the recreation assessment also can help change some aspect of resident behavior such as attitudes, skills, knowledge, resistance, defensiveness, stress, and abilities. The goal of the recreation assessment is to place the resident in the right intervention programs that have been developed specifically to manage their leisure-related needs.

General Requirements

The activity program designed for each resident should provide the intervention needed to:

- Stimulate

- Comfort

- Promote physical health

- Improve cognitive health
- Support emotional health
- Aid self-expression
- Encourage choice

The resident's activity plan should be versatile to allow activity at any time and not be limited to formal activities provided by the facility. The overall activities program must be directed by a qualified therapeutic recreation professional who is licensed or registered and eligible for certification, if not already certified.

The individual care plan for each resident must address appropriate activities as reflected in the comprehensive assessment. The progress notes contained in the health record should document the activities, the resident outcomes, and individual interventions.

The formal activity program should indicate:

- Schedules, options, and resident rights
- Convenient hours
- Waking hours (that is, early morning, late afternoon, evening, and such)

The program should appeal to:

- Cultural and religious aspects of the residents
- Both male and female residents
- All age groups

The therapeutic recreation assessment must reflect:

- Resident's name and health record number
- Resident's history
- Diagnoses
- Information collection: Observation, discussion, chart review, interview, and such
- Social communication skills
- Affect
- Motor skills
  - —Mobility
  - —Balance
  - —Transfer status
  - —Endurance
  - —Hand dominance
  - —Reaching

- —Grasp
- —Manipulating objects
- Cognitive skills
  - —Tracks
  - —Imitates
  - —Follows direction
  - —Attention
  - —Awareness of visual field
  - —Awareness of environment
- Precautions
- Leisure interests
- Behavior
- Plan
- Recommendation
- Comments
- Signature and date

Leisure Activities as a Quality Indicator

QI 23, Prevalence of little or no activity, affects the recreation activity assessment. The QIs that examine resident behavioral symptoms, depression, cognition, physical functioning, and psychotropic drug use also correlate or clinically link to QI 23 and activity.

Documentation in the Health Record

The assessment for therapeutic recreation should occur upon admission to the facility as outlined by facility policy or by state mandates. The MDS comprehensive assessment tool captures an assessment on activities as well.

The therapeutic recreation assessment may be filed in the therapeutic recreation section of the health record in chronological or reverse chronological order. The progress notes may be placed as interdisciplinary team progress notes or filed in the activity section of the resident's health record.

Social Service Assessment

"The facility must provide medically-related social services to attain or maintain the highest practicable physical, mental, and psychosocial well-being of each resident" (CMS 2001a, PP-60). The needs of the resident must be met by the appropriate discipline. Further, "Medically-related social services means services provided by the facility's staff to assist residents in maintaining or improving their ability to manage their everyday physical, mental, and psychosocial needs" (CMS 2001a, PP-60).

The purpose of the social service assessment is to ensure that the resident has help in adjusting to the new environment. The initial assessment is completed at the time of admission with subsequent updates at the time of care planning. The assessment helps identify specific needs of the resident such as:

- Arrangement for adaptive equipment

- Contact with family (with resident's authorization) concerning health status, care plans, and other issues

- Health choices

- Referrals for outside services

- Referrals for outside resources

- Financial and legal needs

- Discharge planning and community services

- Counseling service

- Support for the resident with traditions, needs, preferences, routines, questions, and options

- Support resident's dignity

- Advance directives

- Interventions to drug therapy

- Supporting the grieving resident

- Interventions for resident's physical and emotional requirements

The social service department's personnel are an important contact for the resident. These professionals help clarify the resident's rights and explain financial policies and bed hold policies. Many times, the social service personnel are the staff that help the resident become acclimated to the facility. Social service staff verifies many pieces of the resident demographic and personal choice information. The social service professional helps the resident transition to a new care setting and allows the resident to feel comfortable.

Moreover, the social service professional identifies the medically related psychosocial issues and needs of the resident. The assessment identifies current medically related social and emotional needs, issues, or changes. The assessment defines goals and interventions to facilitate the resident's emotional and psychosocial well-being.

The social service role is to help identify any areas of concern that the resident and family may have with respect to the transition to a long-term care setting. The social service professional works with the nursing staff to enable the resident to attain optimal functioning and emotional support.

General Requirements

"Regardless of the size, all facilities are required to provide for the medially related social services needs of each resident" (CMS 2001a, PP-60).

Following are types of conditions that require social service staff intervention:

- Lack of support systems
- Behaviors
- Chronic conditions and resident deterioration
- Chronic or acute pain
- Socialization
- Legal or financial issues
- Abuse of alcohol or drugs
- Coping
- Emotional support
- Restraints
- Changes in the family unit, functioning ability, and resident health condition
- Need for an advocate

The social service or psychosocial assessment may contain the following information:

- Resident's name and health record number
- Date of assessment
- History and who provides it
- Admission date and source
- Date of birth
- Personal/social history
- Number of children and grandchildren
- Resident's response to admission
- Family plan and attitude
- Response to primary medical conditions
- Biopsychosocial factors
  —Current living arrangement with risk indicated
  —Initial discharge plan with risk indicated
  —Family and social support with risk indicated
  —Formal support service agencies and community involvement
  —Need for additional support
- Past psychiatric history
- Drug and alcohol
- Educational, occupational, and recreational background

- Cultural and spiritual factors
- Mental and emotional status
- Behavioral and social status
- Assessment of strengths and coping mechanisms
- Intervention plans
  —Identified problems
  —Interventions
  —Goals
- Financial and legal concerns
- Discharge plan
- Discharge potential
- Signature and date
- Interim notes

Documentation in the Health Record

The resident record should contain evidence of the means by which the facility staff executes social service interventions to meet established goals. There must be evidence of the mechanism used to monitor the resident's progress in improving physical, mental, and psychosocial functioning. The goals of the resident must be monitored for achievement and the care plan updated appropriately. The documentation should link the goals for psychosocial functioning and well-being to the actual care plan. Documentation of relationships established between facility social service staff and the resident and resident's family members or responsible party should be maintained. The resident's record should show confirmation that social service involvement has effectively concentrated on the resident's need and has connected social support, physical care, and physical environment with identified needs and individualism.

Psychosocial Status as a Quality Indicator

Social service may be required to provide services and interventions to those individuals who are identified in the following QIs:

QI 3   Prevalence of behavioral symptoms affecting others
QI 4   Prevalence of symptoms of depression
QI 5   Prevalence of depression with no antidepressant therapy
QI 7   Incidence of cognitive impairment
QI 17   Incidence of decline in late-loss ADLs
QI 18   Incidence of decline of ROM
QI 19   Prevalence of antipsychotic use in the absence of psychotic or related conditions
QI 20   Prevalence of antianxiety or hypnotic use
QI 21   Prevalence of hypnotic use more than two times in one week
QI 22   Prevalence of daily physical restraints
QI 23   Prevalence of little or no activity

The social service role is important because it involves the planning of interventions to help the resident cope with the long-term care setting. The easy transition into the long-term care facility will help the resident maintain or improve his or her ability to manage everyday physical, mental, and psychosocial needs.

The JCAHO expects that facilities will assess the resident's psychosocial status, including level of functioning, cultural and ethnic factors, current emotional status, social skills, family circumstances, family relationships, current living situation, relevant past history, past roles, and response to current status as well as the resident's spiritual status and needs, and the dying individual's concerns.

Documentation in the Health Record

Social service contact should begin on the day of or just prior to admission to ensure that the resident's physical, mental, and psychosocial well-being is addressed as soon as possible. The change in the resident's day-to-day routine and his or her adaptability to the new environment should be of the utmost importance for the organization to consider. The assessment of the resident's needs should begin on day one of admission.

Typically, social services has its own section in the health record. All documents pertaining to the social service department may be filed in the social services section.

Restorative/Rehabilitative Nursing Assessment

According to the CMS, it should be the goal of long-term care facilities to ensure that "a resident who enters the facility without a limited range of motion does not experience reduction in range of motion unless the resident's clinical condition demonstrates that a reduction in range of motion is unavoidable; and [that] a resident with limited range of motion receives appropriate treatment and services to increase range of motion and/or to prevent further decrease in range of motion" (CMS 2001a, PP-98).

To this end, **restorative nursing care** incorporates resident-specific programs that restore and preserve function to assist in attaining a lifestyle that allows the resident to maximize his or her functional independence and achieve a satisfactory quality of life. Restorative nursing care does not require a physician's order. Physical or occupational therapists can provide the assessment while the nursing staff provides treatments designed to assist the resident to achieve maximum functional ability. This may differ depending on state or facility standards. Some facilities may allow either the therapist or the nurse to complete the assessment. Restorative nursing care does not include procedures or techniques completed by a qualified therapist. For inclusion on the MDS assessment, a rehabilitation or restorative care assessment must include the following:

- Measurable objectives and interventions must be documented in the care plan and in the clinical record.

- Evidence of periodic evaluation by licensed nurse must be present in the clinical record.

- Nurse assistants/aides must be trained in the techniques that promote resident involvement in the activity.

- These activities are carried out or supervised by members of the nursing staff. Sometimes, under licensed nurse supervision, other staff and volunteers will be assigned to work with specific residents.

- This category does not include exercise groups with more than four residents per supervising helper or caregiver" (CMS 2002, p. 192).

The purpose of the restorative assessment and nursing oversight of the care provided is to utilize nursing interventions that help the resident to achieve maximum functional potential. The restorative nursing program does not include programs and services provided by qualified therapists but, rather, is usually accomplished by nurses or nursing assistants based on the restorative assessment completed by a therapist.

The resident's activities of daily living (ADL) do not decrease unless there are circumstances in which the resident's clinical picture demonstrates that decreased function is unavoidable. These ADLs include:

- Bathing

- Dressing

- Grooming

- Transferring

- Ambulating

- Toileting

- Eating

- Communicating

- Psychiatry/psychology interventions and counseling

General Requirements

Prior to beginning the provision of restorative care, there should be an assessment from physical, occupational, or speech therapy for the specific care required by the resident. The restorative assessment should include measurable goals and interventions that are documented in the resident care plan. There should be periodic evaluation by a licensed nurse to ensure that the goals are being met and that the care plan is updated. When nursing assistants provide the interventions, these staff members must be provided education to ensure that the techniques are used properly and that resident involvement continues the activity. The activities are supervised by nursing staff.

Once again, depending upon state or facility practice, the nurse may complete the actual restorative assessment. Areas that the therapy restorative assessment may consider include:

- Active range of motion

- Ambulation

- Bed mobility

- Bowel and bladder retraining

- Communication

- Decline in function

- Device assessments

- Dressing

- Hygiene

- Grooming

- Eating and swallowing

- Feeding

- Gait belts

- Hand rolls

- Joint mobility

- Mobility assessments

- Prosthesis

- Range of motion risk factors

- Skill practice

- Splint or braces

- Toileting

- Transfer

- Walking

If decline is noted, the nursing staff may request therapy intervention that contains:

- Resident's name and health record number

- Date of request

- Date of admission

- Diagnoses

- Evaluation by occupational therapy, physical therapy, or speech language

- Orthotic notification

- Adaptive equipment evaluation

- Comments

- Signature of the nurse and date

Rehabilitation Needs as Quality Indicators

Quality concerns are contained in the following QIs:

QI 2   Prevalence of falls

QI 8   Prevalence of bladder or bowel incontinence

QI 9   Prevalence of occasional or frequent bladder or bowel incontinence without a toileting plan

QI 10   Prevalence of indwelling catheters

QI 11   Prevalence of fecal impaction

QI 16   Prevalence of bedfast residents

QI 17   Incidence of decline in late loss of ADLs

QI 18   Incidence of decline in ROM

The clinical links to these QIs are as follows:

- Accidents

- Behavior and emotional patterns

- Clinical management, use of nine or more medications

- Cognitive patterns, incidence of cognitive impairment

- Elimination and incontinence

- Infection control and urinary tract infection

- Nutrition and eating

- Physical functioning

- Psychotropic drug use

- Quality of life

- Skin care

Again, this area of assessment takes into consideration all eleven clinical indicators. Facilities must pay careful attention to the QI reports generated from MDS and correlate information from these reports to provide insight into problem areas within the resident population. Actively focusing on optimal physical, mental, and psychosocial functioning will improve resident care outcomes. Establishing mechanisms to compare QI indicator reports with assessments can help identify problem areas that may require more intensive restorative care. Indications of fall risks and increased accidents may be indicators of resident decline, which possibly could be corrected with a formal restorative care program for that resident.

The restorative assessment may be filed in the nursing restorative care section of the resident's health record. Depending on facility policy, these documents may be filed in the nursing or therapy section or other designated area of the record.

Documentation in the Health Record

The restorative assessment is captured in the care-planning process and through the MDS comprehensive assessment. Any supporting documentation should be filed in the health record. The capture of restorative care differs from facility to facility. Some institutions may require that nursing restorative care be documented on rehabilitation treatment records; others may develop flow sheets or data capture forms that are specific to restorative care provided at the nontherapy level. Regardless of the method used to capture the documentation, periodic progress notes or assessments should be included that coincide with the care plan updates. The initial restorative care assessment provides the baseline of restorative functions so that improvements or declines can be measured over time.

Integration of Assessment with the Resident Assessment Instrument

The content of resident assessment instruments (RAIs) is specified by each state. RAIs are used to conduct comprehensive assessments and collect information for the Minimum Data Set for Long-Term Care (MDS). It includes the utilization guidelines and the resident assessment protocols (RAPs).

The quality concerns discussion in each assessment area discussed in this chapter has brought out important data to indicate that the assessments need to be integrated with the RAI process. This can be accomplished through automated documentation systems that would support the RAI, decrease duplicity, and improve correlation and quality outcomes reporting.

In the manual process, time and effort are required to ensure that the assessments are completed accurately, that documentation is not contradictory, and that the MDS RAI matches the resident's health record and true medical, physical, and emotional picture. Integrating these assessments and correlating them to the QI will not only help improve clinical outcomes but also will ensure monitoring of resident goals and updating of the resident's care plan. "Many MDS items will not be documented elsewhere in the clinical record, and the completed MDS may ultimately be the single source of documentation about these issues" (CMS 2002).

Integration of the resident's assessments provides a holistic picture of his or her needs physically, emotionally, and functionally. The integration of the documents and flow of information will assist the interdisciplinary team in managing and providing for the resident.

According to the RAI questions-and-answer document, "The MDS is a clinical assessment. As such, it is a primary source document and is considered part of the clinical record by federal regulation. There is no further requirement for a second source of documentation elsewhere in the record to substantiate the resident's status for each and every MDS item" (CMS 2001b). However, those areas of assessment not covered on the MDS must be addressed by the facility and the facility must ensure that the resident's full health status picture is assessed and treatment plans developed for identified concerns or problems. This will differ according to both state and facility standards. From this quote, however, the CMS is not mandating supportive documentation.

The RAI contains valuable resident health status information that should be used as the foundation of the resident's assessment process and ultimate care plan. All other documentation would supplement this RAI and provide the ability to demonstrate the ongoing monitoring and reassessment, constant vigilance in documentation practice, and quality clinical outcomes. The duplication of documentation effort would be decreased, and staff could provide more hands-on care. With the MDS and RAPs as the primary assessment tools, all other assessments could support the collection of information that is required to supplement the comprehensive assessment rather than reiterate the data.

Documentation of the provision of care in the long-term facility is intricate and can at times be difficult to complete because of time constraints. Integrating the assessment with the RAI process could help speed documentation time and provide better-quality documentation. The RAI gathers vast resident data that describe the resident's full health status and supports the care-planning process. With supporting documentation in the form of reassessments of goals and interventions and flow sheets of day-to-day resident status, the RAI becomes the principal documentation tool for the resident's functional capacity and health status.

Supporting documentation would include those areas not specified in the RAI. Further assessment and reassessments would support periodic updates that would be required between annual RAI assessments. "The scope of the RAI does not limit the facility's responsibility to assess and address all care needed by the resident" (CMS 2001a, PP-69). The facility also must ensure that the resident's needs are addressed at the "moment of admission."

RAI Assessments

The following assessments are addressed in the RAI:

- Fall assessment

- Skin assessment

- Bowel and bladder assessment

- Physical restraint assessment

- Self-administration of medication

- Nutrition assessment

- Activities/recreation/leisure interest assessment

- Social service

- Mental and psychosocial functioning

- Restorative/rehab nursing assessment

By integrating the RAI with the assessment process, the facility can streamline its documentation practice. The interdisciplinary team assessment process that would utilize the RAI would become the basis for the process rather than a supplemental document of the process. The QIs are driven from the RAI assessment submission, and so it makes sense to ensure that the data quality of the RAI is the most efficient, while providing supplemental documents to support its creation. This would ensure that the facility and clinical staff have control over the resident's overall health status and the QI process as well.

Summary

Facilities have developed a number of different types of assessments for evaluating the care needs of nursing home residents in support of the RAI process and in support of the federally mandated Minimum Data Set. The assessment process gathers information about the resident's health status that is used to determine the interventions and services that would best meet his or her needs. Maintenance of such documentation in the long-term care setting is driven by federal and state regulations as well as accreditation standards. For example, the JCAHO requires the facility to have a process in place for assessing and reassessing residents on a regular basis and that a registered nurse oversee the assessment process.

Generally, facilities begin with a preadmission assessment used to determine whether an individual requires skilled nursing care in an institutional setting. The preadmission assessment includes the Preadmission Screening Assessment and Annual Resident Review (PASARR), which is a requirement under the Omnibus Budget Reconciliation Act of 1987 to screen for mental illness and mental retardation.

When a resident is accepted into the long-term care facility, he or she completes an admission assessment, which is the initial nursing assessment. The federal government also requires the facility to complete a resident assessment instrument (RAI) within a certain period of the resident's admission. The JCAHO requires initial assessments to be completed within fourteen days after the resident's admission to the facility.

The types of assessments performed typically include a skin assessment, a fall assessment, a bowel and bladder assessment, a physical restraint assessment, a psychotropic medication assessment, and so on. Each area being assessed may be looked at as a quality indicator, which is an additional source of information the facility can use to evaluate its performance in the provision of care to its residents. Additionally, each assessment and its resultant care planning must be documented in the resident's health record in detail.

Finally, each resident's assessments must be integrated with the RAI process . RAIs are used to perform comprehensive assessments and to gather data for the Minimum Data Set for Long-Term Care. Integration of assessments with the RAI process sometimes cuts down on the time required to document patient care. It also contributes to better-quality documentation. In essence, the facility's overall assessment documentation process can be streamlined.

References

Centers for Disease Control. www.cdc.gov.

Centers for Medicare and Medicaid Services. 2001a (October 31). Guidance to Surveyors—Long-Term Care Facilities, appendix PP in *State Operations Manual.* Available at www.cms.gov.

Centers for Medicare and Medicaid Services. 2002 (December). *RAI Version 2.0 Manual.* Available at http://cms.hhs.gov/medicaid/mds20/man-form.asp.

Centers for Medicare and Medicaid Services. 2002 (September). State Medicare Manual, Part 4: Services. Available at http://www.cms.hhs.gov/manuals/pub45pdf/smm4t.asp.

Centers for Medicare and Medicaid Services. 2001b (March). *RAI Version 2.0 Questions and Answers.* Available from http://www.hcfa.gov/medicaid/mds20.

Joint Commission on Accreditation of Healthcare Organizations. 2004. *Comprehensive Accreditation Manual for Long-term Care.* Oakbrook Terrace, Ill.: JCAHO.

University of Wisconsin—Madison. 1999. Facility Guide for the Nursing Home Quality Indicators. Available from http://cms.hhs.gov/medicaid/ltcsp/manual.pdf.

Chapter 7

Resident Assessment Instrument

Every long-term care facility must complete a comprehensive assessment of every resident's needs by using the resident assessment instrument (RAI) specified by the state in which the facility operates. The RAI is a three-pronged approach consisting of a standard Minimum Data Set (MDS), resident assessment protocols (RAPs), and utilization guidelines. Any state-specific items are included in an optional section of the document (Section S).

The **resident assessment instrument** was initially developed by the Centers for Medicare and Medicaid Services (CMS, then known as the Health Care Financing Administration) to fulfill the requirements of the **Omnibus Budget Reconciliation Act of 1987** (OBRA). The first version of the RAI was introduced in 1991, and the current version was introduced in 1995. The instrument's purpose is to standardize the collection of patient data and establish assessment protocols in skilled nursing facilities (SNFs) and nursing facilities (NFs). It includes version 2.0 of the **Minimum Data Set for Long-Term Care** (MDS 2.0). Electronic submission of MDS data was mandated in 1998.

The RAI is used to evaluate new admissions to long-term care facilities within fourteen days of admission. Thereafter, evaluations are conducted every quarter, every year, and whenever there is a significant change in the resident's status. The completion schedule for residents who are eligible for Medicare benefits is slightly different than the schedule for other residents and is shown in table 7.1.

According to the CMS, a significant change is any "decline or improvement in the resident's status that will not normally resolve itself without further intervention by staff or by implementing standard disease-related clinical interventions, that has an impact on clinical

Table 7.1. Medicare assessment schedule

Assessment Type	Assessment Window	Maximum Days	Payment Days
5-day	Days 1–8*	14	1–14
14-day	Days 11–14	16	15–30
30-day	Days 21–29	30	31–60
60-day	Days 50–59	30	61–90
90-day	Days 80–89	10	91–100

* When a patient expires or transfers to another facility before the 5-day assessment is complete, the facility must still prepare a Minimum Data Set (Transmittal 372).

interventions, that has an impact on more than one area of the resident's health status, and requires interdisciplinary review or revision of the care plan, or both" (2001, p. 73). Periodic evaluations are performed on a regular basis and whenever there are significant changes in the resident's condition to ensure that the most recent assessment accurately represents the resident's current health status.

Using an RAI enables the clinical interdisciplinary team to assess each resident according to a standardized data set at specific times in his or her stay. It also ensures that the facility conducts all required assessments and completes the reassessments in compliance with state and federal regulations. Although the RAI is a comprehensive assessment tool, other pertinent information may be identified during a resident's stay and must be considered during the care-planning process in addition to the information gathered through the required RAI. Although the regulations state that a comprehensive assessment must be completed within fourteen days of admission, the facility must develop an interim care plan to manage the resident's physical and emotional health status at the moment of admission.

Minimum Data Set for Long-Term Care

The MDS must be maintained by long-term care facilities that are certified to participate in the Medicare and Medicaid programs. It constitutes the first portion of the RAI. It is used to gather information concerning specific health status factors and incorporates information about specific risk factors in the resident's care. This information is used to plan the ongoing care and treatment of the resident in the long-term care facility.

The backbone of the RAI, the MDS is a "core set of screening, clinical and functional status elements, including common definitions and coding categories, that forms the foundation of the comprehensive assessment for all residents of long term care facilities" (CMS 2002). It is a comprehensive tool used to gather resident-specific information concerning health status. The facility should explore opportunities to correlate and integrate the comprehensive assessment with all assessments, evaluations, and the resident's care plan. Integration of all these key components of documentation concerning the resident's needs, desires, preferences, and abilities provides a mechanism to ensure that the facility addresses all of the resident's care requirements and current health status.

The three components—the MDS, the RAPs, and the utilization guidelines—provide a comprehensive tool for the assessment of each resident. "The RAPs are problem-oriented frameworks for additional assessment based on problem identification items (triggered conditions). They form a critical link to decisions about care planning. The RAP Guidelines provide guidance on how to synthesize assessment information within a comprehensive assessment. The Triggers target conditions for additional assessment and review, as warranted by MDS item responses; the RAP Guidelines help facility staff evaluate 'triggered' conditions" (CMS 2002).

These components of the comprehensive assessment provide valuable data on the resident's overall well-being. The comprehensive assessment strengthens resident care and ultimate quality of life. It provides detailed, individualized care planning focusing on the specific resident requirements. The tool facilitates communication and enhances documentation practice.

General Requirements

The comprehensive assessment, which includes the MDS and RAPs, must be completed according to established guidelines. Each resident must have a comprehensive assessment and additional assessments completed according to regulations, accrediting agencies, and facility policy.

Although the MDS and RAPs contain many valuable data points concerning the resident, the facility must develop a process to ensure that problems or issues identified outside the MDS and RAP assessments are incorporated in the care-planning process. Facilities should not be complacent with the MDS or RAP assessments but, rather, should integrate other assessments into the process as well. Diligence in correlating all assessment data into the care-planning process is important to ensure that the highest level of well-being can be obtained for each resident.

On April 2, 2003, the CMS published the draft of the MDS Version 3.0, which is available at http://www.cms.hhs.gov/providers/nursinghomes/nhi/draftmds30.pdf. The implementation date for the MDS 3.0 has not been established. "Due to our strong interest in quality assurance and our ongoing research efforts related to outcome measures for quality, as well as MDS accuracy, new payment and classification systems, and new assessment instruments across postacute care settings, it is certain that, over time, the scope and content of items included on all MDS assessment instruments will change. For example, we are planning to modify the full MDS in order to simplify some items and update others, according to clinical practices. This modification will be the MDS 3.0, which we expect to complete in 2004. Similarly, we are engaged in a significant effort to develop tools to help providers educate staff and assure the accuracy of their MDS assessments" (DHHS 2002).

The content of the MDS Version 2.0 is collected on the following documents:

- *Basic assessment tracking form:* Section AA contains the identification information. The form is completed with a full assessment, quarterly assessment, and state-mandated assessments.

- *MDS version 2.0 full-assessment form:* This form comprises MDS sections A through R. Section S may be contained in the MDS assessment depending on individual state requirements. It also includes background (face sheet) information at admission and sections AB, AC, and AD, which are included only at the initial admission to the facility.

- *MDS version 2.0 quarterly assessment form:* This is a required subset of MDS assessment information from sections A through R. Specific states may require that an extended quarterly assessment form, Optional Version for RUG-III, be completed on a quarterly basis.

- *RAP summary form:* Section V was developed to capture triggered RAP documentation.

- *Discharge tracking form:* This form collects section AA, items 1 through 9, with selected information from item 8 and items AB 1 and 2, A6, and R 3 and 4. It is completed at the time of resident discharge from the facility.

- *Reentry tracking form:* This form collects section AA, items 1 through 9, with selected information from item 8 and items A 4a and b and A6. It is completed at the time of resident reentry to the facility.

The comprehensive assessment must be coordinated by a registered nurse, who also must sign and certify completion and accuracy of the assessment. The federal regulations mandate that the comprehensive assessment be coordinated through those professionals who are involved in the resident's evaluation, care, and planning. The attending physician also should participate in the comprehensive assessment process as part of the interdisciplinary team involved in the evaluation of each resident. Depending on facility standards or policies, the physician's participation may be in the form of physician order and renewal of the care plan. Each facility should determine how physician involvement should be accomplished.

The Centers for Medicare and Medicaid Services (CMS) began requiring electronic submission of the MDS on June 22, 1998.

Importance of the MDS

The MDS is part of the comprehensive assessment tool mandated for all long-term care facilities that render care to Medicare residents. It was developed as required by the OBRA to enhance and improve the quality of care for each resident in a long-term care setting.

Under the **prospective payment system** for skilled nursing facilities (PPS SNF), which was defined in 1998, Medicare reimbursement began to be based on the acuity of care provided to the residents in long-term care facilities with adjustments for regional economic differences. Under this PPS system, the CMS determined that Medicare payments to nursing homes would decrease and cost savings for the Medicare system would result.

"Congress mandated in Section 314 of the Benefits Improvement and Protection Act that the Office of Inspector General review the Medicare payment structure for services classified within the rehabilitation resource utilization groups (RUGs) no later than October 1, 2001" (DHHS 2001, p. 3).

Resource utilization groups are divided into seven major categories: special rehabilitation, extensive services, special care, clinically complex, impaired cognition, behavior problems, and reduced physical function. Each RUG is associated with a payment rate based on a number of factors such as the need for therapy and the level of functioning measured in terms of activities of daily living (ADL). Medicare reimburses SNFs for residents coded only in the first four categories. Residents requiring physical or occupational therapy are assigned to a RUG in the special rehabilitation category. There are five special rehabilitation subcategories: ultra-high, very high, high, medium, and low. Each resident is classified in a subcategory depending on the number of therapy minutes required as indicated on the MDS in the last seven days (DHHS 2001, p 7).

Under the PPS, SNFs are required to assign residents to one of forty-four RUG categories. Facilities are required to capture acuity levels through the computerized MDS forms. RUGs are assigned to resident care needs, which determine payment. The highest-rated RUG is the ultra-high rehabilitation category for residents who need more resources. The lowest-rated RUGs provide payment reimbursement for residents who do not need as many resources, as much assistance with physical function, or aggressive rehabilitation services. The RUGs category that a resident is reimbursed under is derived from the MDS data submission. It is imperative that facilities have adequate MDS processing in place because the MDS not only provides data for quality and the QIs, but it also can affect reimbursement.

The documentation of the MDS and other assessments drives Medicare reimbursement (and Medicaid in some states) for facilities. The process of accurately capturing the MDS data and assessment information is a vital component for facility reimbursement. Ensuring that the MDS accurately reflects the resident's current health status and that other supporting documents and assessments corroborate the MDS assessment data allows the faculty to be thoroughly prepared in documentation practice that will support reimbursement. Documentation practice is key to ensuring accurate MDS submissions and proper reimbursement.

Documentation in the Health Record

The following documents are required to be completed and kept as permanent documents in the resident's health record as determined by established time frames:

- All tracking forms
- MDS full assessments

- MDS quarterly assessments

- RAP summary forms

- All other assessments and supporting documents generated to ensure complete and proper care and treatment of the resident

The full assessment is completed at admission, annually, and when the resident has a significant change in health status, as required by the Medicare PPS. The MDS Version 2.0 quarterly assessment form is completed no less than every three months within the required yearly full assessment. A comprehensive assessment must be completed within fourteen days after the facility has determined that there has been a significant change in the resident's physical or mental condition.

The MDS and RAPs are often placed in the comprehensive assessment and care-planning section of the resident's health record. Typically, they are filed in chronological order by MDS with trigger RAPs.

At a minimum, the RAI specified by each state must include the CMS MDS form and contain the following information:

- Identification and demographic data

- Resident-specific customary routine

- Cognitive patterns

- Communication

- Vision

- Mood and behavior patterns

- Psychosocial well-being

- Physical functioning and structural problems

- Continence

- Disease diagnosis and health conditions

- Dental and nutritional status

- Skin conditions

- Activity pursuit

- Medications

- Special treatment and procedures

- Discharge potential

- Documentation of summary information through the RAPs

- Participation in assessment

Figure 7.1 details the information contained in sections AA through V of the MDS. Appendix F provides a copy of the MDS.

Figure 7.1.   Information contained in the MDS by section

Section AA: Identification
Name, gender, date of birth, race, Social Security number, facility number, Medicaid number, reason for admission, signatures, title and date of persons entering data

Section AB: Demographic data
Date of entry, admitted from, living arrangements, occupation, language, mental health history, conditions

Section AC: Resident-specific customary routine
Daily routines, eating patterns, ADL routines, daily involvement, signatures, title and date of persons entering data

Section A: Identification and demographic data
Resident's name, room, assessment reference date, date of entry, marital status, health record number, payment sources, reasons for admission, responsible party, advance directives

Section B: Cognitive patterns
Comatose, memory, memory recall, cognitive skills, awareness, change in cognition

Section C: Communication
Hearing, communication devices, means of expression, communicating to others, clarity of speech, understanding others, changes

Section D: Vision
Limitations, appliances

Section E: Mood and behavior patterns
Depression, anxiety, mood, length of mood problems, mood changes, behavioral issues, change in behavior

Section F: Psychosocial well-being
Involvement, unstable relationships, past lifestyles and relationships

Section G: Physical functioning and structural problems
Bed mobility, transfers, walking, movement from place to place, dressing, eating, toileting, hygiene, bathing, balance, limits in range of motion, appliances used for movement, transfer needs, task division, ADL functioning potential, changes

Section H: Continence
Bowel and bladder continence, bowel routine, toileting programs and needs, changes in urine self-control

Section I: Disease diagnosis and health conditions
Specified diagnosis that may be considered a risk factor for decline in residents

Infections

Section J: Health conditions
Identified problem, pain assessment, accidents, stability

Section K: Oral and nutritional status
Problems, height, weight, weight change, nutritional issues, approaches, intake considerations

Section L: Dental and oral
Problems, oral condition

Section M: Skin conditions
Ulcers, kind of ulcer, history of problems, other skin conditions, treatments, foot issues

Section N: Activity pursuit
Time spent: awake, in activities, chosen activities, general activities, changes in activities

Section O: Medications
Number of medications, new medications, injections, and number of days in which specified medications were received

Section P: Special treatment and procedures
Specific special treatments, procedures, or services, mood and behavior interventions, nursing restorative care needs, restrictive devices, hospital stays, emergency treatment, doctor visits and orders, abnormal laboratory results

Section Q: Discharge potential
Potential for discharge and change in needs

Section R: Participation, signatures, title and date of persons entering data

Section T: Therapy supplement for Medicare PPS

Special treatments and walking performance

Section U: Medications

Section V: RAPS summary

Quality Improvement

The RAI process should be monitored to ensure the compliance accuracy of the data as well as completion schedules and timeliness of submission. The following audits may be required:

- Tracking forms are completed and signed as required.
- MDS is complete and correct.
- MDS face sheet is complete with signatures and dates.
- A-3 **assessment reference date** (ARD) is correct.
- R-2b information is not prior to the A-3 date.
- Staff completing the MDS use titles when completing the instrument.
- Triggered RAPs are contained in section V, as appropriate.
- RAPs triggered are documented correctly and completely.
- Date in VB2 is correctly entered.
- Date in VB3 is correctly entered.
- RAPs are done on or before the VB2 date.
- All relevant RAPs are addressed on the resident's care plan.
- Significant change assessments are completed as required.
- Business office notification of any corrected MDS form for adjustment of bills is completed.
- The validation report is examined after each submission and follow-up is conducted on identified errors.

The MDS-based quality indicator (QI) system was developed to help facilities examine quality improvement efforts for resident care. The twenty-four QIs are provided in figure 7.2.

Eleven domains are captured within the MDS assessment, and these domains contain clinical links or connections to several assessment areas within the MDS comprehensive assessment tool. (See figure 7.3.)

Additional quality requirements include:

- The MDS assessments must accurately depict the resident's care needs.
- All assessments must be submitted according to established time frames.
- Any resident who experiences a change in status must have a significant change form submitted.
- RAPs are completed, supplemental information is gathered, and care plans incorporate the identified data.
- MDS documentation corresponds with other assessments and observations and interviews conducted with the resident, family, or responsible party.
- MDS assessments are filed according to established guidelines and available to staff as required.
- MDS documents are safely filed and can be easily assembled.
- The MDS forms contain the identification and credentials of the professionals who are caring for the resident.

Figure 7.2.   Quality indicators

QI 1   **New fractures, incidence**
Residents who have fractures that are new since the last MDS assessment.

QI 2   **Falls, prevalence**
Residents who have been coded on the MDS with a fall within the past 30 days.

QI 3   **Behavior affecting others, prevalence**
Residents who have shown any type of problem behavior toward others on the most recent MDS assessment.

QI 4   **Symptoms of depression, prevalence**
Residents with symptoms of depression on the most recent MDS assessment.

QI 5   **Depression with no antidepressant therapy, prevalence**
Residents with symptoms of depression and do not have antidepressant therapy on the most recent MDS assessment.

QI 6   **Use of nine or more medications**
Residents who receive nine or more different medications as indicated on the most recent MDS assessment.

QI 7   **Cognitive impairment, incidence**
Residents with the onset of cognitive impairment over the past two MDS assessments.

QI 8   **Bladder or bowel incontinence, prevalence**
Residents who were coded as incontinent or frequently incontinent on the most recent MDS assessment.

QI 9   **Bladder or bowel incontinence, no toileting plan, prevalence**
Residents who are assessed as occasionally or frequently incontinent and who do not have a toileting plan documented on the most recent MDS assessment.

QI 10   **Indwelling catheters, prevalence**
Residents with an indwelling catheter documented on their most recent MDS assessment.

QI 11   **Fecal impaction, prevalence, *sentinel event***
Residents who have fecal impaction coded on their most recent MDS assessment.

QI 12   **Urinary tract infection, prevalence**
Residents with urinary tract infection coded on their most recent MDS assessment.

QI 13   **Weight loss, prevalence**
Residents with a weight loss (5% in 30 days or 10% in 6 months) documented on the most recent MDS assessment.

QI 14   **Tube feeding, prevalence**
Residents who have feeding tubes documented on the most recent MDS assessment.

QI 15   **Dehydration, prevalence, *sentinel event***
Residents who have the condition of dehydration documented on the most recent MDS assessment.

QI 16   **Bedfast residents, prevalence**
Residents who have been coded as bedfast on the most recent MDS assessment.

QI 17   **Decline in late-loss ADLs, incidence**
Residents with decline in ADL functioning over the past two MDS assessments. These late-loss ADLs are considered to be the last to decline such as eating, bed mobility, transferring, and toileting.

QI 18   **Decline in range of motion, incidence**
Residents who have had a decrease in function or increase in functional limitations in range of motion (ROM) over the past two MDS assessments.

QI 19   **Psychotropic drug use, prevalence**
Residents who are receiving antipsychotic medications on the most recent MDS assessment.

QI 20   **Antianxiety/hypnotic use, prevalence**
Residents who receive antianxiety medications or hypnotics on the most recent MDS assessment.

QI 21   **Hypnotic use greater than two times per week, prevalence**
Residents who have received hypnotic medications more than twice in the past week on the most recent MDS assessment.

QI 22   **Daily physical restraints, prevalence**
Residents who were restrained using trunk, limb, or chair restraints on a daily basis on the most recent MDS assessment.

QI 23   **Little or no activity, prevalence**
Residents who had little or no activity documented on the most recent MDS assessment.

QI 24   **Pressure ulcers, prevalence, *sentinel event***
Residents who have been assessed with pressure ulcer(s) stage 1 to 4 on the most recent MDS assessment.

Figure 7.3.   QI domains and their clinical connections

Accidents

QI 1   New fractures

QI 2   Falls

QI 6   Use of nine or more medications

QI 13   Weight loss

QI 15   Dehydration

QI 17   Decline in late-loss ADLs

QI 19   Psychotropic drug use

QI 22   Daily physical restraints

Behavioral and emotional problems

QI 6   Use of nine or more medications

QI 7   Cognitive impairment, incidence

QI 11   Fecal impaction, prevalence

QI 12   Urinary tract infection, prevalence

QI 13   Weight loss, prevalence

QI 15   Dehydration, prevalence

QI 16   Bedfast residents, prevalence

QI 19   Psychotropic drug use, prevalence

QI 22   Daily physical restraints, prevalence

QI 23   Little or no activity, prevalence

Clinical management, use of nine or more medications

QI 2   Falls, prevalence

QI 4   Symptoms of depression, prevalence

QI 6   Use of nine or more medications

QI 7   Cognitive impairment, incidence

QI 8   Bladder or bowel incontinence, prevalence

QI 9   Bladder or bowel incontinence, no toileting plan, prevalence

QI 11   Fecal impaction, prevalence

QI 13   Weight loss, prevalence

QI 15   Dehydration, prevalence

QI 17   Decline in late-loss ADLs, incidence

QI 19   Psychotropic drug use, prevalence

QI 20   Antianxiety/hypnotic use, prevalence

Cognitive issues

QI 3   Behavior affecting others, prevalence

QI 4   Symptoms of depression, prevalence

QI 5   Depression with no antidepressant therapy, prevalence

QI 11   Fecal impaction, prevalence

QI 12   Urinary tract infection, prevalence

QI 13   Weight loss, prevalence

QI 15   Dehydration, prevalence

QI 17   Decline in late-loss ADLs, incidence

QI 19   Psychotropic drug use, prevalence

QI 22   Daily physical restraints, prevalence

QI 23   Little or no activity, prevalence

Elimination and incontinence

QI 6   Use of nine or more medications

QI 12   Urinary tract infection, prevalence

QI 15   Dehydration, prevalence

QI 16   Bedfast residents, prevalence

QI 17   Decline in late-loss ADLs, incidence

QI 19   Psychotropic drug use, prevalence

QI 20   Antianxiety/hypnotic use, prevalence

QI 21   Hypnotic use greater than two times per week, prevalence

QI 22   Daily physical restraints, prevalence

QI 24   Pressure ulcers, prevalence

Infection control

QI 3   Behavior affecting others, prevalence

QI 6   Use of nine or more medications

QI 7   Cognitive impairment, incidence

QI 8   Bladder or bowel incontinence, prevalence

QI 9   Bladder or bowel incontinence, no toileting plan, prevalence

QI 10   Indwelling catheters, prevalence

QI 15   Dehydration, prevalence

QI 16   Bedfast residents, prevalence

QI 24   Pressure ulcers, prevalence

Nutrition and eating

QI 4   Symptoms of depression, prevalence

QI 5   Depression with no antidepressant therapy, prevalence

QI 6   Use of nine or more medications

QI 7   Cognitive impairment, incidence

QI 11   Fecal impaction, prevalence

QI 12   Urinary tract infection, prevalence

QI 16   Bedfast residents, prevalence

QI 17   Decline in late-loss ADLs, incidence

QI 19   Psychotropic drug use, prevalence

QI 20   Antianxiety/hypnotic use, prevalence

QI 21   Hypnotic use greater than two times per week, prevalence

QI 22   Daily physical restraints, prevalence

QI 24   Pressure ulcers, prevalence

(Continued on next page)

Figure 7.3.   (Continued)

Physical functioning

QI 1   New fractures, incidence

QI 2   Falls, prevalence

QI 4   Symptoms of depression, prevalence

QI 5   Depression with no antidepressant therapy, prevalence

QI 6   Use of nine or more medications

QI 7   Cognitive impairment, incidence

QI 8   Bladder or bowel incontinence, prevalence

QI 9   Bladder or bowel incontinence, no toileting plan, prevalence

QI 10   Indwelling catheters, prevalence

QI 11   Fecal impaction, prevalence

QI 12   Urinary tract infection, prevalence

QI 13   Weight loss, prevalence

QI 15   Dehydration, prevalence

QI 19   Psychotropic drug use, prevalence

QI 20   Antianxiety/hypnotic use, prevalence

QI 21   Hypnotic use greater than two times per week, prevalence

QI 22   Daily physical restraints, prevalence

QI 23   Little or no activity, prevalence

QI 24   Pressure ulcers, prevalence

Psychotropic drug use

QI 2   Falls, prevalence

QI 3   Behavior affecting others, prevalence

QI 4   Symptoms of depression, prevalence

QI 5   Depression with no antidepressant therapy, prevalence

QI 6   Use of nine or more medications

QI 7   Cognitive impairment, incidence

QI 8   Bladder or bowel incontinence, prevalence

QI 9   Bladder or bowel incontinence, no toileting plan, prevalence

QI 10   Indwelling catheters, prevalence

QI 13   Weight loss, prevalence

QI 17   Decline in late-loss ADLs, incidence

QI 18   Decline in range of motion, incidence

QI 19   Psychotropic drug use, prevalence

QI 20   Antianxiety/hypnotic use, prevalence

QI 21   Hypnotic use greater than two times per week, prevalence

QI 22   Daily physical restraints, prevalence

QI 23   Little or no activity, prevalence

Quality of life

QI 2   Falls, prevalence

QI 3   Behavior affecting others, prevalence

QI 4   Symptoms of depression, prevalence

QI 5   Depression with no antidepressant therapy, prevalence

QI 13   Weight loss, prevalence

QI 15   Dehydration, prevalence

QI 16   Bedfast residents, prevalence

QI 17   Decline in late-loss ADLs, incidence

QI 18   Decline in range of motion, incidence

QI 19   Psychotropic drug use, prevalence

QI 20   Antianxiety/hypnotic use, prevalence

QI 21   Hypnotic use greater than two times per week, prevalence

QI 22   Daily physical restraints, prevalence

QI 24   Pressure ulcers, prevalence

Skin care

QI 1   New fractures, incidence

QI 8   Bladder or bowel incontinence, prevalence

QI 9   Bladder or bowel incontinence, no toileting plan, prevalence

QI 10   Indwelling catheters, prevalence

QI 13   Weight loss, prevalence

QI 15   Dehydration, prevalence

QI 16   Bedfast residents, prevalence

QI 22   Daily physical restraints, prevalence

QI 23   Little or no activity, prevalence

QI 24   Pressure ulcers, prevalence, *sentinel event*

Those areas on the MDS that contribute to the QIs are indicated in figure 7.4. The scoring in each of these indicators creates the trigger for the QI. (Refer to the MDS Version 2.0 User's Manual for specific entry requirements.)

When facilities begin to examine the QI reports, the MDS criteria presented in figure 7.4 can be compared to documentation in the record to ensure that accuracy in reporting was achieved. The facility needs to ensure that when the QIs demonstrate that issues are present, systems and processes are in place to further examine resident-identified problems. The entire RAI process needs to encompass not only the assessment and care-planning phases of the process, but also quality analysis, development, and reporting mechanisms. The state QIs provide each facility with valuable data to determine if the systems and processes should be continued or refined to better service the resident and the community.

Resident Assessment Protocol

Resident assessment protocols (RAPs) are triggers that provide further clarification or instruction on specified MDS assessment data points. They identify conditions for further consideration and

Figure 7.4.   QIs and MDS data points

Quality Indicator	MDS Data Point
QI 1 New fractures, incidence	J4c, J4d
QI 2 Falls, prevalence	J4a
QI 3 Behavior affecting others, prevalence	E4bA, E4cA, E4dA
QI 4 Symptoms of depression, prevalence	E2 = 1,2 & 2 or more E1a, E1n, E4eA, E1o, E1p, E1j, N1d N1 and B1, E1g, K3a
QI 5 Depression with no antidepressant therapy, prevalence	O4c
QI 6 Use of 9+ medications	O1
QI 7 Cognitive impairment, incidence	B2a and B3e and B4
QI 8 Bladder or bowel incontinence, prevalence	H1b or H1a
QI 9 Bladder or bowel incontinence, no toileting plan, prevalence	H3a, H3b
QI 10 Indwelling catheters, prevalence	H3d
QI 11 Fecal impaction, prevalence	H2d
QI 12 Urinary tract infection, prevalence	I2j
QI 13 Weight loss, prevalence	K3a
QI 14 Tube feeding, prevalence	K5b
QI 15 Dehydration, prevalence	J1c, I3
QI 16 Bedfast residents, prevalence	G6a,
QI 17 Decline in late-loss ADLs, incidence	G1aA, G1bA, G1hA, G1iA
QI 18 Decline in range of motion, incidence	G4a–f
QI 19 Psychotropic drug use, prevalence	O4a
QI 20 Antianxiety/hypnotic use, prevalence	O4b or d
QI 21 Hypnotic use greater than two times per week, prevalence	O4d
QI 22 Daily physical restraints, prevalence	P4c, P4d, P4e
QI 23 Little or no activity, prevalence	N2
QI 24 Pressure ulcers, prevalence	M2 or I3

assessment. The RAI version 2.0 contains eighteen RAPs. The RAPs include the principal components of a long-term care resident's care plan. They are used to further define the resident's care-planning needs and treatment. Moreover, they are used in conjunction with the MDS to ensure that the resident's assessment is comprehensive and the care-planning process is complete.

The RAP is "a component of the utilization guidelines, the RAPs are structured, problem-oriented frameworks for organizing MDS information, and examining additional clinically relevant information about an individual. The RAPs help identify social, medical and psychological problems and form the basis for individualized care planning" (DHHS 2002).

RAPs are used to examine the MDS assessment conclusion and determine if the clinical decisions are correct. They provide a more in-depth look at identified MDS assessment results and allow the interdisciplinary team to determine if:

- The resident has a problem that requires further assessment.

- The resident's functional status may be enhanced or at minimum remain constant with no deterioration.

- The resident may have problems or issues that could jeopardize health status and cause deterioration.

- The resident's care at the end of life focus on comfort and dignity.

RAPs work in correlation with the MDS to enhance the care-planning process by triggering the interdisciplinary team to identify problems or issues. They also provide alerts to reevaluate the existing resident's care plan. Moreover, RAPs allow the interdisciplinary team to further understand any problems or issues that may be present upon completion of the MDS assessment. The MDS comprehensive assessment and RAPs provide the foundation for the care-planning process for each resident assessed.

RAPs contain the following four parts:

Section I, problems: The eighteen defined RAPs

Section II, triggers: Answers to the problems

Section III, guidelines: Actual guidelines for determining if problems may lead to resident limitations or risks

Section IV, RAP key: A reexamination of the RAP and summary

As the team begins to examine the RAPs triggers that are the result of the MDS assessment, they can begin to determine if correlations exist between problem and risks. In examining the QI for accidents, the team may be able to correlate the accident to one of the QI indicators with further examination. For example, upon closer examination of the RAPs for a fall, the team determines that the resident has nine or more medications, one of which is a psychotropic drug. In the fall, the resident also fractured a leg. Since the resident incurred the fracture, the significant change MDS indicates that the resident has excruciating pain, weight loss, and decreased activities. The RAPs for each of these conditions trigger to remind staff to further investigate the resident's health status. In this example, a correlation emerges between the fall, the fractured leg, decreased activity, and the pain. The team needs to look further into the resident's condition and documentation to determine if there is a correlation of these problems to the weight loss. RAPs assist in the decision-making process, providing help in determining whether the trigger requires a care plan.

Figure 7.5 is a screen example of a computerized RAP summary sheet that indicates on the left-hand side where problems may exist. The RAPs sheet provides the interdisciplinary team with possible and identified problems and possible and identified risks that allow the team to then investigate each RAP trigger in more detail to determine if a problem does exist. The center column provides an area for notes. The care-planning column provides a mechanism to track completion of the care-planning process for each area. The final column provides a quick help reference to refer the team back to the area on the MDS that is triggering this RAP.

General Requirements

The RAP features the following eighteen problems:

- Delirium

- Cognitive loss and dementia

Figure 7.5. Computerized RAP summary sheet

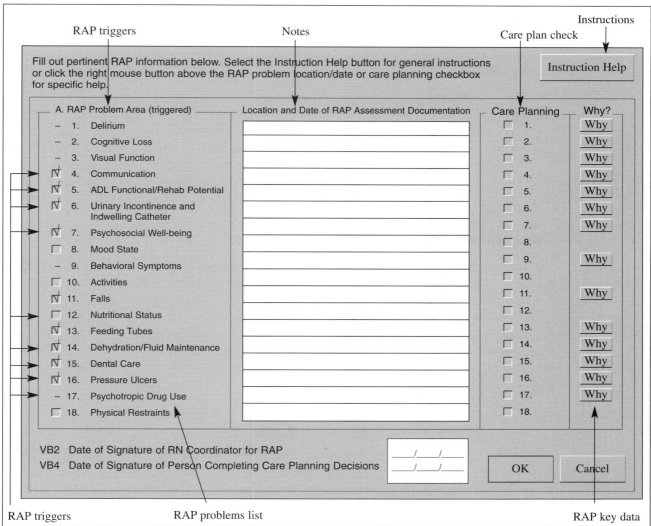

- Visual function

- Communication

- ADL function and rehabilitation

- Urinary incontinence and indwelling catheters

- Psychosocial well-being

- Mood state

- Behavioral symptoms

- Activities

- Falls

- Nutritional status

- Feeding tubes

- Dehydration and fluid maintenance

- Dental care

- Pressure ulcers

- Psychotropic drug use

- Physical restraints

The actual RAPs are listed in worksheet fashion for the interdisciplinary staff to use to begin examining identified problems in more detail.

RAPs help the interdisciplinary team to reexamine identified resident-specific problems and further evaluate the effect of those problems on the resident's functional and health status. If a pressure ulcer is documented in the MDS, the pressure ulcer RAP will provide further assessment capability to ensure that the resident's condition is examined in detail and that the care plan also is documented with proper intervention and treatment options.

Documentation in the Health Record

The RAP is the required documentation for the RAPs triggers. It provides further explanation on where to find specific assessments or problems areas within the resident's health record and indicates whether the problems were addressed in the care-planning process.

RAPs have the same completion time frames as the MDS assessments described earlier in the chapter. Many facilities file RAPs in the comprehensive assessment and care-planning section of the resident's health record, directly behind the appropriate MDS assessment. This system ensures that the MDS and RAP that correspond are filed together. The RAPs trigger legend, guidelines, or RAP key are not filed in the resident's health record.

RAPs should contain the following types of information:

- *Summary:* Summarizes the triggers that have been identified by the MDS assessment data entry. This document must be signed and dated by the registered nurse responsible for coordinating the resident's MDS assessment.

- *Trigger legend:* Displays pertinent information concerning the eighteen RAPs and specific MDS data points of the assessment process. It shows in graphic format which MDS data points trigger a RAP. (See figure 7.6.)

Figure 7.6.   RAP trigger legend

```
Legend Key

•  Indicates one point will trigger the RAP      * One of three in addition to at least one other point
❷ Means two points needed to trigger the RAP    ≅ When both ADL triggers, maintenance is primacy
```

- *Guidelines:* Discuss the identified problem in detail.

- *Key:* Provides a crosswalk between the triggered RAP and the MDS assessment form. It allows the interdisciplinary team to examine each data point that may trigger the particular RAP.

Quality Improvement

The QI domains provide the facility and the interdisciplinary team insight into areas on the MDS and RAPs triggers to determine whether correlations exist in the resident's current health status and the ever-changing health status that comes with the aging process. RAPs were developed to help facilities dig deeper in the assessment process and work to ensure that the resident achieves the highest practicable physical, mental, and psychosocial well-being.

Other Pertinent Information

The facility should have a well-defined process for completing the MDS. Each facility may differ in its approach to completing and submitting the MDS assessment. Steps in the RAPs process may include the following considerations:

- MDS assessments and other assessments are completed.

- RAPs triggers are identified electronically after MDS assessment data entry completion.

- An interdisciplinary team investigates the RAPs triggers completely and does further assessment, as indicated, to establish the type of problem and recognize the cause.

- Findings are noted on the RAP comment section to include:

  —Characteristics of the condition

  —Complications and risk

  —Action plan

- Teams determine if the problem contributes to the resident's health status and a care plan is required.

- The care plan is completed, corrected, and updated according to input from the team, resident, resident's family, or responsible party.

Summary

Federal regulations mandate the use of a comprehensive assessment. The RAI to be used to complete the comprehensive assessment is specified by each state. The RAI consists of the MDS and RAPs, which are required in facilities that are certified to participate in Medicare and Medicaid programs.

The comprehensive assessment is used to collect data on health status factors, incorporating risk factors, which are used to plan the overall care of each resident. The RAPs triggers help clarify specific MDS data. These protocols trigger the interdisciplinary team to further consider and assess identified areas of concern.

The RAI provides detailed comprehensive assessments for the evaluation of resident status, care requirements, and resident declines or improvements. The MDS process is mandated to be electronic. When the MDS assessments are completed, they must be submitted to the state.

QI reporting, derived from MDS data submission, provides a mechanism for each facility to further examine identified problem areas. Contained within the QIs are sentinel event indicators of fecal impaction, dehydration, and pressure ulcers. Facilities should develop mechanisms to provide thorough follow-up when these specific problems are triggered. Proactive examination of MDS data points should be considered to ensure that the MDS comprehensive assessment is completed accurately and completely prior to submission.

References

Centers for Medicare and Medicaid Services. 2001 (October 31). Guidance to Surveyors—Long-Term Care Facilities, appendix PP in *State Operations Manual*. Available at www.cms.gov.

Centers for Medicare and Medicaid Services. 2002. CMS Version 2.0 Manual, p. 4-1. Available at http://cms.hhs.gov/medicaid/mds20/man-form.asp.

Centers for Medicare and Medicaid Services. 2000. RUG-III Version 5.12 Calculation Worksheet 44 Group Model. Available at http://www.cms.hhs.gov/medicaid/mds20/mds44ws2.pdf.

Department of Health and Human Services. 2002. *Federal Register* 67, no. 105, May 31.

Department of Health and Human Services, Office of Inspector General. 2001. Trends in the assignment of resource utilization groups by skilled nursing facilities. OEI-02-01-00280. Available at http://www.hhs.gov/oig/oei.

University of Wisconsin—Madison. 1999. Facility Guide for the Nursing Home Quality Indicators. Available at http://cms.hhs.gov/medicaid/ltcsp/manual.pdf.

Chapter 8

Care Plan

"The facility must develop a comprehensive care plan for each resident that includes measurable objectives and timetables to meet a resident's medical, nursing, and mental and psychosocial needs that are identified in the comprehensive assessment" (CMS 2001, p. 82). Although state and accrediting bodies may have specific requirements for the care plan criteria, the care plan must be not only completed, but also updated as the resident's care and treatment needs change over time. The care plan is the "living and breathing" document that drives the resident's ultimate attainment and achievement of the highest practicable physical, mental, and psychosocial well-being.

Importance of the Care-Planning Process

The **care plan** is the basis for all care and treatment modalities the resident requires. It directs the interdisciplinary team to the care and treatment needed for each resident. Moreover, it is the primary source for ongoing documentation of the resident's care, condition, and needs.

Through the assessment process, the resident has been evaluated and problems have been identified. It is not good enough to simply identify resident problems; the interdisciplinary team must develop programs and interventions to assist the resident in maintaining health status and/or attaining improved health status. In those instances where the resident's health status is declining, the care plan identifies areas in which to focus care on comfort and quality of life.

The care-planning process includes the following key components:

- Comprehensive assessment, which is the Minimum Data Set (MDS)
- Other assessments as outlined in chapter 6
- Resident assessment protocols (RAPs)
- Care plan development
- Care plan implementation
- Ongoing evaluation and updates

The resident-specific care plan considers the resident's needs, desires, preferences, and abilities to achieve the highest physical and emotional functioning and well-being. Each care plan is individualized and can easily identify the resident's problems and needs.

"Planning includes creating an initial plan for care, treatment, and services appropriate to the resident's specific assessed needs and then revising or maintaining the plan based on the resident's response. Planning for care, treatment, and services is individualized to meet the unique needs and circumstances of the resident. Performed by qualified individuals, planning for care, treatment, and services involves using an interdisciplinary approach and involving the resident to the extent possible" (JCAHO 2004, PC-17).

General Requirements

The care plan must include the services required for residents to achieve the outlined goals on the plan. It must indicate transitional steps if those steps will enable the resident to achieve the outlined goals. When the care contains priority interventions, they must be noted on the care plan itself or in the resident's health record. The care plan must include the needs, strengths, and preferences that are recognized on the comprehensive resident assessment.

Should a resident refuse an intervention, the health record must reflect the resident's wishes. The federal regulations allowing a resident the right to refuse treatment interventions do not provide for the right of the resident or family to request any medical treatment the facility believes to be unsuitable.

An interdisciplinary team must prepare the care plan. The team includes those professional disciplines, as appropriate, required to care for the identified needs and interventions gathered on the resident from the assessment process. Team members include:

- The attending physician

- The registered nurse with responsibility for the resident's care

- Other appropriate professionals as indicated by the resident's needs and to the extent that the resident can accomplish participation in identified interventions

- The resident's family or legal representative

The facility develops a process for resident care planning that incorporates an interdisciplinary team approach. Documentation should provide evidence that the care plan is routinely reviewed by the team following each reassessment, evaluation, or as the resident's status changes based on his or her response to care and treatment.

The importance of the care-planning process cannot be overstated. The care plan incorporates the many data elements of the comprehensive assessment with other assessment processes to develop one document that supports resident care and treatment. The care plan enhances the resident's quality of life and ensures that he or she will achieve the highest practicable physical, mental, and psychosocial well-being.

Documentation in the Health Record

The actual care plan must be a detailed written plan. A comprehensive assessment must support the interdisciplinary care plan as well as all other assessments that have been developed during the assessment and care-planning stages of the resident's stay in the facility. The care plan itself must contain quantifiable goals that are developed to ensure that the resident reaches the highest level of functioning. These goals are used to measure the resident's progress. There must be evidence of ongoing assessments and evaluations of the resident's current health status and updates to the existing care plan document.

Quality Improvement Requirements

The care plan must be accurate and reflect the resident's current health status. It must be updated in a timely manner and must adequately demonstrate the resident's problems and the interventions the resident requires.

The JCAHO requires the following in PC.4.10:

- The care plan is individualized.

- It is appropriate to resident's needs, strengths, limitations, and goals.

- Assessment findings are integrated into the final care plan.

- Care plans are reviewed and revised as needed.

- The resident and resident's family or responsible party are involved in the planning process.

- The goals, interventions, and objectives are reasonable and measurable.

- The interdisciplinary team collaborates to develop the plan.

Indicators for success for care planning may contain the following criteria:

- The care plan is complete and contains all current identified resident-specific problems.

- The care plan is updated as appropriate.

- The care plan is accurate.

- The care plan identifies specific barriers for completion.

- The care plan identifies the resident's preferences, needs, and abilities.

- The care plan demonstrates the resident's current health status and health issues and concerns.

- The care plan provides effective care options and demonstrates goal achievement.

- The goals are reasonable and measurable.

- The care plan integrates resident assessments.

- The care plan is interdisciplinary.

Indicators for the planning process may include the following:

- There is evidence of an interim care planning and process development.

- The facility follows its care-planning policies and procedures.

- The care-planning process outlines how care will be provided.

- The facility process ensures involvement of the resident, family, or responsible party.

"A comprehensive care plan must be developed within 7 days after the completion of the comprehensive assessment" (CMS 2001, p. 82.2). The plan must be reviewed and updated periodically. Although no time frames are identified, at a minimum this should correlate with the comprehensive assessment schedule. This means at the following intervals:

- Admission

- Quarterly reviews

- Annually

- At significant change in condition

The JCAHO requires that "an individualized, interdisciplinary plan of care, treatment, and services is developed by an interdisciplinary team representing all appropriate health care professionals as soon as possible after admission, but no later than 7 calendar days after completion of the comprehensive assessments" (JACHO 2004, CAM PC.4.10).

The JCAHO subacute requirements are that "The interdisciplinary care plan is completed no later than 72 hours after comprehensive assessments are completed (which occurs within 72 hours of admission)" (JACHO 2004, PC.4.10).

The resident care plan is filed in the care-planning section of the resident's record. It is filed in chronological order, or the facility policy may specify that a discontinued care plan may be filed in the resident's overflow chart kept in the facility's health record department. This will eliminate any confusion and ensure that the resident's most current care plan is utilized.

Contents of the Care Plan

At a minimum, the care plan must contain or meet the following guidelines as outlined from the CMS *State Operations Manual* (CMS 2001)

- Identify problems

- Set measurable goals. For example:

    —Resident will remain free from skin breakdown for the next three months.

    —Resident will remain free from infection for the next three months.

    —Resident will transfer by self prior to discharge to home.

- Establish timetables to meet goals

- Contain services to be provided

- Furnish goals to attain or maintain highest practicable physical, mental, and psychosocial well-being

- Be completed within seven days after the comprehensive assessment

- Interdisciplinary

- Be reviewed and revised periodically

- Resident participation

- Resident may refuse treatment modalities

At the time of admission, the facility should develop a temporary initial care plan that outlines care needs until the comprehensive assessment and care plan are completed.

Because the care plan is an extremely important document and is required at the federal, state, and accreditation levels, it should be updated as warranted and appropriate dates and signatures should be added to verify authenticity and time and date of review and revision. This process should follow the proper legal documentation guidelines on authentication and timing of health record entries. The process is completed each time there is a new entry, a change in entry, or when an entry is discontinued.

Care-Planning Process

There are five steps in the care-planning process:

1. Actual assessment

2. Problem or nursing diagnosis and analysis

3. Plan development

4. Implementation

5. Evaluation of outcomes

The care plan may be computerized, handwritten, or typed in grids or columns to capture the items required for care planning. (See figure 8.1 through figure 8.3.) The content of the care plan may include the following information:

• Resident name

• Health record number

Figure 8.1.   Sample resident care plan A

Resident Care Plan

Resident Name: _____   Health Record Number: _____   Date: _____

Age:_____   Sex:_____   Room Number: _____

Admission Diagnosis/History: _____

_____

Goal:_____

Diagnosis Problem	Measurable Outcome/ Goal	Interventions	Rationale	Progress	Discipline	Date
Potential for skin breakdown	Resident will remain free from skin breakdown.	Assist to turn/ position Q2 hrs Assess for skin breakdown Q shift Meds as ordered	Helps with mobility to decrease likelihood of skin breakdown	Resident has remained free from skin breakdown.	Nurse/CNA	1/01/2003

- Date

- Age and sex

- Diagnosis

- Goals

- Evidence of the diagnosis

- Problems

- Identified risk

- Measurable outcomes

- Interventions/action

- Rationale for intervention

- Discipline responsible

- Review date/completion of goal date

Figure 8.2.   Sample resident care plan B

Resident Care Plan

Resident Name: _____ Health Record Number: _____ Date: _____

Age:_____ Sex:_____ Room Number: _____

Admission Diagnosis/History: _____

_____

Nursing diagnosis/problem	Nursing actions or interventions	Resident outcomes of care
Potential for skin breakdown	Assist to turn/position Q2 hrs Assess for skin breakdown Q shift Meds as ordered	Resident remained free from skin breakdown.

Figure 8.3.   Sample resident care plan C

Resident Care Plan

Resident Name: _____ Health Record Number: _____ Date: _____

Age:_____ Sex:_____ Room Number: _____

Admission Diagnosis/History: _____

Problem	Goal	Approach	Discipline
Potential for skin breakdown due to resident immobility Incontinence of bowel and bladder	Resident will not develop any skin breakdown.	Assist to turn/position Q2 hrs Assess for skin breakdown Q shift Meds as ordered	Nurse/CNA Nurse/CNA Nurse

Care Conference Summary

Although not required by federal regulation, the care conference summary provides an overview of the resident's care-planning sessions. It provides a mechanism to demonstrate that the planning process was interdisciplinary and that the resident and resident's family or responsible party were involved in the process. Facility practice will drive this process.

At the end of the care conference, changes, additions, or achievements are identified and the plan rewritten to ensure that it is easy to read and implement. This provides an effective mechanism to ensure that each resident's care plan is updated according to regulations and requirements. The care conference summary is the mechanism that demonstrates that the process is complete.

The interdisciplinary team should include all those individuals who would be expected, based on assessment criteria and findings, to be involved in the care of each resident. In reviewing chapter 6, those professionals involved in the assessment process may include the following departments listed alphabetically:

- Case management
- Consultants
  - Dental
  - Podiatry
  - Urology
  - Ophthalmology/optometry
  - Psychiatry/psychology
  - Others as specific to the resident's needs and requirements
- Discharge planners
- Infection control
- Nursing
- Nursing assistants
- Nutrition
- Occupational therapy
- Pastor care
- Pharmacy
- Physical therapy
- Physician
- Physician extender
- Resident and family
- Respiratory therapy
- Social service
- Speech language pathology
- Therapeutic recreation

The care conference summary may be handwritten, a typed report, or computerized, and should be filed in the comprehensive assessment and care-planning section of the resident's health record.

Attendance or Attendee Records

A signed attendance or attendee record is not mandated by federal regulations but is used by many facilities. (See figures 8.4 and 8.5.) Such a record is the mechanism used to identify that the care-planning process is interdisciplinary and includes the resident or resident's family or responsible party. The attendance or attendee record contains all the signatures of those individuals who attended the care conference. This document is filed with the care conference summary in the comprehensive assessment and care-planning section of the resident's health record.

Summary

The care-planning process is a key component of the resident's stay in the long-term care facility and identifies resident-specific problems, needs, preferences, and ability to meet the care plan interventions and goals. It involves several key components such as the Minimum Data Set, resident assessment protocols, and so on, and the input of an interdisciplinary team consisting of the attending physician, the registered nurse with primary responsibility for the resident's care, other appropriate professionals, and the resident's family or representative.

The resident's care plan is the road map that the facility's interdisciplinary team will use to ensure that the resident ultimately attains and achieves the highest practicable physical, mental, and psychosocial well-being while in the long-term care facility.

Figure 8.4.   Care plan attendee sign-in sheet

XYZ Organization
Anytown USA 00000

Care Plan Attendee Sign-In Sheet

Resident Name: _____   Health Record Number: _____

Date	Attendee	Discipline or Relationship to Resident (self, daughter, son, etc.)

Figure 8.5.   Care plan meetings signature documentation

XYZ Organization
Anytown USA 00000

Care Plan Meetings

Signature Documentation

Date	Attendee	Date	Attendee

References

American Health Information Management Association. 2001. Long-Term Care Health Information Practice and Documentation Guidelines. Available at www.ahima.org.

Centers for Medicare and Medicaid Services. 2001 (October 31). Guidance to Surveyors—Long-Term Care Facilities, appendix PP in *State Operations Manual.* Available at www.cms.gov.

Centers for Medicare and Medicaid Services. 2002 (December). *RAI Version 2.0 Manual.* Available at http://cms.hhs.gov/medicaid/mds20/man-form.asp.

Joint Commission on Accreditation of Healthcare Organizations. 2004. *Comprehensive Accreditation Manual for Long-term Care.* Oakbrook Terrace, Ill.: JCAHO.

University of Wisconsin—Madison. 1999. Facility Guide for the Nursing Home Quality Indicators. Available at http://cms.hhs.gov/medicaid/ltcsp/manual.pdf.

Chapter 9

Narrative Charting and Summaries

Documentation is an extremely important function for clinical staff to perform. It should be second only to providing high-quality care. Narrative charting provides a mechanism for the clinical staff to document the care being provided to the resident. It is a common charting method for documentation practice.

Techniques for Narrative Charting

The health record houses the chronologically documented information gathered on the resident's progress. Many different types of narrative charting techniques are available, and the style depends on the facility's policies, procedures, and practices. Narrative charting requires typical sentence structure to capture and organize the treatment and care of the resident in a time frame specified by facility policy or other mandates. Time frames may be specified as every shift, daily, on exception, or as needed, or indicated by the resident's condition. They are supplemented with graphic sheets of check-off summaries to enhance data capture and provide a vivid picture of each resident's past, present, and future care and treatment plans.

Narrative charting is documented as progress notes, either interdisciplinary or discipline specific. Interdisciplinary progress notes have formatted columns to identify the date and time, discipline, and note content, and are signed at the end of the note. (See figure 9.1.) The notes are written consecutively in date order. Areas left blank should contain an X to ensure that the documentation flows chronologically.

Discipline-specific notes have columns for date and time, the note section, and the section for the discipline completing the form. (See figure 9.2.) Signatures on any type of narrative note must identify the writer and also contain the writer's credentials.

Some formats for facility-specific narrative charting may include more columns to identify treatment, observations, and comments as well as the date and time and signature requirements. Narrative charting requires time to document the note. Interruptions can occur at any time, and clinical professionals documenting in the resident's record must be diligent in completing notes and signing them. Because of the time requirement needed to handwrite narrative notes, legibility can become an issue.

"Clinical records on each resident in accordance with accepted professional standards and practices that are complete, accurately documented, readily assessable, and systematically organized" (CMS 2001).

Figure 9.1.   Sample interdisciplinary progress note

XYZ Organization Anytown USA		
Interdisciplinary Progress Notes		
Date/Time	**Discipline**	**Progress Note**
1/1/00 1pm	Nursing	Resident slept well. . . . . **Signature of Nurse**
1/2/00 8am	PT	Resident ROM within normal limits . . . **Signature of PT**
1/3/00 3pm	MD	Resident has no change in status . . . . . **Signature of MD**
1/3/00 4pm	Nursing	Resident fell, no injury reported. . . . **Signature of Nurse**

Figure 9.2.   Sample discipline-specific note

XYZ Organization Anytown USA		
Nurse Notes		
Date/Time	**Progress Note**	**Signature of Nurse**
1/1/00 1pm	Resident slept well	*Doe RN*
1/2/00 8am	Resident ROM within normal limits	*Doe RN*
1/3/00 3pm	Resident has no change in status	*Doe RN*

Purpose of Narrative Charting

The purpose of narrative charting is to provide a mechanism for clinical staff to communicate the resident's health status, health status changes, interventions, and health status progress over time. The resident's health record is the legal record for the facility. If care is not documented, it did not happen regardless of the quality of care provided. Similarly, if the documentation is not legible, the care did not occur. It is extremely important that all clinical staff ensure the legibility of their documentation. The resident's health record also serves as a tool used to communicate from discipline to discipline and from shift to shift. Legibility of documentation is a key factor in the entry of the narrative note.

The resident's health record must have adequate data "to identify the resident, support the diagnosis, justify the treatment, document the course and results, and promote continuity of care among health care providers" (JACHO 2004, IM Standards). As seen in earlier chapters, documentation practice and interdisciplinary team approaches to resident care are extremely important to ensure that the resident achieves the highest practicable physical, mental, and psychosocial well-being. The health record is constrained by ethical considerations to provide facts about the resident in a clear and concise manner, and records care as it occurs. The legal system takes the position that the information contained within the health record is true and that unrecorded events did not happen.

Narrative charting provides the ability to track the resident over time and gives a true picture of the resident's needs, wants, desires, and preferences on a day-to-day basis. This charting style provides another mechanism for the facility to demonstrate that its professional staff is fully aware of the resident's status and that the documentation in the record is factual. It supplements the care-planning process and supports the documentation of the results of the care provided by the team. Narrative notes are a means of capturing the resident or family's response to care, any change in condition, and recommendations for changes in treatment plans.

An advantage to narrative charting is its versatility for use in many different settings. It also is the best-known documentation style, flexible, and used widely in healthcare. Narrative charting provides detailed information of the resident's care over time.

Narrative charting has its disadvantages, too. Documentation is placed in individual sections of the resident's record. It takes a great deal of effort to find various pieces of the episode of care. It may be more difficult and time-consuming to track a problem from beginning to end and locate all the disciplines contributing to the resident's care. The narrative resident health record can be extremely extensive and may contain much duplication. The sequence of events cannot be easily determined. General requirements for documentation are provided in figure 9.3.

Formats for Narrative Charting

Several different types and formats of narrative notes are discussed in this chapter. Each is specific in its requirements and format. Some of the areas covered are:

- Types of notes

    —Admission/readmission: Notes documented when the resident is admitted or readmitted, which provide a baseline for that stay

    —Interdisciplinary: Notes completed by a team consisting of nurses, therapists, and other allied health professionals, depending on facility practice

    —Noninterdisciplinary, or discipline specific: Discipline-specific notes such as the nurses' handwritten entries. Each discipline involved in the resident's care contributes its own section of narrative notes.

    —Monthly summary: A monthly synopsis of the resident's improvements or decline as specified by facility policy

Figure 9.3.   General documentation requirements

- There must be a record for each resident.
- Notes must be objective, accurate, and precise.
- Notes should be entered as close to the time of care as reasonably possible.
- Notes must be recorded chronologically.
- Notes must contain only approved facility abbreviations.
- Notes are dated with the month, day, and year to help identify the actual occurrence of the provision of care. Although there is no regulation for timing documentation entry, timed entries are extremely important to help determine provision of care.
- Discipline signatures should include first name, middle initial, and last name as well as credential.
- Notes should not be obliterated when incorrect but, rather, corrected according to the error correction policy of the facility.
- If an addendum is needed, sound documentation practices are followed per facility policy.
- Notes must be legible and written in ink. (There is no specification of color of ink; however, black is the industry standard to ensure quality of documentation when producing copies.)
- Notes should never be destroyed when entered into the resident record.

- Formats of notes

  —Narrative: Handwritten notes that describe the resident's condition, treatments, or interventions, and response to care

  —Data, action, and response (DAR): This format provides a focused style of documentation that provides headings of data, action, and response. Its characteristics offer a problem-oriented documentation style.

  —**SOAP** or problem-oriented method: This format provides a problem-focused style of documentation, as does the DAR charting. The acronym *SOAP* stands for subjective findings, objective findings, assessment of the resident, and plan of action.

  —**SOAPIER** method: Soapier notes begin the same as SOAP notes, then add the implementation, the evaluation, and any revision in the course of action or plan of care.

  —**Focus** format: The focus format utilizes a data-action-response style of documentation.

  —Problem, intervention, evaluation (PIE) format: The PIE format utilizes a problem-intervention-evaluation style of documentation where the problem is listed, followed by any interventions identified and an evaluation of the resident.

  —Charting by exception (CBE): This format is charting by exception in which only exceptions to normal care or normal findings are documented.

The form the narrative note is written in makes little difference as long as it captures the essence of general documentation guidelines. Any form designed to better facilitate the documentation of the narrative note is acceptable as defined by facility guidelines. The narrative note should be clear, concise, and not duplicative. Staff must remember to update care plans when narrative notes indicate that change has occurred with the resident. This is an important step in ensuring that the documentation throughout the resident's record accurately reflects the care needed.

Quality Improvement Requirements

Proper documentation practice is important for high-quality resident care. In an effort to provide the critical information about the resident to other healthcare providers, the health record must be properly completed to include:

- The care and services provided

- The resident's response to care

- Outcomes of the treatments and interventions

Proper documentation practice also ensures that should the record be examined by the legal system, it will reflect the true and accurate picture of the resident's complete medical treatment.

Quality issues include:

- Write the documentation in ink, preferably black, with no "white-out" or obliterations.

- Handwritten notes should be legible.

- Indicate date and time on all entries.

- Chronicle entries regardless of the format of the final health record; information should flow in sequence.

- There should be no blank spaces. These can lead to entries placed out of sequence.

- The documentation should show the full signature of the writer, complete with credential(s).

- Cosignatures should appear, as required by facility policy and practice.

- Only approved abbreviations should be used.

- Addendum should be added and identified as outlined in facility policy.

- Personal and subjective opinion concerning the resident should never be documented.

- Documentation should be objective.

- Document facts. (Statements that may be taken as a guarantee of improvement should not be entered.)

Timeliness of Documentation

The narrative note should be charted as soon as possible. Charting in this manner ensures that the chart reflects a true picture of the resident and that all care considerations and observations were noted as appropriate.

The narrative note should be placed in the section of the chart that is defined in the facility policy. (See the discussion on interdisciplinary and noninterdisciplinary narrative notes.)

For those facilities that would like the "story of the resident" to flow in book fashion, the notes are filed in chronological order. For those facilities that would prefer to have the latest information at the front of each section, the narrative note would be filed in reverse chronological order.

Admission/Readmission Documentation

Upon admission to the facility, an admission note should be entered into the resident's health record that includes the date and time of admission, how the resident arrived at the facility (for example, by ambulance), the reason for the admission, and the resident's current condition and health status. State regulations include specific requirements for admission documentation, time frame for completion, and other specified requirements.

The purpose of the admission note is to identify the moment the resident enters the healthcare facility, and it provides the baseline information from which to begin the interim care plan and the assessment process. The admission note prepares and helps inform the facility's clinical staff of the resident's needs, preferences, abilities, and desires for care.

Upon admission to the facility, the nursing staff is usually the first clinical staff to meet the resident. The staff notes how the resident arrives, immediate care needs, appliances, and level of initial functioning. The admission note is not an in-depth assessment like the admission assessment; rather, it provides a clear, crisp snapshot of the resident as he or she enters the facility's system. In many cases, it provides the first visual assessment of the new admission. For readmission, it allows the staff to determine the resident's immediate care issues or new conditions or problems. The admission note establishes care needs promptly.

This baseline assessment or narrative admission and readmission note provides information on the resident's physical, functional, and emotional status as he or she becomes acclimated to new surroundings. It conveys the first impression of the resident to other clinical staff who will manage his or her care during the stay. It also allows the facility to determine whether outcomes have been met over time. This initial admission note can and should be used in the assessment process for the resident care planning and treatment management, as appropriate. This does not mean that the admission note should be duplicated in the initial assessment but, rather, that important information is gathered on admission that should be utilized to properly assess the resident's care needs.

There is no federal or JCAHO requirement for an admission or readmission note; however, the information gathered on admission is vital to development of the care-planning process.

Depending on facility policy, the admission note may contain the following information:

- Date and time of arrival
- Mode of arrival
- Person who accompanied the resident, if applicable
- Station/unit and room number
- Resident status, condition, diagnosis, extenuating circumstances: Tubes, catheters, IVs, equipment, emotional and functional status, and so on
- Comments on resident acclimation to environment and documentation of orientation to environment as appropriate
- Notation of any ancillary orders such as therapy, X rays, follow-up appointments, and such

The content of the admission note is important to the interim care-planning process and the resident's introduction to the care-planning team.

Assessment criteria for any narrative note could include the following:

- Note is written, dated, and signed.
- Note is objective.
- Note is comprehensive as defined by facility requirements.

The admission or readmission note must be written as soon after the resident's admission to the facility as is feasibly possible.

The narrative note may be entered in the progress note section of the interdisciplinary chart or in the nursing section of the resident's record if the documentation process is noninterdisciplinary.

Monthly Summary

There are no federal requirements for a summary note; however, state laws may be more specific. (See figure 9.4.) (It is important that each facility review state regulations for licensure or reimbursement purposes.) The monthly summary provides a concise monthly update of the resident's condition and health status. It may be written as a problem-oriented summary addressing each problem individually or as a narrative summary of the month's events.

Figure 9.4.   **Sample monthly summary**

MONTHLY SUMMARY				
Resident Name:			**Health Record Number:**	
Date	**Shift**	**Narrative Summary**		**Signature**

The monthly summary supports further assessment of the resident and the care-planning process, and supplements the resident's record. It does not replace further assessment criteria or narrative charting but, rather, enhances the entire documentation process.

The monthly summary should correlate with the resident's care plan. It should reflect any changes in the resident's condition and health status. Should the resident exhibit changes from the prior monthly summary or if those changes are not addressed in the care plan, the summary should depict the resident's current health status and the reasons determined for the change. The care plan must be updated accordingly to ensure that the resident's needs are planned for adequately. The monthly summary should reflect the resident's condition over the prior month. This enhances and clarifies treatments and helps ensure that the interdisciplinary team has captured all healthcare needs for that particular resident in the care-planning process.

If the monthly summary consists of check boxes or checklists, there also should be areas for narrative comments to help clarify any checked area. It is vital that nursing staff understand that all areas in a check box or checklist format must be addressed, even when the area is not applicable. When the area is not applicable, this should be indicated with the term *not applicable* or an approved abbreviation of N/A.

Flow sheets that consist of check boxes supplement the care plan and narrative charting practices but do not stand alone as a prime source of the resident's condition or health status. Each time a resident's condition changes, the change warrants an update to the care plan and should include a narrative note to identify the change, provide the reasons for the change, and identify the interventions the team will use to manage or maintain the change. The resident's status may change for the better, and those changes should be documented as well. The purpose behind documenting and care planning is to provide a full and accurate accounting of the resident's health status.

The monthly summary process helps correlate the resident's addressed needs, treatments, desires, preferences, and care-planning process to ensure that the resident is viewed from a holistic approach. It helps tie the documentation and assessment processes together and provides a concise, complete picture of the resident's status and condition on a monthly basis. Moreover, it supplements the comprehensive assessment process and should trigger staff to incorporate resident changes into the care-planning process. Facilities should check state-specific requirements for the need for a monthly summary.

Documentation in the Health Record

In some facilities, the monthly summary may be formatted in a manner to capture identified problems on separate pages. (See figure 9.5.) This would allow the interdisciplinary team to document one problem on each page so that all comments on the page concern that particular problem. The problem number would correlate to the care plan to enhance the care-planning process.

The quality concerns inherent in the monthly summary process are those already mentioned for documentation accuracy and care planning. If the monthly summary suggests resident decline or change and the care plan does not reflect such change, the facility will have quality issues with the documentation. The resident's assessments, care plans, monthly summaries, and narrative notes should correlate and clearly depict his or her current health status.

Sample criteria that could be monitored for the monthly summary may include:

- Monthly summary document is charted.

- Monthly summary identifies change with narrative explanation of change and action plan, as appropriate.

- Monthly summary findings correlate with the care plan.

Figure 9.5.   Sample monthly summary organized by problem

MONTHLY SUMMARY			
Resident Name:		Health Record Number:	
Problem Number 1			
Date	Shift	Narrative Summary	Signature

MONTHLY SUMMARY			
Resident Name:		Health Record Number:	
Problem Number 2			
Date	Shift	Narrative Summary	Signature

The monthly summary should be completed once every month on every resident as defined by facility policy and philosophy. It is important to determine schedules for each resident and stay on schedule to ensure that the documentation is completed.

The monthly summary is placed in the care plan section of the record to ensure that the summary and the care plan correlate.

Interdisciplinary versus Noninterdisciplinary Progress Notes

At the beginning of the chapter, the interdisciplinary format was compared to the noninterdisciplinary format. The interdisciplinary format is used in many acute care and long-term acute care hospitals. It provides a mechanism for the information to flow in sequenced order and more easily demonstrates the resident's progress and treatment over time because all notes are entered in the health record one after the other. There are no separate sections for each discipline; instead, all notes are kept in the progress note section and incorporated with physician documentation as well. The whole resident health status can be determined by reading one section of the chart instead of flipping through many different sections to determine resident health status, needs, and treatments. Interdisciplinary charting provides one longitudinal record of the resident's stay in the facility.

Interdisciplinary notes are integrated narrative notes entered sequentially in the health record by each discipline treating the resident, including the physician. Noninterdisciplinary notes are progress notes documented as narrative notes in discipline-specific sections of the resident's health record.

The purpose of each kind of note is to provide well-documented resident care that supports the assessment, care planning, and monthly summary process.

Where interdisciplinary narrative notes provide the benefit of having the documentation flow in sequential fashion, noninterdisciplinary narrative notes allow the reader to focus on one area of the record at a time. If the person reviewing the record wants to examine all activity records, he or she simply turns to the activity section of the record to see the sequential documentation of the activity staff.

There are pros and cons to each form of narrative documentation. Facility practice and philosophy drive the documentation practice for the organization. Both interdisciplinary and noninterdisciplinary charting can be problem focused depending on the documentation format chosen by the facility.

Health Record Formats

Formats for health record content can be source oriented, problem focused, and integrated.

- *Source-oriented format:* This format provides a section for each department, and the record is assembled in reverse chronological order. This allows the sources of the documentation to be housed together. The source-oriented format works well with noninterdisciplinary charting practice.

- *Problem-focused, or POMR, format:* This format contains four basic sections.

    —Database contains a set of data gathered on each resident.

    —Problems list is located at the beginning of the progress note section and provides a detailed list of all of the resident's problems.

—Initial plan provides the treatments and modalities to be used for resident care.

—Progress notes are the narrative outcomes and progress of each resident.

The problem-focused format lends itself well to long-term care facilities because of the MDS comprehensive assessment and care-planning process. Along with the monthly summary written as problem-focused summaries, the system produces a clear picture of the resident's overall health status, problems, and outcomes.

- *Integrated format:* This format provides for the strict chronological order of the resident's health record. It places the documents written on each episode of care together in the health record.

The interdisciplinary chart lends itself well to integrating the resident's health status. The individual disciplines must work together to achieve the goals of the care plan. The documentation flows from one discipline to another so that the record contains evidence that the resident is cared for by the whole team. The entire team focuses on problems, and episodes of care can be more easily determined.

The problem with interdisciplinary charting is that individual discipline notes are not together for discipline-specific review of issues. The entire set of entries must be read to determine discipline-specific areas of documentation.

Importance of Documentation

The general requirements for interdisciplinary narrative notes include the fact that each discipline documents in the progress note section of the chart in sequential order. There are no separate sections for discipline narrative notes. Other general requirements include all those discussed for proper documentation practice.

The general requirements for noninterdisciplinary charting include maintaining proper documentation practice within individual sections for the resident's record.

The importance of documentation cannot be overemphasized. The professional disciplines responsible for charting in each resident's record must ensure that the record is updated in a timely and accurate fashion. Each individual charting on the resident's care needs and outcomes must follow the facility policy on documentation style and content.

The resident's health record is the legal record for the facility and must always be current and reflect the resident's needs, care, and treatment plan. The importance of documenting the narrative note, whether it is interdisciplinary or noninterdisciplinary, ensures that the events of the notes are conveyed to other disciplines, across shifts and over time.

Federal, state, and accrediting agencies require that residents be monitored and assessed periodically as defined by facility policy. The narrative documentation practices of the professional staff help meet this requirement. The narrative progress note documents progress, identifies problems, and charts outcomes to achieve requirements.

Formats for Progress Notes

SOAP, SOAPIER, and focus or DAR narrative notes are problem-oriented documentation styles. Each type of narrative note discusses or addresses the specific problems of the resident.

As mentioned earlier, the letters in the acronym SOAP stand for a section of the note:

Subjective
Objective
Assessment
Plan

The letters of the SOAPIER documentation style stand for:

Subjective
Objective
Assessment
Plan
Implementation
Evaluation
Revision

The focus style of documentation is known as a DAR note and contains the following:

Data: Subjective or objective information about the problem of focus. The *D* is omitted if no new data exist.

Action: Intervention planned. If there are no actions planned, the *A* is omitted.

Response: Resident's response to the intervention and goal attainment. If there is no response to care provided, the *R* is omitted.

The purpose of a facility-chosen documentation format is to provide standardization for the health record kept in the organization and to provide professional staff with guidelines for documenting to ensure consistency.

These problem-focused formats for narrative writing provide systematic approaches to documentation practice for the facility to follow. Problem-focused or SOAP narrative notes focus on the resident's unresolved problems. This provides yet another means for the facility to ensure correlation of the assessments, care plans, monthly summaries, and narrative notes into one complete care plan for the resident's stay.

Focused- or problem-oriented documentation decreases charting times, providing a format for the writer to follow and stay on track of the unresolved problem or issues. The narrative problem-oriented note is resident centered. The format centers on unresolved problem recognition and outcomes in a concise manner.

The problem-focused documentation style can be used in charting by exception. However, charting by exception captures only significant findings or exceptions to standards or normal patterns of care instead of all unresolved problems.

The problem-focused documentation style does support both interdisciplinary and non-interdisciplinary narrative notes. It enhances care planning and provides documentation on outcomes.

General Requirements

The requirements of each type of narrative note covered in this chapter include the need to address each area in the format. For instance, a SOAP note would include the subjective, objective, assessment, and plan. The only exception is that the DAR style may not require each area to be addressed.

The facility policy on documentation format and style should be followed at all times to ensure consistency and compliance.

The SOAP, SOAPIER, and focus styles of charting provide standardized methods to capture narrative documentation. The professional can clearly see the identified problems and objective data used to determine the actions and the plan of care. These types of narrative notes enhance communication among professionals across all shifts.

Quality Improvement Requirements

Whether the narrative notes are interdisciplinary or noninterdisciplinary, the content must be consistent with facility philosophy and policy. The quality of the SOAP, SOAPIER, and focus notes are extremely important for compliance initiatives. They should be easy to read and should reflect the resident's status and current condition. Moreover, the notes should be legible and written in ink as mentioned earlier in the chapter.

Each area of the particular style is addressed as appropriate:

- Notes are objective.
- Notes identify the problem or outcome.
- Notes are dated and signed with credentials.
- If errors occur, the documentation is corrected according to facility policy.
- Addenda are appropriately documented according to facility policy.
- If problems are identified, the care plan is updated as appropriate.

Documentation in the Health Record

The SOAP, SOPIER, and focus narrative notes are filed according to facility policy. If the notes are interdisciplinary, they are filed in chronological order in the progress note section of the resident's record. If they are noninterdisciplinary, they are filed in each discipline's section of the resident's record.

Other Pertinent Information

Charting by exception (CBE) is a type of charting system whereby only important findings or exceptions to established standards of care are documented. This type of charting utilizes flow sheets and/or check boxes to assess and evaluate residents. Should exceptions occur, they are identified with an asterisk. The asterisk notation also indicates that a narrative note has been documented to further explain the exception.

Other disciplines use narrative charting to demonstrate the provision of care. The following disciplines may have narrative charting included in their documentation practice:

- Nursing
- Physicians (progress notes)
- Consultants
- Nutrition
- Physical therapy
- Occupational therapy
- Respiratory therapy
- Social services
- Speech–language therapy
- Therapeutic recreation

Summary

Narrative charting provides a mechanism for capturing resident-specific health information that is not captured on other forms or documents. These notes support the care-planning and comprehensive assessment process for the resident's overall care requirements. The documentation of narrative notes may be either interdisciplinary or noninterdisciplinary. The interdisciplinary narrative notes place all healthcare providers' progress notes in one section written in chronological order. Using noninterdisciplinary narrative notes places each discipline's notes in a separate section of the resident's health record.

Upon admission or readmission to the facility, an admission note should be recorded in the resident's health record to include specified criteria as outlined by facility policy. This supports the baseline assessment done at the time of admission and provides further details on the resident's needs, preferences, abilities, and desires for care.

Facility policy defines the need for a nursing monthly summary. The monthly summary is a precise summary of the resident's health status. It is a recap of what has occurred over the past month.

The format for the narrative is outlined in facility policy for documentation practice and expectations. The style may differ from facility to facility. Options for narrative notes include SOAP, SOAPIER, focus, and DAR. Narrative notes provide the ability to capture additional information concerning the resident's current health status and function.

References

Centers for Medicare and Medicaid Services. 2001 (October 31). Guidance to Surveyors—Long-Term Care Facilities, appendix PP in *State Operations Manual*. Available at www.cms.gov.

Joint Commission on Accreditation of Healthcare Organizations. 2004. *Comprehensive Accreditation Manual for Long-term Care*. Oakbrook Terrace, Ill.: JCAHO.

Chapter 10

Medicare Documentation

The federal government requires accurate, timely, and complete health record documentation of the skilled nursing and therapeutic services provided to Medicare beneficiaries. The resident's health record must substantiate the clinical indications and medical necessity for Medicare part A coverage as well as the skilled services required and the resident's continued need for coverage. "Documentation that supports skilled services were medically reasonable and necessary is required for all charges submitted on the UB-92" (CMS 2002).

Medicare Reimbursement for Long-Term Care Services

"The Balanced Budget Act of 1997 mandates the implementation of a per diem prospective payment system (PPS) for skilled nursing facilities (SNFs) covering *all* costs (routine, ancillary and capital) related to the services furnished to beneficiaries under Part A of the Medicare program. Major elements of the system include:

- *Rates:* Federal rates are set using allowable costs from FY 1995 cost reports. The rates also include an estimate of the cost of services for which, prior to July 1, 1998, payment had been made under part B but furnished to SNF residents during a Part A covered stay. FY 1995 costs are updated to FY 1998 by a SNF market basket minus 1 percentage point for each of fiscal years 1996, 1997 and 1998. Providers which received new provider exemptions in FY 1995 are excluded from the data base. Exceptions payments are also excluded. The data is aggregated nationally by urban and rural area to determine standardized federal per diem rates to which case mix and wage adjustments apply.

- *Case-mix adjustment:* Per diem payments for each admission are case-mix adjusted using a resident classification system (Resource Utilization Groups III) based on data from resident assessments (MDS 2.0) and relative weights developed from staff time data.

- *Geographic adjustment:* The labor portion of the federal rates is adjusted for geographic variation in wages using the hospital wage index.

- *Annual updates:* Payment rates will be increased each Federal fiscal year using a SNF market basket index (minus one percentage point in FY 2000 through FY 2002).

- *Transition:* A three-year transition that blends a facility-specific payment rate with the federal case mix adjusted rate will be used. The facility-specific rate includes allowable costs (from FY 1995 cost reports) including exceptions payments. Payments associated with 'new provider' exemptions will be included but limited to 150 percent of the routine cost limit. It will also include an add-on for related Part B costs similar to the federal rate.

- *Effective date:* The PPS system [was] effective for cost reporting periods beginning on or after July 1, 1998" (CMS 2002).

The PPS for skilled nursing facilities applies to all costs of covered SNF services provided to beneficiaries for Part A Medicare. **Resource utilization groups, version III** (RUGs III), based on the use of the MDS are used to provide reimbursement to the SNF. "RUGs III classification is based, in part, on the beneficiary's need for skilled nursing care and therapy" (DHHS 2001, p. 39563).

Payment rates established under the PPS "cover all the costs of furnishing covered skilled nursing services (routine, ancillary, and capital-related costs) other than costs associated with approved educational activities" (DHHS 2001, p. 39564).

The Link between Documentation and Reimbursement

The assessments, reassessments, narrative notes, and data obtained from observation and interviews all contribute to development of a comprehensive assessment and completion of the Minimum Data Set (MDS) for Long-Term Care. The computerized MDS software calculates the resource utilization group (RUG) payment level for Medicare beneficiaries based on the data entered in the assessment form. To ensure proper compliance with Medicare billing, the resident's record must contain all ancillary services provided to the resident and billed to Medicare. To include these services for billing purposes, documentation within the resident's record must demonstrate that the services were provided and were medically necessary.

Fiscal intermediaries (FIs) and other payers may have local requirements that apply to documentation practices for billing. It is advisable to check with the local FI for exact local specifications concerning supporting and source documentation.

The purpose of any documentation system is to ensure that the facility follows basic documentation practices recording all assessments and reassessments, treatments and interventions, orders, and care provided for each resident. Documentation supports reimbursement of the resident's care. Without documentation of these care provisions, a claim for payment cannot be substantiated. Documentation of the resident's health status and care requirements ensures that:

- A legal record exists for each resident.
- Assessments, reassessments, narrative notes, and other supporting documentation correlate to the care-planning process.
- Care is provided as planned.
- Care is interdisciplinary.
- A physician is involved in the process.
- A device exists to allow communication among caregivers working on different shifts.
- Proof of care is provided.
- Federal, state, and accreditation standards are met.

Documentation for the Medicare process should follow general documentation principles, but specific documents also are required by the Medicare program, such as the MDS assessments, physician certifications, and evidence of "skilled" nursing and therapy care. Documentation is important no matter who pays for healthcare services. This discussion should not be understood to suggest that Medicare documentation is more important or more mystifying than general documentation principles and practice; it is not. However, Medicare stipulates that the facility must demonstrate that the services were actually provided and were medically necessary. There is no better proof than through use of proper documentation techniques to show that the facility understands these requirements and strives to ensure that the resident achieves the highest practicable physical, mental, and psychosocial well-being.

The federal requirement for documentation (F514) states that "the facility must maintain clinical records on each resident in accordance with accepted professional standards and practices that are complete, accurately documented, readily accessible and systematically organized" (CMS 2001, PP-197). These records, the required documentation of the resident's stay, contain the link that supports submission of reimbursement information.

The complete resident record represents the factual encounters of the resident while in the facility. It must include enough information to demonstrate that the facility understands the resident's status. Additionally, there needs to be evidence of satisfactory plans of care and a demonstration of the efficacy of the care given to the resident. The resident's record must contain a complete "picture of the resident's progress, including response to treatment, change in condition, and changes in treatment," thereby ensuring that the facility documentation supports the payment received for care provided to each resident (CMS 2001, PP-197).

The facility must determine the frequency of documentation other than that done for the resident assessment instrument (RAI) process as well as documentation of functional and behavioral goals and changes toward meeting those goals. Through this determination, the facility provides a systematic schedule to capture the resident's progress in sustaining or gaining functional abilities and mental and psychosocial status, and the facility demonstrates more consideration that staff has enough data to manage the resident's progress with less emphasis on time frames for data collection.

Improper documentation practices and principles have a significant impact on quality, care, costs, and reimbursement. When documentation is missing or incomplete, the resident may not receive the care required. Clinical staff can become frustrated with lack of information. Services may be billed, but charges will be denied because of insufficient documentation. Regulations cannot be met when resident services and care are not documented. Poor documentation can lead to incorrect MDS assessments, which reflect in the QI reports and RUG categories causing significant lost revenue. Documentation must support the care provided to the resident. Good documentation practices throughout each resident's stay lead to proper MDS assessments, which produce appropriate RUG category assignments and the highest reimbursement allowed under PPS. The flowchart in figure 10.1 illustrates the effects of correct documentation on reimbursement.

Figure 10.1.   Effects of good documentation practices

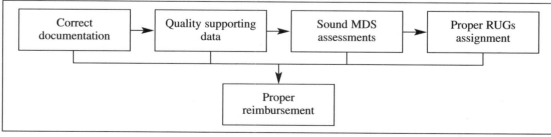

"The RUG-III classification system has seven major classification groups: Rehabilitation, Extensive Services, Special Care, Clinically Complex, Impaired Cognition, Behavior Problems, and Reduced Physical Function. The seven groups are further divided by the intensity of the resident's activities of daily living (ADL) needs, and in the Clinically Complex category, by the presence of depression. One hundred and eight (108) MDS assessment items are used in the RUG-III Classification system to evaluate the resident's clinical condition" (CMS 2002). Figure 10.2 provides a detailed description of the seven classification groups of the RUG-III classification system.

The MDS comprehensive assessment drives reimbursement of the facility through the RUGs calculations. The MDS is based on other supporting assessments completed on the resident on a periodic basis. These assessments together with the narrative notes and the resident care-planning process support the MDS assessment documentation, which indicates the treatments and services the resident has received. Therapy documentation also becomes a key piece of the RUGs calculation as does nursing restorative care. (Rehabilitation documentation is discussed in chapter 11; restorative nursing is discussed in chapter 6.)

"The SNF PPS establishes a schedule of Medicare assessments. Each required Medicare assessment is used to support Medicare PPS reimbursement for a predetermined maximum number of Medicare Part A days. To verify that the Medicare bill accurately reflects the assessment information, three data items derived from the MDS assessment must be included on the Medicare claim:

Assessment reference date (ARD): The ARD must be reported on the Medicare claim. If no MDS assessment was completed, the ARD is not used and the claim must be billed at the default rate. CMS has developed mechanisms to link the assessment and billing records.

The RUG-III Group: The RUG-III group is calculated from the MDS assessment data. The software used to encode and transmit the MDS assessment data calculates the RUG-III group. CMS edits and validates the RUG-III code of transmitted MDS assessments. Facilities cannot submit Medicare Part A claims until the assessment has been accepted into the CMS database, and they must use the RUG-III code as validated by CMS when bills are filed.

Health Insurance PPS (HIPPS) codes: Each Medicare PPS assessment is used to support Medicare Part A payment for a maximum number of days. The HIPPS code, also known as an

Figure 10.2.   RUG-III classification groups

1. **Rehabilitation Residents** receiving physical, speech or occupational therapy.

2. **Extensive Services Residents** receiving clinical interventions that include IV feeding or medications, suctioning, tracheostomy care, ventilator/respirator and comorbidities.

3. **Special Care Residents** receiving complex clinical care for conditions including multiple sclerosis, quadriplegia, cerebral palsy, respiratory therapy, ulcers, stage III or IV pressure ulcers, radiation, surgical wounds or open lesions, tube feeding and aphasia, fever with dehydration, pneumonia, vomiting, weight loss or tube feeding.

4. **Clinically Complex Residents** receiving complex clinical care requiring skilled nursing management and treatments for burns, coma, septicemia, pneumonia, foot/wounds, internal bleeding, dehydration, tube feeding, oxygen, transfusions, hemiplegia, chemotherapy, dialysis, physician visits/order changes.

5. **Impaired Cognition Residents** demonstrating difficulty in decision-making, recall and short-term memory.

6. **Behavior Problems Residents** who demonstrate behaviors including wandering, verbally or physically abusive or socially inappropriate, or who experience hallucinations or delusions.

7. **Reduced Physical Functions Residents** requiring assistance with activities of daily living and general supervision. (CMS's RAI Version 2.0 Manual CH 6).

Assessment Indicator, must be entered on each claim, and must accurately reflect which assessment is being used to bill the RUG-III group for Medicare reimbursement" (CMS 2002).

The skilled nursing facility HIPPS modifiers or assessment type indicators are as follows:

01   5-day Medicare-required assessment/not an admission assessment

02   30-day Medicare-required assessment

03   60-day Medicare-required assessment

04   90-day Medicare-required assessment

05   Readmission/return Medicare-required assessment

07   14-day Medicare-required assessment/not an admission assessment

08   Off-cycle other Medicare-required assessment (OMRA)

11   5-day (or readmission/return) Medicare-required assessment and admission assessment

17   14-day Medicare-required assessment and admission assessment

18   Other Medicare-required assessment (OMRA) replaces 5-day Medicare-required assessment (CMS 2002a).

19   Special payment situation: 5-day assessment

28   OMRA replaces 30-day Medicare-required assessment

29   Special payment situation: 30-day assessment

30   Off-cycle significant change assessment (outside assessment window)

31   Significant change assessment replaces 5-day Medicare-required assessment

32   Significant change assessment (SCSA) replaces 30-day Medicare-required assessment

33   Significant change assessment replaces 60-day Medicare-required assessment

34   Significant change assessment replaces 90-day Medicare-required assessment

35   Significant change assessment replaces a readmission/return Medicare-required assessment

37   Significant change assessment replaces 14-day Medicare-required assessment

38   OMRA replaces 60-day Medicare-required assessment

39   Special payment situation: 60-day assessment

40   Off-cycle significant correction assessment of a prior assessment (outside assessment window)

41   Significant correction of a prior assessment (SCPA) replaces a 5-day Medicare-required assessment

42   Significant correction of a prior assessment replaces 30-day Medicare-required assessment

43   Significant correction of a prior assessment replaces 60-day Medicare-required assessment

44   Significant correction of a prior assessment replaces 90-day Medicare-required assessment

45   Significant correction of a prior assessment replaces a readmission/return assessment

47   Significant correction of a prior assessment replaces 14-day Medicare-required assessment

48   OMRA replaces 90-day Medicare-required assessment

49   Special payment situation: 90-day assessment

54   90-day Medicare assessment that is also a quarterly assessment

78   OMRA replaces 14-day Medicare-required assessment

79   Special payment situation: 14-day assessment

00   Default code

When the MDS data are completed and "export ready" in an electronic assessment software form, the RUGs are calculated. RUGs can be calculated and recalculated at any time. Their values are not saved until the assessment is locked. This allows the interdisciplinary team to verify data entry and ensure that the required documentation is accurately reflected in the MDS prior to final RUG calculation.

Quality Considerations

Because the documentation contained in the MDS is so vital to the facility from a quality and reimbursement perspective, consideration for accurately reflecting the resident's health status, care needs, treatment, and diagnosis should be a major initiative for a long-term care facility. The tying together of all of the various pieces of the resident's care must be a highly visible process that all caregivers fully understand. Documentation practice should not be considered a *task* but, rather, an integral part of the overall process to ensure that the resident's well-being is maintained and improved.

Documentation to support the resident's care and treatment must be maintained for reasons of legality, quality initiatives, reimbursement, and resident outcomes. A flowchart of the MDS process to include documentation integral to the care-planning process may help facilities to see how all the parts of the resident's health record create the QI reports, the RUGs categories, and the resident's outcomes.

The flowchart should be specific to the facility. When flowcharting the MDS process, the facility may consider the information contained in figure 10.3.

From a Medicare documentation perspective, the quality requirements include the QI reports that are generated for more advanced quality initiatives. Examining those areas on the MDS that trigger QIs is an important step in the quality process. Results of audits should be tracked and trended over time so that the facility can determine where potential problems exist and whether they are real after further investigation. The results would determine if the process was in control. Correlating the QI reports to existing internal auditing criteria or reporting mechanisms would help the facility better understand the quality issues of documentation.

QIs were developed to serve as a method to identify potential problems with resident care, which required more comprehensive review and follow-up. Although QIs are a measure of quality, they should not be used to make determinations about the quality of care without further examination. The QI report is a tool to be used within the organization to help in evaluating the quality of care. It provides a means to begin looking at quality of care in a more detailed manner.

Facilities may include some of the following assessment criteria in quality initiatives:

- Accurate MDS assessments

- Inconsistencies in the data (comatose residents cannot walk)

- Resident outcomes

- Resident outcomes changes

- Care plan reflective of MDS outcomes

- Chart reflective of MDS outcomes

- Identified problems accompanied by action plans

Figure 10.3.   Flowchart of the MDS process

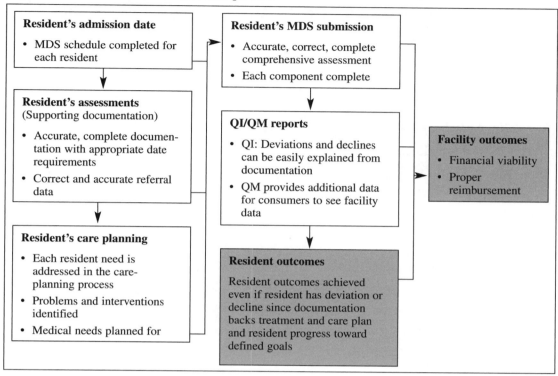

- Appropriate use of RAPs

- RUGs helping define resident population categories

- MDS process flow and process improvement opportunities

Supporting Documentation for the MDS

The MDS is the required assessment used for RUG categories and facility reimbursement activity. The resident's health record is required to justify the answers on the MDS for the time period identified by the assessment reference date. State-specific documentation may be identified as source data to back up the MDS data. (Check with existing state regulations for documentation required to support MDS data.)

Supporting documentation for the MDS includes those documents that justify the MDS comprehensive assessment. Although the MDS is a primary source document, some processes that support resident care and treatment are integral to the documentation practice that helps clarify and strengthen MDS responses.

The purpose of supporting documentation is to contribute to and help clarify MDS data entry. In reality, if treatment time is not documented, the entry in this section of the MDS would be a best-guess response. Because the health record must be an accurate reflection of the resident's health status and needs, a best-guess philosophy would not be acceptable. Another purpose of supporting documentation is to provide a means to begin to look further into any identified potential problems that may be uncovered during the MDS process. Supporting documentation provides insight and detail required to follow up on potential issues.

To complete an accurate, comprehensive assessment, information must be gleaned from many different reference points within the resident's record. The MDS full assessment covers the following areas:

- Cognition
- Communication
- Vision
- Mood and behavior
- Physical functioning
- Bowel and bladder function
- Diagnosis
- Health conditions
- Nutritional status
- Oral and dental status
- Skin
- Activities
- Medications
- Special treatments
- Discharge potential

In an effort to accurately reflect the resident's condition or status in all of these areas, several assessments, consultations, narrative notes, or supporting documents must exist and be used as justification for the MDS data. The information within the MDS must be valid. Using the supporting document that contains information concerning these areas of the resident's health and treatment ensures that the MDS is thorough and meets the requirement to be accurate.

RUG calculations are derived from the MDS assessment criteria. Depending on the resident's condition and supporting documentation, the MDS is completed and the RUGs category is calculated. Each RUG calculation is specific to the resident but can be determined using the RUGs-III 44 Group Model Calculation Worksheet for SNFs. Because each RUG calculation depends on the documentation of the MDS, it is difficult to provide a listing of each specific data point used to calculate the final RUGs scores. However, those sections of the MDS that affect the RUGs calculation are as follows:

ADL score	Sections G and K
Rehabilitation	Sections P and T
Extensive services	Sections B, C, E, H, I, J, K, M, and P
Special care	Sections I, J, K, M, and P
Clinically complex	Sections B, G, I, J, K, M, P, and E
Impaired cognition	Sections B C, H, and P
Behavior problems	Sections E, J, H, and P
Reduced physical functions	Sections H and P

Refer to chapter 6, Medicare SNF PPS, in the CMS *RAI Version 2.0 Manual,* for the calculation worksheets for specific data points used for RUG calculations. These are discussed further in the section on therapy treatment time in this chapter.

Supporting documentation may include:

- Therapy treatment time, frequency, duration, and plan
- ADL charting
- Mood and behavior documentation
- Hospital documentation
- Medicare certification/recertification
- Nursing restorative care
- Assessments
- Nursing notes

Quality of Documentation and QI Reports

It is ultimately the quality of the documentation that leads to proper Medicare reimbursement. Facilities must understand that ensuring sound supportive documentation within the MDS assessment cycle provides a mechanism to ensure high-quality care planning, sound reimbursement, and high-quality resident outcomes. The resident is the focus behind the entire process of documentation and quality. The best documentation drives the best communication and produces the best resident outcomes the facility can achieve. This in turn ensures accurate reimbursement for the facility.

The QIs provide a method for facilities to identify potential problems and investigate and resolve them, ensuring that the resident's needs are met and outcomes obtained. Linking the documentation, the MDS cycle, and incorporation of QI reports help the facility better understand how reimbursement may be affected.

The QIs are presented to the facility after submission of the MDS to the state. The MDS assessment process should provide the interdisciplinary team the opportunity to begin looking at potential problems well before the QIs have been received by the facility. In examining the supporting documentation of the MDS process, the team can certainly determine inconsistencies within the resident health record. Documentation that is inadequate or inconsistent should be examined thoroughly. Inconsistencies should be examined and validated before the MDS is submitted. Proper documentation practice and staff diligence will help provide the caliber of supporting documents required to produce high-quality outcomes. This in turn ensures that the facility has met the Medicare documentation standards and provides the best possible reimbursement allowed.

Supporting documentation should be completed as soon after treatment as possible. Documenting soon after the treatment session allows the writer to more easily remember what occurred and the resident's outcomes from the session.

The supporting documentation used for an MDS must be dated within the time frame of the assessment reference date as well. Outdated information should not be used for the MDS assessment.

Therapy Treatment Time

The time the resident spends in therapy must be entered on the MDS assessment. This includes individual and group therapy treatment minutes for each resident. The minutes are documented in the resident's health record along with dates for which treatment was provided. When this information is entered into the MDS and completed for export, the RUGs level is calculated. (See chapter 11 for an example of a therapy treatment form to document minutes spent in treatment.)

The therapy treatment time is the actual time spent treating the resident's care needs. This time does not include documentation time. The documentation of minutes is shown in figure 10.4.

The unit signifies each fifteen-minute interval of treatment time when documented in the resident's record. Minutes are tracked on the MDS. Units as defined above are documented in the record and may be used for billing purposes. The CMS guidelines for therapy times also are included in chapter 11.

The purpose of documenting therapy treatment time is to ensure that the resident's record includes an accurate accounting of care provided. The documentation of therapy time supports the completion of the MDS and RUGs assignment for reimbursement.

Therapy treatment time may be provided by therapists from specific disciplines, such as occupational therapy, physical therapy, or speech therapy. The supporting documentation in the resident's health record provides evidence that the services identified and received by the resident were provided. The record must contain evidence that the resident received a skilled service for therapy. Every treatment should be documented in the resident's record.

The resident's condition and health status as well as identified needs dictate the frequency of documentation. The framework for the documentation for therapy treatment should include the medical reason for the service and, as always, should be objective and include a plan of care with measurable goals and expected outcomes.

Medicare provides worksheets that provide clarity for calculating RUGs scores. These worksheets provide a mechanism to determine useful and pertinent documentation of interventions, treatments, problems, and the resident's response to the care given. A complete discussion of the use of these worksheets can be found in chapter 6 of the CMS *RAI Version 2.0 Manual* available at www.cms.hhs.gov.

The documentation contained in the resident's health record should be consistent across all disciplines to support Medicare benefits. The nursing documentation must demonstrate that the interventions implemented and functional skills taught in therapy are used on a daily basis and continue to be reinforced after the resident has returned from therapy sessions.

A variety of forms and formats to capture the documentation of therapy treatment and times may be used by facilities. This book has discussed narrative formats, flow sheets, checklists, and various other mechanisms to ensure data capture and accurately documented health records. The documentation practice should follow the facility's philosophy, but, most important, the health record must contain the data to support the resident's needs, treatments, care plans, and outcomes.

General Documentation Requirements

To receive Medicare reimbursement, the health record must contain evidence showing that the resident required and received skilled services such as therapy or nursing as ordered. For a claim to be submitted for payment, the health record also must show evidence of the reason for

Figure 10.4. Minutes rounded to increments

1 unit = >7 minutes to <23 minutes	5 units = >68 minutes to <83 minutes
2 units = >23 minutes to <38 minutes	6 units = >83 minutes to <98 minutes
3 units = >38 minutes to <53 minutes	7 units = >98 minutes to <113 minutes
4 units = >53 minutes to <68 minutes	8 units = >113 minutes to <128 minutes

treatment. "The definition of 'skilled service' for SNFs can be found in the Code of Federal Regulations 42CFR §409.31. The beneficiary must meet eligibility requirements, services billed must be ordered by a physician, and the beneficiary must require the skills of a technical or professional healthcare personnel on a daily basis. The services provided must be of a skill level that can only be provided on an inpatient basis at a SNF" (CMS 2002).

Because the Medicare system requires specific documentation, there is evidence that the process for documenting therapy treatments is important. In examining the RUGs worksheets, it is evident that the documentation process within the facility can provide opportunities to increase reimbursement as well as providing a valid, accurate picture of the resident's progress toward goals and outcomes of interventions. The entire process for documentation of the resident's condition, treatments, interventions, and outcomes is valuable not only for the facility, but also for the resident's well-being and further functional gains.

To be eligible for Medicare coverage, the beneficiary must meet technical and clinical eligibility requirements. "Under SNF PPS, beneficiaries must meet the established eligibility requirements for a Part A SNF-level stay" as follows:

- Technical eligibility requirements

  —Beneficiary is enrolled in Medicare Part A and has days available to use.

  —There has been a three-day prior qualifying hospital stay.

  —Admission for SNF-level services is within thirty days of discharge from an acute care stay.

- Clinical eligibility requirements

  —A beneficiary is eligible for SNF extended care if all the following requirements are met:

    –The beneficiary has a need for and receives medically necessary skilled care on a daily basis, which is provided by or under the direct supervision of skilled nursing or rehabilitation professionals.

    –As a practical matter, these skilled services can only be provided in an SNF.

    –The services provided must be for a condition for which the resident was treated during the qualifying hospital stay, or arose while the resident was in the SNF for treatment of a condition for which he or she was previously treated in a hospital.

Physician Certification

"A physician or a clinical nurse specialist or nurse practitioner employed by a physician (and not employed by the SNF) must certify and then periodically re-certify the need for extended care services in the nursing facility" (CMS 2002).

The physician's order must include the frequency, duration, and scope of treatment. The resident's health record should include a treatment plan with long- and short-term goals and progress notes indicating the medical necessity of the treatments and services. The resident's medical record must demonstrate that he or she has the ability to cooperate and make gains. The documentation also should demonstrate that the resident has the ability to retain and use education provided by the nurse or therapist during therapy. The resident's health record must meet general documentation practice standards as well as discipline-specific documentation practice standards.

To ensure accurate documentation of the therapy minutes for resident care, the resident's health record should be updated at the end of the treatment session. The therapy treatment time is placed in the discipline-specific section of the health record.

Quality Improvement Considerations

Therapy treatment time must be recorded accurately in the health record. The total therapy treatment time helps calculate the final RUGs score and reimbursement for the facility. The accuracy of documentation must be maintained, and monitors should be in place to ensure that the resident's bills are submitted correctly.

"A calculation worksheet was developed in order to provide clinical staff with a better understanding of how the RUG-III classification system works. The worksheet translates the software programming into plain language to assist staff in understanding the logic behind the classification system. A copy of the calculation worksheet for the RUG-III Classification system for nursing facilities can be found at the end of this section" (CMS 2000). To ensure proper assignment of the RUGs category, the facility can utilize the RUGs calculation worksheet. These worksheets assist the facility in achieving quality MDS submission and thus better reimbursement outcomes. Before using the RUGs worksheet, the facility should double-check "out-of-range" MDS data points. These are MDS data entries that may be invalid.

The time spent in treating the resident's needs also must be accurate. The facility must follow Medicare guidelines on documentation standards for time spent treating the resident. For example, if the treatment time is less than seven minutes, no time should be recorded.

The following criteria can be used to ensure proper documentation of therapy treatment time:

- Physician order should be present, including:
  - Frequency
  - Duration
  - Scope of treatment
  - Dated and signed
- Skilled services are required.
- Treatment plan should have long- and short-term goals.
- Progress notes should indicate the medical necessity of the interventions and treatments.
- Resident's ability to cooperate and make gains should be noted in the documentation.
- Resident's ability to retain and use education noted should be included in therapy documentation.

Medicare guidelines for documentation of times are utilized. Documentation reflects proper notations of time spent in treatment.

Other Pertinent Information

The documentation of therapy minutes is important to the RUGs calculation. Figure 10.4 gives assistance in rounding minutes into increments.

Charting of Activities of Daily Living

The charting of activities of daily living (ADL) is the process of documenting the resident's functional status. Functional ability can be divided into the following categories:

- Bed mobility
- Transfer
- Walking
- Locomotion
- Dressing
- Eating
- Toilet use
- Personal hygiene
- Bathing

Those areas included on the RUGs calculation for ADL charting are bed mobility, transfer, eating, and toilet use, which are late-loss ADLs. It has been determined that late-loss ADLs were "more predictive of resource use" and that early-loss ADLs did not substantially change the hierarchy of the RUGs categories. The purpose for ADL charting is to help support the MDS process and to better explain the resident's activity on a day-to-day and shift-to-shift basis.

The ADL section—section G of the MDS—provides data that will affect every RUG category for Medicare reimbursement. The resident's health record must demonstrate justification for the scoring of the ADL section. The health record documentation as well as observation and interviews with staff and the resident provide the required justification for the completed ADL section. When observation and interview are utilized to help support the ADL functioning of the resident, notation of the process must be entered in the resident's record to demonstrate the justification of the data points in the ADL section of the MDS.

The resident's medical record is the communication device that allows clinical staff to share the information recorded on the resident's condition, treatments, interventions, and outcomes of care provided. This shared information abstracted from all three shifts should be used to assist in defining the resident's ADL functioning during the past seven days. Documentation discrepancies concerning the resident's ADL functioning status should be noted in his or her health record to further explain the ADL scoring on the MDS assessment.

ADL charting is required of the nursing assistants or therapy aides who care for the resident on a daily basis. These assistants are the individuals who provide the majority of the care for the residents, and ADL charting allows them to capture the work they accomplish. ADL charting requires that the assistants write down exactly what they did for each resident during their shift. ADL charting captures the personal care provided to the resident.

ADL charting looks at how the resident functions or performs daily activities. It indicates whether the residents can provide for themselves, need supervision, require limited assistance, need extensive assistance, or require total assistance. Obviously, the higher the score (the more intense the resource use), the higher the RUG category. ADL charting also documents the ADL support required for each resident. These indicators examine the assistance the resident needs for setup or physical help such as setup only: one person assist or two or more person assist. The nursing assistants or the rehabilitation aides provide the care involved in the aspects of the resident's care. The documentation is generally captured on flow sheets or check-off sheets to help streamline the documentation process for the assistants who provide the care.

The MDS and ADL Charting Connection

There is no requirement for ADL charting at the federal level, but the MDS must reflect accurate and complete care of the resident. Therefore, it is implied that ADL charting is an important function to complete. This documentation then supports the MDS assessment process and ensures that the resident's health status and functioning level are adequately captured for the resident's record.

The nursing staff is responsible for overseeing the ADL charting process. Most of the care provided within the long-term care facility includes the ADL of the resident. It is the information gathered from the ADL charting process that is crucial in maintaining the resident's health, safety, and dignity. The ADL charting documentation provides the details of the resident's care needs on a daily basis. Often a certified nursing assistant indicates that the care required is completed by placing his or her initials on the ADL charting form. This process documents that the care was provided and the form can be used as reminder of what care is required. The documentation indicates the resident's functioning ability on a shift-by-shift basis, and, as such, it is easy to see the importance of such documentation for maintaining the quality of care for the resident. Moreover, the documentation is an excellent source for communicating the resident's status and functioning ability to other care providers.

ADL charting captures the resident's basic care requirements. In essence, it is evidence of the resident's daily functioning ability. The data are valuable for the entire interdisciplinary team. Promoting accurate ADL documentation and reporting is crucial to the MDS assessment process and general documentation practices. (See figure 10.5 for a sample ADL documentation record.)

The ADL charting should be completed as close to providing care as possible. The documentation should not wait until the end of the shift to be completed as this may reflect inaccurate or systematic checking rather than actual events. The ADL charting documentation is often

Figure 10.5.   Sample ADL documentation record

XYZ Organization Anytown USA 00000																							
ADL Flow Sheet																							
Resident name: _____ Health record number: _____																							
Month and year: _____																							
ADL scoring: **Self-performance** 0 = independence 1 = supervision/cueing 2 = limited assist 3 = extensive assistance 4 = total assistance 8 = did not occur **Support needed** 0 = none 1 = setup 2 = one person 3 = 2 or more people 8 = did not occur																							

ADLs		**Sun**			**Mon**			**Tues**			**Wed**			**Thur**			**Fri**			**Sat**		
		N	D	E	N	D	E	N	D	E	N	D	E	N	D	E	N	D	E	N	D	E
Bed mobility	Self-support																						
Transfer	Self-support																						
Walk in room	Self-support																						
Walk in corridor	Self-support																						

placed in the nursing section of the resident's health record because nursing staff is required to oversee ADL charting.

Quality Considerations for ADL Charting

The accuracy of the documentation must be ensured. Completion of the documentation also must be accomplished. The certified nursing assistant is extremely important to the ADL charting process, but this individual has many job functions and tasks to accomplish on a daily basis. Time requirements to complete the documentation should be kept to a minimum (a requirement that led to the concept of the checklist or flow sheet).

Educating certified nursing assistants on the entire MDS process would be beneficial to ensure that they completely understand the importance of comprehensive and accurate documentation and their role from a documentation perspective. The certified nursing assistant also should understand basic quality concepts and the integration of documentation of the resident's complete health record.

ADL charting may include the following indicators:

- The ADL charting form is complete.

- Areas that are not applicable are so indicated.

- Documentation is initialed when completed.

- ADL charting reflects MDS assessment criteria accurately.

Charting of Mood and Behavior

Mood and behavioral problems and scoring of these criteria on the MDS affects the final RUGs categories. The criteria that drive this RUG calculation are captured in sections E, J, H, and P of the MDS and can be found in the clinically complex RUG and the behavior problem RUG. Mood and behavior charting captures the mood of the resident over the past thirty days. Behavioral system data points examine the behavioral symptom frequency during the past seven days. Mood and behavior charting helps support the MDS assessment process by providing more in-depth documentation of mood or behavioral issues or concerns.

When assessing the resident, it is essential to include what was observed during the assessment period. Staff needs to address the resident's mood and behavior in the health record.

The certified nursing assistant can help document behavioral or mood issues on a check-off list or behavior flow sheet or behavioral log. Identification of behavioral issues then can be transferred to the MDS. Behavioral and mood charting becomes an important supporting documentation record for the MDS process.

"Behavioral symptoms are often seen as a source of danger and distress to the residents themselves and sometimes to other residents and staff. It is important to address behavioral symptoms for several reasons. Behaviors are often the only means some residents have for communicating health problems, discomfort, personal needs, preferences, or fears. To ignore such communication attempts by the resident may further isolate someone already burdened by the physical and cognitive losses associated with Alzheimer's disease or other types of dementia. Residents with behavioral symptoms represent a risk to other residents and staff and are much more likely to be abused or neglected." (CMS 2002). Behavioral and mood problems or symptoms may be an area of concern because residents may be more difficult to manage.

Those areas to monitor for behavioral and mood supporting documentation that affect RUGs scoring include:

- Wandering
- Verbal abuse
- Physical abuse
- Inappropriate behavior
- Resistance to care
- Delusions
- Hallucinations

Behavior Logs

The supporting documentation should include monitoring of the above areas of concern. The behavior log could include check boxes to identify these assessment criteria or could be a narrative format. (See figure 10.6.)

A behavioral log should include the following information:

- Resident name and health record number
- Time, date, place, and people who witness the event
- Description of the behavioral event
- Environmental factors present
- Observation of causative factors, intervention (treatment), and effectiveness or ineffectiveness of treatments/intervention

When mood or behavioral issues arise, this type of charting should be completed as soon after the event as possible. Behavioral and mood documentation may be placed in the comprehensive assessment and care-planning section of the resident's health record to support the appropriate MDS assessment.

Supporting documentation for those residents who have been identified with behavioral or mood issues must be complete to ensure completion of an accurate MDS assessment. The quality of the assessment helps provide the needed criteria for the MDS reporting period.

Figure 10.6.   Sample behavioral log

ORGANIZATION				
Resident name: _____			Health record number: _____	
Date/time	**Behavior**	**Witnesses**	**Factors**	**Signature**

Hospital Documentation

Specific areas within the MDS assessment form include hospital services provided to the resident. These services may affect the RUGs categories and impact reimbursement. The records indicating the hospital services that were delivered are used as supporting documentation for the care provided to the resident. The preadmission assessment that captures hospital services and dates of delivery as well as any follow-up services should be used to support the MDS.

Hospital documentation that could be considered supporting records for the MDS may include:

- Preadmission assessment (completed by the facility after communication with hospital staff)
- Discharge summary
- Operative notes
- Emergency department notes
- Procedure notes
- Special treatment record such as dialysis, chemotherapy, radiation therapy
- Medication administration record (MAR)

The purpose of hospital documentation is to support the MDS assessment process. These records contain valuable data such as hospital stay information, diagnosis, and special treatment considerations.

The MDS assessment contains information requirements for special treatments and procedures as well as hospital stay information and emergency department visits. These MDS data points are located in sections B, G, I, J, K, M, and P. To support the MDS assessment documentation, it is important to include the resident's hospital treatment documentation in the process. Those areas identified in the MDS that include the hospital information also affect the final RUGs score and reimbursement.

All hospital documents used to justify the MDS assessment should be included in the resident's health record. Hospital records used for MDS justification become a permanent part of the resident's record and should be treated the same as documents created at the facility.

The following RUGs categories may be affected by a hospital visit or stay: extensive services, special care, and clinically complex.

- Diagnosis
- Dehydration
- Internal bleeding
- Tube feeding
- Burns
- Infections
- Ulcers and wounds
- Chemotherapy
- Dialysis

- IV medication
- Oxygen therapy
- Transfusion
- Ventilation
- Hospital stay
- Emergency department visits

Any hospital stay that occurs within the MDS assessment period that would support the MDS should be retained as a permanent part of the resident's health record. The hospital's documentation becomes an important part of the justification for MDS assessment criteria and needs to be available to ensure that the resident's health status and condition are accurately reflected in his or her health record.

Any hospital visit records that indicate hospital stay, resident condition, special treatments, emergency department visits and procedures, or testing or other notes indicating resident health status are required to indicate or facilitate the following:

- Resident's needs and care requirements
- Further assessment for the resident
- Care planning for the resident
- Communication of resident's current requirements and health status
- Resident medical condition
- Hospital stay verification
- Support for an accurate MDS assessment

The resident's hospital information is a valuable part of the MDS assessment process. The facility must have a process to ensure that it receives the necessary information from the acute care setting.

Documentation from the acute care facility should be sent with the resident when he or she returns to the facility. In instances such as surgery when a typed operative note is not immediately available, the handwritten operative note should accompany the resident on return to the facility. Follow-up by the nursing department or the health records department can be accomplished to ensure receipt of the final operative summary.

The initial admission hospital information and subsequent hospital information received by the facility should be filed in the designated section of the resident's health record.

Certification/Recertification

Each Medicare resident must have a Medicare part A certification and recertification executed and signed by the physician who knows the resident's care and treatment requirements. **Certification/recertification** include the reasons for Medicare coverage and those skilled services that will be provided. Certification is mandated upon admission; recertifications are mandated for as long as the resident continues to receive Medicare part A benefits. The recertification also would be required when the resident returns to the long-term care facility after a temporary acute care hospital stay as long as the resident still qualifies for Medicare coverage.

The exact requirements are as follows:

- Certifications are required at the time of admission or as soon thereafter as is reasonable and practicable (42 CFR 424.20),

    —The initial certification certifies, per the existing context found in 42 CFR 424.20, that the resident meets the existing SNF level of care definition, or

    —Validates that the beneficiary's assignment to one of the upper RUG-III (Top 26) groups is correct through a statement indicating the assignment is correct.

- Re-certifications are used to document the continued need for skilled extended care services.

    —The first re-certification is required no later than the 14th day.

    —Subsequent re-certifications are required no later than 30 days after the first re-certification.

NOTE: These certification statements have no correlation to requirements specifically related to the plan of treatment for therapy that is required for purposes of coverage (CMS 2002).

"Payment for covered posthospital extended care services is made if a physician certifies and where services are furnished over a period of time, recertifies the need for them" (CMS 2002, p. 2-24.1).

The purpose of the certifications and recertifications is to attest that the resident does indeed require the skilled level of care and qualifies for Medicare coverage.

The certification and recertification documentation process is an important step in the Medicare documentation process. Without these certifications and recertifications, the facility cannot bill Medicare for services rendered.

Certification Format and Procedure

"There is no requirement for a specific procedure or form as long as the approach permits verification that the certification and recertification requirement is met" (CMS 2002, p. 2-24.1). Certifications and recertifications can be incorporated in "forms, notes, or other records" that the physician would typically sign when providing care for the resident, or there may be a separate form contained in the resident's health record.

If the facility is unable to obtain a certification or recertification, the covered services should not be billed to Medicare. "Your provider agreement precludes you from doing so" (CMS 2002, p. 2-24.1).

The attending physician or a physician who knows the resident's case and care requirements must sign the certification and recertification. Moreover, the certification must include the reasons and need for skilled nursing or rehabilitation care. Finally, it must be completed on admission or as soon after admission as possible.

Certification of ambulance services required by the long-term care facility also is required. It indicates that the ambulance service was medically necessary.

Recertification must include the reason for continued services, an estimated length of stay in the facility, and an appropriate plan for home care needs

The long-term care facility is "expected to obtain timely certification and recertification statements. However, delayed certifications and recertification will be honored where, for example, there has been an oversight or lapse" (CMS 2002, p. 2-26). These delayed "certifications and recertification must include an explanation for the delay and any medical or other evidence which the SNF considers relevant for purposes of explaining the delay" (CMS 2002, p. 2-26).

There is no stipulation for the format or form for the certification. The recertification must contain the items indicated. However, the certification and recertification do not have to be a separate form. They may be documented in the progress notes or other areas within the resident's health record as long as they comply with the standards established.

The first recertification must be completed no later than the fourteenth day of the resident's stay. Subsequent recertifications must be completed every thirty days but can be completed sooner.

The certification and recertification must be maintained in the admission section of the resident's health record.

Summary

There must be a clinical record for each resident in a long-term care facility. The federal government mandates accurate, timely, and complete documentation for each Medicare beneficiary admitted into the long-term care facility. The MDS comprehensive assessment is the documentation tool that Medicare requires to be completed for each resident and submitted according to a defined schedule. Supporting documentation in the form of assessments, reassessments, narrative notes, and other mechanisms also are required. General documentation principles should be followed when documenting resident health record information.

Complete documentation is crucial to high-quality care outcomes. Lack of documentation can lead to frustration and poor outcomes not only for the resident, but also for the facility. The documentation must support the care given to each resident. Documentation of the MDS comprehensive assessment has a far-reaching impact on each long-term care facility if the data are not accurate or reflective of the care provided.

The MDS submissions trigger QI reports that test the quality of the care given to each resident. Accuracy of the MDS assessment is a key component in Medicare documentation.

Completion of the MDS leads to RUG scores that predetermine reimbursement for the care provided. Supporting documentation such as ADL charting, mood and behavior records, and therapy time contribute to the assignment of the RUGs category. If the documentation is not accurate, a correct RUGs assignment will not occur. MDS data must be reported accurately and in a timely manner, which affects the overall reimbursement for the facility.

Hospital documentation also is a key component of the long-term care health record. Documentation that is sent from the acute care hospital helps determine services and interventions for the resident upon admission to the long-term care facility.

Each Medicare resident must have a Medicare part A certification and recertification completed by the physician to authorize Medicare coverage for his or her stay. The certification must be complete by day fourteen and recertifications must be done every thirty days thereafter until Medicare benefits exhaust.

Documentation is important for payment to the facility. It is important to ensure that accurate and timely documentation is completed for each resident regardless of payment source because proper documentation practice leads to better-quality outcomes for all concerned.

References

Centers for Medicare and Medicaid Services. 2001 (October 31). Guidance to Surveyors—Long-Term Care Facilities, appendix PP in *State Operations Manual*. Available from www.cms.gov.

Centers for Medicare and Medicaid Services. 2002. Medicare Skilled Nursing Facility Prospective Payment System, chapter 6 in *RAI Version 2.0 Manual*. Available from www.cms.hhs.gov.

Centers for Medicare and Medicaid Services. 2003 (May). Skilled Nursing Facility Manual. Available at http://cms.hhs.gov/manuals/12_snf/SN00.asp.

Department of Health and Human Services. 2001. *Federal Register,* volume 66, no. 147, July 31.

Chapter 11

Documentation of Rehabilitative Therapy

Rehabilitative therapy comprises those services provided by licensed therapist staff. These individuals are allied health professionals in physical therapy, occupational therapy, speech–language therapy, and respiratory therapy. Rehabilitative therapy should not be confused with nursing restorative care, which is discussed in chapter 6.

The federal government sets stringent standards for nursing homes "to attain or maintain the resident's highest practicable physical, mental, and psychosocial well-being." It mandates that should the comprehensive assessment and care plan determine that a resident needs specialized rehabilitation services, the facility must provide them. "Specialized rehabilitative services are considered a facility service and are, thus, included within the scope of facility service" (CMS 2001, PP-156).

The following general items refer to physical, occupational, and speech–language therapies. For all of their pertinent information, see the respiratory therapy section.

Importance of Rehabilitative Therapy Documentation

Therapy documentation is a means to communicate the resident's functional level, impairments and limitations, goal achievement, progress, and therapy activity to other clinical staff and the physician. It justifies the therapy care and appropriate reimbursement for all services provided. The therapy documentation focuses on the resident's functional abilities. It helps support the plan of care and overall treatment of the resident. Therapy documentation must follow the standards of documentation established by federal, state, and accrediting bodies including the Joint Commission on Accreditation of Healthcare Organizations (JCAHO) and the Commission on Accreditation of Rehabilitation Facilities (CARF).

The therapy documentation supports the interdisciplinary care of each resident who receives therapy services. Therapy services documentation helps improve resident outcomes. Therapists are responsible for the P and T sections of the MDS. These sections also help define the RUGs assignment for the resident and triggers reimbursement levels for the facility

Purpose of Rehabilitative Therapy

The purpose of therapy discussed in this chapter is to prevent avoidable physical deterioration and to help residents achieve or maintain the highest practicable level of functional and psychosocial well-being. This therapy documentation reflects a complete and accurate account of the therapy services administered, supports the assessment and reimbursement process, and provides a communication mechanism to ensure that the interdisciplinary team is knowledgeable and aware of therapy services, progress, and outcomes. Further, therapy documentation provides instruction, information on resident status, the resident's ability to function, and support for therapy care and appropriate reimbursement for services that have been provided. It captures the resident's functional limitations and impairments, and supports care planning while creating timed, measurable goals and expected outcomes. Therapy services encompass examinations, evaluations, treatment plans, and interventions provided to the resident.

Rehabilitative Therapy Standards of Practice

Documentation is the chief way to communicate with and support the interdisciplinary care team. The rehabilitation department has a set of established standards that it practices within the facility. If rehabilitative services are provided by an outside service, that service may provide the standards of clinical practice for the organization. These standards provide the foundation for therapy practice within the facility and should be readily available for reference. These practice standards also guide documentation practice and facilitate communication among members of the interdisciplinary team.

The standards of practice may include the following components:

- Referrals to therapy

  —How they are received

  —Timeliness of response

  —Referral after discharge

- Assessments and evaluations

  —Types of assessments and evaluations

  —Time frames for completion of the assessments

  —Procedure for prioritizing resident assessments

  —Communication methods

  —Discharge or readmission assessment criteria for documentation

- Screenings of residents

  —Defined by facility policy

- Documentation required

  —Daily

  —Weekly

  —Biweekly

  —Quarterly

  —Forms

    –Care plans

   –Progress notes

   –Grids

   –Flow sheets

   –Education flow sheets

   –Assessment, evaluation

   –Pathways

   –Productivity sheet

   –Exercise booklets

—Student documentation and signature guidelines

—Temporary licensed therapists

—Signature guidelines for therapists

—Supervision and oversight of assistant staff such as COTAs, PTAs, and rehab aides

Rehabilitative Therapy Assessments and Evaluations

The attending or covering physician must order services for therapy. The specified therapy must be medically necessary, reasonable, and appropriate for the therapy treatment program. Therapy documentation must reflect the legal standards of documentation practice including completeness, accuracy, legibility, and ethical practices. The resident's health record must contain a clear and concise reflection of the resident's health status, any therapy provided, and the outcomes of the specific therapy session.

The therapist begins the assessment as soon as possible after admission as prescribed by the physician. Those residents who are not admitted for therapy are regularly reassessed by the nursing staff or through therapy screenings as defined by facility policy. These reassessments determine that therapy may be necessary to allow the resident to maintain or improve function. Should nursing determine the need for therapy, it will request a therapist to complete the therapy screening assessment. When it is determined through the therapy-screening tool that therapy is needed, the therapist asks the nurse to obtain an order from the physician for such treatment. Referrals from the nursing department are sent to the rehabilitation department for implementation.

Referrals from nursing include:

• Resident name and health record number

• Date

• Diagnosis

• Date admitted

• Therapy request (physical therapy, occupational therapy, speech for such things as communication or swallowing)

• Specific interventions requested (orthotic, adaptive equipment)

• Comments to further describe the order

• Signature of the nurse and date of the request

The therapy team must respond appropriately, and in a timely manner, to all referrals.

Therapy documentation consists of screenings, evaluations and reevaluations, assessments, intervention plans and interventions, progress notes, flow sheets, discharge summaries, and documents to prove supervision and oversight of therapy assistants. Each form may have a specific format according to the type of document needed. Progress notes may be narrative notes or interdisciplinary notes and would be entered into the resident's record as facility practice dictates.

Each specific therapy session must be documented to ensure continuity of care and proper reimbursement practices. The referral or order for the therapy must be written and signed by the physician and be included in the resident's health record. The use of flow sheets augments the therapy section to help capture individual treatments and minutes of treatment provided.

The therapist is responsible for assisting with the completion of section P and T of the MDS comprehensive assessment and subsequent RUGs reimbursement assignment.

Therapy documentation should be completed as close to the time of service as possible. Documentation is an important aspect of the long-term care arena because it ties into the legal record for the facility, coding, reimbursement, the survey process, and compliance. Documenting treatment for the resident as soon as it is delivered also helps facilitate communication within the interdisciplinary team.

The JCAHO sets time frames for completion of subacute physical therapy documentation to be initiated within twenty-four hours and completed within forty-eight hours of referral.

Quality Concerns and Assessment Criteria

The following assessment criteria may be used for therapy documentation:

- Order is present.
- Order is complete.
- Therapy was initiated in a timely manner.
- Therapy documentation is complete.
- Therapy interventions are contained within the plan of care.
- Plan of care for therapy is updated per policy.
- Goals are measurable and timed.
- Orders are renewed every thirty days or as required.

At discharge, the following components may need to be addressed:

- Criteria for discharge
- Current physical and functional status
- Goals and outcomes achieved or degree of achievement
- Discharge plan
- Signature date and credential

The requirements for documentation standards should be followed in therapy, which includes completeness, accuracy, and timeliness of the treatments provided. Forms used within the therapy department to capture resident treatment and care should be completed in their entirety. The resident's care plan should accurately reflect the specific therapy interventions and services being provided to the resident. A quality check of the therapy documentation in conjunction with the care plan should provide insight into the accuracy of this documentation in the care-planning process.

Therapy-specific documentation should be peer reviewed to determine the quality of the data. Peer review provides a mechanism for therapists to monitor themselves and provides opportunities for improvement in documentation practice.

Therapy documentation supports the resident's assessment, care planning, and MDS processes. The resident's health record must be consistent with the MDS assessment to ensure proper reimbursement for the facility. Rehabilitation is captured in sections P and T of the MDS. The documentation contained in the resident's health record should correlate to the MDS and the bill that is submitted for reimbursement. As discussed in chapter 10, documentation of therapy treatment time is a quality concern as well. (See figure 11.1.)

Physician orders should be written and signed in the resident's health record for each requested therapy referral. A cross-check of this requirement may be done for quality purposes. Physician orders for therapy should contain the following data elements:

- Resident name
- Date
- Diagnosis pertinent to the request as required
- Therapy requested: Physical therapy (PT), occupational therapy (OT), or speech therapy
- Specific service needed, evaluate and treat, swallowing evaluation
- Frequency and duration of the treatment
- Physician signature, credentials, and date

Other Pertinent Information

Claims for physical therapy, occupational therapy, and speech therapy must include specific procedures performed and appropriate ICD-9-CM coding assignment.

Physical Therapy

Physical therapy is the field of study that focuses on physical functioning of the resident on a physician-prescribed basis. Physical therapists focus on basic gross mobility skills and can provide orthotics and prosthetics, lower extremity therapy, and adaptive mobility devices and training. Gait training is an important part of physical therapy, and loss of mobility should be brought to the therapists' attention. Physical therapy can provide for increased mobility

Figure 11.1.   Translation of minutes to units

1 unit = >7 minutes to <23 minutes	5 units = >68 minutes to <83 minutes
2 units = >23 minutes to <38 minutes	6 units = >83 minutes to <98 minutes
3 units = >38 minutes to <53 minutes	7 units = >98 minutes to <113 minutes
4 units = >53 minutes to <68 minutes	8 units = >113 minutes to <128 minutes

through transfer training, gait training, wheelchair mobility, car transfers, stair training, balance, and adaptive devices. Family education in these areas also can allow for greater resident mobility, including trips to relatives' homes, restaurants, and so forth.

When facilities use interdisciplinary care plans or interdisciplinary data capture techniques, it is important that the physical therapist examine the content of the forms to ensure that the requirements for physical therapy documentation are included as directed by federal, state, and accrediting agencies such as the JCAHO, CARF, and the **American Physical Therapy Association** (APTA). Guidelines for physical therapy documentation are available at www.apta.org.

Physical therapy services encompass the following evaluation and treatment areas:

- Mobility and functional training

- Therapeutic exercise such as strength, coordination, endurance, energy conservation, range of motion, balance, cardiopulmonary function, and pain

- Posture and positioning

- Posture mechanics

- Sensory

- Neurodevelopment and motor programs

- Accessibility and equipment

- Casting and orthotics

- Modalities of heat, cold, hydrotherapy, biofeedback, electrical muscle stimulation, transcutaneous nerve stimulation, ultrasound, traction, mobilization, massage, and manual techniques

- Pulmonary rehabilitation

- Aquatic therapy

Placement of Physical Therapy Documentation in the Health Record

Typically, physical therapy documentation is placed in a section specific to physical therapy. With the exception of care plans and any integrated notes required in facility policy, all physical therapy documentation is contained in this specific section of the resident's health record.

Requirements for Physical Therapy Documentation

Federal regulations require facilities to provide specialized rehabilitation services to their residents as identified in the assessment process, which includes not only physical therapy, but also occupational therapy and speech–language pathology. If the facility does not have residents who need specialized rehabilitation services, it is not required to provide the services as long as resident assessments continue to indicate that those services are not required to its resident population.

Surveyors are guided to examine the following areas in the physical therapy documentation:

- Did the resident's muscle strength improve?

- Did the resident's balance improve?

- Were assistive devices explored?

- Is the resident encouraged to use the assistive devices required?

Physical therapy orders must be renewed every thirty days or as needed. Usually, because the physician is not required to visit the resident this often, the physical therapist faxes or mails the treatment plan to the physician for signature. The physician then signs the treatment plan and returns it to the facility for inclusion in the resident's health record. This signifies renewal of physician orders. This process provides physician oversight of the resident's medical care and ensures the continuity of care for the resident's needs.

The content of the physical therapy evaluation is presented in figure 11.2.

Occupational Therapy

Occupational therapy involves treatment of residents who have physical disabilities and/or psychosocial needs. This therapy uses constructive activities planned to help restore the resident's ability to carry out needed activities of daily living and improves or maintains the resident's functional ability. "Occupational therapy is the therapeutic use of self-care, work, and play activities to increase independent function, enhance development, and prevent disability; may include adaptation of task or environment to achieve maximum independence and to enhance quality of life" (AOTA 1998). Occupational therapists can provide special splints, hand/upper extremity (arm) therapy, and work hardening/work conditioning programs.

Occupational therapists usually focus on activities of daily living—the ability to bathe, toilet, dress, cook, clean, and manage safely in the home environment—as well as strengthening

Figure 11.2.   Documentation content for physical therapy

• Resident name and health record number	• Test and measures appropriate to resident care:
• Referral mechanism	—Arousal, attention, and cognition
• History of problem	—Neuromotor development and sensory integration
• Current complaints	—Range of motion
• Precautions	—Muscle performance
• Pertinent diagnosis and comorbidities	—Ventilation and respiration
• Medical history	—Posture
• Applicable psychological, social, and environmental considerations	—Gait, locomotion, and balance
	• Clinical judgments
• Relevant current physical therapy	• Plan of care
• Resident's information about the problem	• Interventions
• Appropriate goals and expected outcomes that are measurable	• Equipment required
	• Changes in resident status
• Review of systems, including:	• Adverse reactions
—Cardiopulmonary	• Conditions that affect treatment schedules
—Integumentary	
—Musculoskeletal	• Consultation with resident, family, responsible party, as appropriate
—Neruomuscular	
• Resident's commutation methods, affect, cognition, language, and learning style	• Signature, date, and credential

activities, splinting, and work-related activities. Occupational therapy documentation is a key component of the interdisciplinary team care-planning process and RUGs reimbursement assignment. It supports and enhances the resident's functional ability.

Documentation Standards

Occupational therapy documentation standards are driven by federal, state, and accreditation agencies such as the JCAHO, CARF, and the **American Occupational Therapy Association** (AOTA). Guidelines for occupational therapy documentation are available at www.aota.org. The facility should develop clinical practice standards for the occupational therapy department. As with physical therapy, if the facility hires outside services for the delivery of occupational therapy, the outside service should provide these practice standards.

Occupational therapy practice standards should be similar to physical therapy practice standards in that they outline the referral assessment and evaluation and documentation requirements of the occupational therapy services.

Occupational therapy encompasses the following areas:

- Activities of daily living
- Home management or home visits programs for residents
- Safety training
- Sensation such as pain, temperature, light touch, stimuli of muscles, tendons, and other internal tissues, identification of forms by touch, and implications of these problems
- Transfers
- Positioning
- Posture and body mechanics
- Splinting
- Upper extremity function such as passive and active range of motion, strength, coordination, tone, hand function, and edema
- Compensatory techniques
- Vocational skills
- Visual perception
- Accessibility
- Ergonomics
- Cognition such as orientation, attention, spatial perception, problem solving, judgment, abstract thinking, and safety awareness
- Modalities
- Education

Placement of Documents in the Health Record

Documentation from occupational therapists is placed in a special section denoted for this service. This section contains all the occupational therapy documentation forms that are required for the resident with the exception of the care plan and integrated progress notes.

Requirements of Occupational Therapy

Occupational therapy services must have a plan of treatment signed by the physician. The plan must be determined before treatment can begin. It must be filed in the resident's health record and be readily available to the interdisciplinary team for review. The occupational therapy plan of care must be reviewed and acknowledged by the physician every thirty days or as required. This means the physician must sign and date the plan of care as proof of medical oversight.

Surveyors would look to occupational therapy to determine the following:

- What was done to decrease the amount of assistance needed for the resident to complete tasks?

- Were behavioral symptoms decreased?

- Were gross and fine motor skills addressed and improved?

- How was sensory awareness addressed?

- Did the facility work to improve problem solving, attention span, and recognition of safety issues?

The content of the occupational therapy evaluation is presented in figure 11.3.

Speech–Language Therapy

Speech–language therapy comprises resident communication behavior and disorders, swallowing functions and disorders, and cognition. Speech–language pathology programs encompass dysphagia or swallowing evaluations and treatment, cognitive, and communication services including hearing ability and memory for residents. The function of the speech–language therapy department is to improve or enhance the resident's ability to communicate and/or swallow, thereby improving the quality of the resident's life in general. The speech–language therapist works to improve the resident's function through compensatory techniques.

The speech–language pathologist helps improve communication, swallowing, and evaluates cognition to enhance the resident's overall functional ability. Documentation for the speech–language therapy department includes evaluations and assessment, programs, and services provided to the resident supporting clinical decision making and the care-planning process. Guidelines for speech–language pathology documentation are available at http://professional.asha.org.

Figure 11.3.   Documentation content for occupational therapy

• Resident name and health record number	• Contraindications
• Resident's significant past medical history	• Resident awareness and understanding of the diagnosis and prognosis, as appropriate
• Diagnosis required for ongoing occupational therapy	• Treatment goals
• Related physical orders	• Summary of treatment provided and results achieved
• Goals and potential for achievement of the goals subject to reasonable time frames: —Type —Amount —Frequency —Durations —Reasonable and necessary	• Signature and credential of the completing therapist and date • Signature of the physician and date

The services provided by the speech–language pathologist support the resident's basic needs. As a member of the interdisciplinary team, the speech–language pathologist provides valuable insight into the resident evaluation and assessment process, which drives the care-planning requirements of each resident.

Speech–language therapy services include the following areas of practice:

- Speech

- Language, oral and written

- Swallowing

- Cognition such as attention, memory, and problem solving

- Sensory awareness associated with communication and swallowing

- Augmentative and alternate communication methods

- Hearing loss and hearing screening (may be accomplished by audiology services)

- Videofluoroscopy examination

- Prosthetics for communication or swallowing

- Education and counseling

- Safety awareness

The facility must have clinical practice standards for speech–language pathology with data elements similar to those in the physical and occupational therapy practice standards.

Placement of Documents in the Health Record

Speech–language therapy documentation is placed in the resident's health record in a specific section denoted for this service. Documents are filed according to guidelines and policy established by the facility. They are typically filed in chronological order with the exception of the resident care plan and integrated progress notes.

Requirements for Speech–Language Therapy

Speech–language therapy services must have orders for service signed by the physician. The plan of care must be completed prior to treatment, and the treatment plan must be kept in the resident's health record. The speech–language pathology plan of care must be reviewed and acknowledged by the physician every thirty days or as needed, which requires the signature of the physician and date the plan was signed. This process ensures that the physician has knowledge of the resident's progress and demonstrates medical supervision of the resident's total plan of care.

Those areas that the survey process may include are:

- Auditory skills are improved.

- Speech improvements are documented.

- Expressive behavior is improved.

- Swallowing assessments are complete and recommendations documented.

- Resident demonstrated improved functional ability with hearing.
- Are alternative methods to communicate instituted?

Content of the Treatment Plan

The content of the speech–language pathology treatment plan would be specific to the problem being evaluated, such as swallowing, hearing loss, cognitive skills, or communication skills. Each form may differ among facilities but, at a minimum, should address the information provided in figure 11.4.

Respiratory Therapy

Respiratory therapy encompasses the practice involved in enhancing respiratory function for the resident. Respiratory therapy activities include diagnostic evaluation, therapy, and education of the resident and family members. Respiratory therapy is provided to residents under the direction of the physician. The respiratory therapy professional is a valuable member of the interdisciplinary and care-planning team in long-term care.

Definitions

"Respiratory Care is the health care discipline that specializes in the promotion of optimum cardiopulmonary function and health. Respiratory Therapists apply scientific principles to prevent, identify, and treat acute or chronic dysfunction of the cardiopulmonary system" (AARC 1999). Respiratory therapy provides direct and indirect pulmonary care and services to each resident who requires intervention.

Purpose of Respiratory Therapy Documentation

The purpose of respiratory therapy documentation is to provide mechanisms to enhance resident outcomes and to enhance communication among members of the interdisciplinary team.

Respiratory therapy services include the assessments, education, treatments, management, control, rehabilitation, diagnostic evaluation, and care of each resident with respiratory deficits and atypical respiratory function. Respiratory care may be required by licensed respiratory therapists twenty-four hours a day, seven days a week, but must be ordered by a physician. Skilled, trained nursing staff may provide some aspects of respiratory care.

Figure 11.4.   Documentation content for speech–language therapy

• Resident name and health record number	• Contraindications
• Resident's significant past medical history	• Resident awareness and understanding of the diagnosis and prognosis, as appropriate
• Diagnosis required for ongoing speech–language therapy	• Treatment goals
• Related orders	• Summary of treatment provided and results achieved
• Goals and potential for achievement of the goals subject to reasonable time frames: —Type —Amount —Frequency —Durations —Reasonable and necessary	• Signature and credential of the completing therapist and date • Signature of the physician and date

Requirements for Respiratory Therapy

Unlike physical, occupational, and speech–language therapies, no specific order exists to request respiratory service. Instead, orders for a nebulizer, other medication treatments, and ventilator or respiratory interventions will trigger the respiratory therapists to treat the resident.

Those residents admitted to the facility on ventilator support will have respiratory care follow-up and services. The respiratory therapist will complete a respiratory assessment prior to services being rendered that will take into consideration any do not resuscitate (DNR) orders or other advance directive criteria that are established by the resident and/or his or her family in conjunction with the physician.

The facility should have an established scope of service for the provision of respiratory therapy service, which may include the following aspects:

- Specimen collections and analysis of blood
- Interpretation of physiological data
- Tests and studies of the cardiopulmonary system for diagnostic, monitoring, and treatment purposes
- Administration of respiratory medications
- Ventilator management
- Chest physiotherapy
- Breathing exercises
- Respiratory rehabilitation
- Cardiopulmonary resuscitation
- Maintenance of natural airways
- Maintenance of artificial airways
- Observation and monitoring of respiratory care and treatment
- Evaluation, treatment, and implementation of respiratory care services as prescribed
- Transcription of written and signed and verbal orders for respiratory care as ordered by the resident's physician
- Education

The documentation required for respiratory services is defined by facility policy, and requirements may differ depending on state-specific requirements. System safety checks also are defined in facility policy and respiratory therapy standards of care. Figure 11.5 presents typical documentation content for respiratory therapy.

Documentation may be captured on the following forms:

- Interdisciplinary flow sheets
- Ventilator flow sheets
- Progress notes
- Resident family education flow sheet
- Tracheostomy tube changes
- Treatment or intervention flow sheets

Figure 11.5.   Documentation content for respiratory therapy

• Resident name and health record number	• O_2 sat and FiO_2
• Breath patterns and sounds	• Precautions
• Clinical observation	• Resident information and observation
• Color notation of resident	• Respiration rate
• Diagnostic test results	• Respiratory pattern
• Equipment and supplies	• Response to care
• Examination of chest	• Secretions
• Functionality of the airway	• Sputum production
• Heart rate	• Suctioning requirements
• Laboratory values and culture results	• Type of tracheostomy tube and size
• Measurements	• Ventilator parameters and alarms

Documented assessments and evaluations should include the following components:

- Resident name and health record number

- Resident's significant past medical history

- Diagnosis required for ongoing respiratory therapy

- Related orders such as ventilation settings and PEEP control, trach size, oxygen, and medication

- Goals and potential for achievement of the goals subject to reasonable time frames

- Indications and contraindications

- Resident awareness and understanding of the diagnosis and prognosis, as appropriate

- Treatment goals

- Summary of treatment provided and results achieved

- Signature and credential of the completing therapist and date

Physician renewal of respiratory orders is completed as per facility policy for medication treatment orders. (See chapter 13 for details on these types of order renewals.)

Residents who are allowed to go out on pass for community service and activities may require that a respiratory therapist accompany them. This should be documented in facility policy and the policy followed. Residents have the right to be as independent as possible.

Those long-term care facilities that provide respiratory therapy services and care should have established standards of respiratory care that outline the policies that will govern the provision of respiratory care services. Those services may include:

- Resident assessments

- Mechanical ventilation

- Airway management

- Therapeutic intervention

- Assessment of oxygenation and ventilation

- Resident and family education

- Discharge planning
- Documentation

Quality Improvement Requirements

Quality requirements for respiratory therapy may be set by state requirements and survey results. Quality concerns for the respiratory therapy department may include:

- Ventilator checks and assessments
- Ventilator circuit changes
- Airway management
- Therapeutic interventions followed and documented
- Overall documentation practice and completion

Assessment Criteria

Assessment criteria may include the following elements:

- Ventilator checks and circuit changes are completed as indicated.
- Assessments are complete and timely.
- Airway management is documented.
- Safety checks are accurate, complete, and done according to policy.
- Therapeutic interventions are relevant and necessary.
- Physician orders are implemented.
- Medication orders are transcribed correctly.
- Medication administration documentation is complete.
- Reassessments are completed as required.

Placement of Respiratory Therapy Documentation in the Health Record

Respiratory therapy documentation may be interdisciplinary or department specific depending on facility policy. If the resident's health record is interdisciplinary, the respiratory progress notes typically will be integrated into the progress note section of the record with the ventilator flow sheets and respiratory flow sheets going into a designated section of the record. The respiratory flow sheet may be integrated with nursing flow sheets to produce an interdisciplinary record. In the noninterdisciplinary resident health record, respiratory therapy is a designated section of the chart, which houses the documentation used as defined by facility policy. Ventilator flow sheets and respiratory flow sheets usually have a dedicated section due to volume and the necessity to be archived more frequently than the other respiratory supporting documentation.

Tracheostomy tube change documentation should remain in the resident's health record at all times. This documentation is typically never archived.

Summary

Physical therapy, occupational therapy, speech–language therapy, and respiratory therapy professionals provide rehabilitative therapy. These services are specialized rehabilitative services that are needed to help ensure that the resident attains or maintains the highest practicable well-being. A long-term care facility must provide these types of services when they are identified as necessary through the comprehensive assessment process.

These types of therapies are provided to prevent avoidable physical deterioration and to help the resident attain or maintain functional ability. Documentation of these services is a chief means to communicate the resident's functional status. The services support the interdisciplinary care team in caring for the resident. Rehabilitative service documentation supports the resident care-planning process.

Each discipline has a well-defined scope of service document that outlines its provision of service practice. If outside providers are used to furnish these services to residents, the service delivery organization will supply the scope of service records to the facility for use.

A physician must order rehabilitative services. Renewal of orders by the physician also is required. These services must be medically necessary, reasonable, and appropriate.

In its reassessment process, nursing may ask to have therapy screenings completed to help determine whether therapy services may be beneficial for the resident. The facility should have a policy and procedure for this type of process.

Physical therapy focuses on the resident's physical functioning. Occupational therapy concentrates on the restoration of activities of daily living. Speech–language therapy examines and treats communication behavior and disorders, swallowing function and disorders, and cognition. Respiratory therapy enhances respiratory function.

Many different documents capture the rehabilitative services provided to the resident. Each document supports the comprehensive assessment and reassessment of each resident. Accurate, complete documentation of rehabilitative services demonstrates residents' needs, gains, or declines and supports the interdisciplinary team care-planning process.

References

American Association for Respiratory Care. 1999. www.aarc.org.

American Occupational Therapy Association, Inc. 1998. Standards of Practice for Occupational Therapy. Available at www.aota.org.

American Occupational Therapy Association, Inc. Guidelines for Occupational Therapy Documentation. Available at www.aota.org.

American Physical Therapy Association. Guidelines for Physical Therapy Documentation. Available at www.apta.org.

American Speech–Language Hearing Association. 2001. *Scope of Practice in Speech-Language Pathology.* Rockville, Md.: American Speech–Language Hearing Association.

American Speech-Language Hearing Association. Guidelines for Speech–Language Pathology Documentation. Available at http://professional.asha.org.

Centers for Medicare and Medicaid Services. 2001 (October 31). Guidance to Surveyors—Long-Term Care Facilities, appendix PP in *State Operations Manual.* Available at www.cms.gov.

Goode, Nancy. 1999. Physical therapy documentation [The reliable resource]. *PT—Magazine of Physical Therapy* 7(9).

Chapter 12

Documentation of Physician Services

"A physician must personally approve in writing a recommendation that an individual be admitted to a facility. Each resident must remain under the care of a physician" (CMS 2001, PP-151). The facility also must guarantee that a physician oversees the medical care of each resident and that another physician has responsibility for the resident's medical care in the event the attending physician is unavailable.

"If the organization has an organized medical staff, the governance approves the medical staff's bylaws and rules and regulations." (JCAHO 2004, LD.1.20). Medical staff bylaws, rules, and regulations are the foundation on which the medical staff provides care in the facility. The facility should have written bylaws for the provision of medical services and oversight within the facility. The medical director's responsibility should be well defined and documented as well.

Definitions

"Supervising the medical care of residents means participating in the resident's assessment and care planning, monitoring changes in resident's medical status, and providing consultation or treatment when called by the facility" (CMS 2001, PP-151). Also included in the oversight of resident care is prescribing orders such as therapy, transfer to an acute care hospital, routine visits, or delegation and supervision of visits by physician extenders. Physician documentation stands as evidence of the physician's knowledge of the resident's health status, functional condition, and medical needs.

Purpose of Documentation of Physician Services

The purpose of physician documentation is to demonstrate that the medical oversight or supervision of care for long-term care residents occurs by a physician who knows the resident's health status. The interdisciplinary team and care-planning process must involve the physician. In the long-term care environment, the physician is not required to visit the resident every day but, rather, as the resident's needs dictate. However, the physician must be informed of the resident's status changes or identified medical problems to ensure that proper care is provided in a timely manner.

Physician documentation begins with the resident's admission to the long-term care facility and continues through discharge. The physician must be involved at regular intervals as federal, state, and accrediting agencies dictate and when the resident's medical condition changes.

Individual states may have requirements for physician services that are more specific than federal regulations. Many facilities also have policies and procedures that more clearly define physician involvement in the resident's care. These may include:

- Medical director role in physician coverage
- Written history and physical
- Renewal of orders
- Time frames for completion of documentation
- Specific orders for treatment options
- Physician-specific documentation requirements
- Physician extender requirements

General Requirements

The physician is required to "Review the resident's total program of care, including medications and treatments, at each visit" (CMS 2001, PP-152). He or she must write, sign, and date progress notes at each visit and sign and date all orders.

"The resident must be seen by a physician at least once every 30 days for the first 90 days after admission, and at least once every 60 days thereafter" (CMS 2001, PP-153). This means that the physician must have face-to-face contact with the resident.

- By federal regulation, a physician's visit may be deemed timely if it happens no later than ten days after the required visit. However, this does not affect the next scheduled visit date. The facility would not need to "specifically look at the timetables" (CMS 2001, PP-153) of the physician's visits except when there is evidence that the physician is providing insufficient medical care.

- The physician visit is expected to occur at the facility unless specific office equipment is required for the visit (CMS 2001, PP-153).

There is no federal requirement stating that there must be a face-to-face physician–resident contact at admission. The decision to admit the resident to the long-term care facility has already precipitated meetings between the physician and the resident culminating in the determination of the resident's care needs and requirements.

If states allow the use of a physician extender, when the initial physician contact has been completed by day thirty, the physician extender may visit the resident in place of the physician at every other required visit. There may be specific state regulations for the levels of treatments and examinations that a physician extender may complete. Each facility should review the state-specific requirements for physician extenders.

When the resident's condition dictates, the physician must make a face-to-face visit. The facility must provide physician services twenty-four hours a day to manage resident care emergencies.

The Joint Commission on Accreditation of Healthcare Organizations (JCAHO) requires that the attending physician or a licensed independent practitioner complete the resident's medical assessment, which includes the medical history and physical examination. They must be completed within required time frames (PC standards).

Physician Involvement in Resident Care

Because of federal, state-specific, and accrediting agency requirements for physician management and supervision, physician documentation becomes important for the facility to demonstrate that the physician is involved in the resident's care. The admission and continuing documentation that the physician provides supports the facility's policies and procedures and ensures that the resident has continued physician involvement in all care requirements.

Because the physician has much more limited visit requirements than acute care or post-acute care hospitals, documentation of physician involvement in care is crucial to verify regulatory compliance. Nursing documentation indicating physician involvement in the resident's care needs also will supplement this requirement. The nursing staff should document calls placed to the physician's office for further clarification of orders, resident care requirements, resident condition change, and resident injuries or accidents as deemed necessary. Ensuring that the physician is well informed about his or her residents helps the facility provide the resident with proper medical care and treatment.

Types of Physician Documentation

The facility may provide several different forms through which the physician documents the care provided. These forms or formats differ according to state-specific requirements, but may include:

- **Certification or recertification** for Medicare services
- History and physical at admission and annually (if required by state laws or accrediting bodies)
- Medication orders
- Treatment orders
- Progress notes
- Consultations
- Discharge summary (if required by state law)
- Discharge order as per state requirements

Quality Requirements

When a resident is diagnosed with dementia, there must be a differential diagnosis. A neurologist, psychiatrist, geriatrician, or other eligible physician may complete assessments of the resident's condition. The Alzheimer's Association can be contacted for the guidelines required for conducting these evaluations (http://www.alz.org). The following must be completed:

- History and physical examination
- Mental status evaluation
- Neurologic examination
- Blood workup
- Psychiatric evaluation

- Neuropsychiatric assessment

- Psychological assessment

- CT/MRI, if needed, as indicated

- Any reversible causes for the presenting symptoms

When these evaluations have been completed prior to admission, the documentation may be requested for the resident's health record.

Based on clinical information provided to the physician, he or she determines whether tests are necessary for the resident. When tests have been completed, the results should be regularly reported to the physician as determined by the resident's health status..

The attending physician orders medical interventions and treatments required for the care of the resident based on current health status and identified need. The interim care plan is established at admission and is based on physician orders, preadmission care requirements, and the assessment completed upon admission to the facility. In order that care may begin promptly, the interim care plan is developed and remains in effect until an interdisciplinary care plan is completed.

The JCAHO philosophy has changed concerning the need for a health record review to be completed on a sample of all open and closed resident records. However, the JCAHO will continue to make available the open and closed record audit tools that it has used for several years. (See table 19.1.) This form is available on the JCAHO Web site (www.jcaho.org). This audit tool looks at any exceptions to compliance of documentation standards. The JCAHO is allowing its continued availability to help assist organizations with continuing quality monitoring of health records.

For those long-term care facilities that are JCAHO accredited, a process should be in place for reviewing the open and closed resident records for the quality of documentation. It is a good idea to incorporate compliance with federal and state standards in this process as well. For those facilities that are not JCAHO accredited, quality audits of documentation practices should be instituted to ensure compliance with standards. The process should outline how the records are to be reviewed, who is responsible for the review, and how the results are reported throughout the organization.

Results from the open and closed audits can support physician credentialing within the facility. The tallied results can be broken down into individual physician **quality assurance** reports that can easily be placed in the specific physician's credential files. The medical director of the facility should receive copies of all individual physician quality assurance reports for review.

Assessment criteria for the JCAHO closed health record for physicians include:

- Initial medical assessment and impressions from the medical history and physical examination (twenty-four hours before or seventy-two hours after admission; forty-eight hours for subacute)

- Record that the required physician visits occurred

- Identification of an alternate physician

- Documentation of the diagnoses

- Reason(s) for admission or treatment

- Orders and renewal of orders for resuscitative services to be withheld or life-sustaining treatment withdrawn

- Discharged record completed (not to exceed thirty days)

- The physician's summary and the resident's final diagnosis if the resident is admitted from a healthcare facility

State-specific requirements may include:

- Chief complaint/reason for admission

- History of present illness

- Past pertinent history

- Family history

- Functional assessment

- Review of systems

- Vital signs

- Cognitive assessment

- Specific test results

Timeliness of Documentation

The physician should document as soon as possible after care has been provided on the day of visit. Please refer to individual physician documentation requirements for specific time frames.

Placement of Physician Documentation in the Health Record

Physician documentation is placed in the appropriate sections of the resident's health record as described in each particular subheading of this chapter and as outlined in chapter 13.

Other Pertinent Information

The resident's health record includes the diagnoses that are pertinent for the current episode of care. The diagnoses are derived from and supported by physician documentation. The diagnosis or problem list, if used in facilities, should indicate the diagnoses on admission to the facility. A diagnosis addendum list, cumulative diagnosis list, or problem list can contain those diagnoses that have developed over time during the resident's long-term care stay. These diagnoses should be addressed on the annual history and physical as well. When the pertinent diagnoses are addressed at the annual evaluation, the diagnoses addendum sheet may be archived and a new list started. The diagnoses or problem list should include the date of onset (if known) of the diagnosis, the applicable ICD-9-CM code, and the resolution date.

The diagnosis and diagnosis addendum sheets should be placed at the front of the resident's health record.

Physician documentation to note the diagnoses may include:

- Written progress notes

- Transfer forms

- Hospital documentation such as the discharge summary

- Consultation reports signed by a physician

- Outside services provided by specialty physicians

When more information is required for diagnosis, a physician query process should be completed to provide the supporting documentation. Unlicensed independent practitioners cannot diagnose or determine diagnoses without first discussing the condition with the physician and securing documentation to justify the diagnoses.

The resident's problem list should be reviewed and updated as established by the facility, and any diagnosis that has resolved should be so noted. Documentation to support the resolution of any diagnosis should be noted by the physician and included in the resident's health record.

Progress Notes

Physician progress notes are written at the time of the physician's visit to the resident. The **progress note** is the means to capture the physician's documentation, continuing care needs, and involvement in the resident's medical health status. The notes outline the resident's progress and provide a mechanism for the physician to provide supporting documentation for the resident's diagnosis and care involvement.

The physician progress note is the documentation of the medical treatment and physician objective findings on each resident. It captures the resident's progress over time and indicates what the treating physician was contemplating and planning with each visit. The progress note also provides a mechanism the physician can use to communicate with other clinical staff and ensures that all shifts know what the physician has determined to be the necessary care and treatment interventions for the resident. Moreover, the progress note is evidence that the physician has visited the resident in a consistent manner according to identified regulations and standards.

The physician's progress note captures the medical necessity of the resident's need for care in the facility. It documents the resident's health status at the time of the physician's visit and serves to identify gains and declines throughout the resident's stay at the facility. Additionally, it provides a means for the physician to provide feedback on consultants and clinical staff treatments and interventions. An important part of the documentation process, the progress note establishes the physician's visits, provides a medical opinion, and objective observations concerning the resident's current health status. Further, it provides insight into the effectiveness of the treatment plan and care-planning process. It provides details of gains and acute episodes of illness or chronic decline as well.

The physician visit includes a review of the resident's medical care. The physician reviews medications and treatments and documents the resident's progress. The facility process for the physician visit should be clearly defined to ensure that documents are prepared for the physician to review. This process should outline who is responsible for:

- Tracking physician visits to ensure that physician renewals are prepared for the physician to review and sign

- Preparing physician order (medication and treatment) renewals

- Determining how the physician receives the documents to review and sign

- Determining when documents are prepared for the physician visit

- Deciding who reviews the documents prior to physician signature

- Filing the signed documents

The nurse may have full responsibility for this process, or the process may be the responsibility of a unit secretary or HIM personnel, depending on facility process and job function. The pharmacy may provide computer-generated medication orders, the unit secretary may prepare the treatment orders for the nursing staff to review prior to physician visits, and HIM staff personnel may track physician visits or physician rounds to ensure that the process is complete and that discharged records are signed. It does not matter specifically how the facility process is defined as long as the process succeeds in ensuring the physician visit and the documentation requirement are achieved.

General Requirements

Federal regulations mandate a physician progress note at each visit. The visit in itself cannot be a *superficial visit* but, instead, must include:

- Evaluation of the resident's status

- Review of the care plan and medical management

- Decisions about appropriate care options

- Review of resident's medications and treatment options

The physician's progress notes clinically justify the need for medical treatment, interventions, and care.

Dictated progress notes provide a more legible alternative to handwritten progress notes. However, the physician should note in the resident's health record that the visit note was dictated. If the visit indicates a significant change in the resident's condition, the physician should handwrite a notation in addition to the dictation in the event that transcription of the declaration is delayed. Dictated progress notes should be completed and filed in the resident's record in a timely manner to ensure continuity of care.

The physician is an integral member of the interdisciplinary team caring for the resident and, in fact, must supervise the medical management needs of the resident. The documentation of progress notes by the physician ensures that:

- Resident care needs are managed.

- Communication to clinical staff is expedited.

- Resident progress is captured.

- Resident status is identified.

- Treatment options and interventions are identified.

- Medical recommendations are recorded.

- Plan of care is clarified.

- Physician oversight of the resident is achieved.

- Regulations are complied with.

Documentation Required

The physician must document each visit in a progress note. The progress note must be written, signed, and dated. It should be objective and reflect:

- Continuity of care

- Resident's mental and physical functioning status

- Resident's progress or problems

- Resident's health status

- Risk factors and underlying factors pertaining to clinical conditions, functional decline, deterioration or possibility for, and lack of, improvement, and whether the conditions are preventable

Quality Requirements

State requirements may include specific criteria for physician visits and progress notes. The facility must incorporate these requirements into the physician documentation process. These criteria can easily be added to the audit assessment tools for monitoring of compliance or regulations for documentation. The facility should have a process in place to monitor receipt of transcribed progress notes.

The physician progress note must be written at each visit. The federal regulations do not require physician renewal of orders but do require physician review of orders. States may have more stringent requirements for renewal of orders so it is important to verify any specific state requirements.

The following indicators could be used to monitor physician progress notes:

- Physician visits are timely.

- Physician documents progress note at each visit.

- Notes are objective.

- Notes are dated and signed (facilities may want to add time to this indicator as appropriate to policy).

- Notes are comprehensive and reflect resident's health status.

- Physician reviews orders and medications at each visit.

Dictated progress notes are received and filed in the resident's health record as per policy or within seven days of dictation. "If a physician dictates a progress note, a brief note should be entered into the record at the time of the visit stating that dictation will follow. If there has been an acute change in the resident's condition, the physician should write a note for the medical record in addition to the dictated progress note. The dictated progress note should be received by the facility and filed in the medical record within seven days. The facility should have a monitoring system to assure that dictated notes are received within the appropriate time period" (AHIMA 2001).

Placement of Progress Notes in the Health Record

Physician progress notes are filed in the progress note section of the resident's health record.

Content

The progress note (shown in figure 12.1) may have different formats depending on the facility's choice of documentation requirements, but typically a physician progress note contains the following components:

- Organization name

- Title (progress notes, physician progress notes)

- Resident name

- Health record number

- Date/time column

- Documentation column

- Signature column

History and Physical/Admission History and Physical

There are no federal regulations requiring a **history and physical** (H&P) at any time during the resident's stay in the long-term facility. However, states may have specific requirements for the H&P as well as specific criteria for an admission H&P and annual requirements for the documentation. Moreover, the JCAHO has requirements for resident H&Ps. The healthcare facility should develop policy and procedures concerning the H&P process based on state regulations and applicable accreditation standards.

Figure 12.1.   Sample progress note

XYZ Organization Anywhere USA 00000 **Physician Progress Note** Resident Name:_____ Health Record Number:_____		
Date/Time	**Progress Summary**	**Signature**

History

The H&P is a detailed recording of an individual's health history by the resident's attending or covering physician. The purpose of the resident's health history is to record pertinent historical medication conditions and treatments rendered over time and the history of any present illnesses. The document provides a detailed accounting of the resident's past health status, functioning ability, and medical interventions at admission and on an annual basis.

The resident's health history is recorded by either the attending or covering physician or the physician extender as allowed by law. In addition to providing a full description of the resident's past medical status and a comprehensive look at the resident's health over time, the health history provides supporting documentation for the MDS assessment as well as for coding and billing processes. The health history at admission and annually contains the resident's diagnoses that will be abstracted for treatment, interventions, medical management, care planning, assessments, and reimbursement. It clarifies the resident's health needs, medical necessity for treatment, and justifies the resident's stay at the facility.

General Requirements

The JCAHO requires that the attending physician or licensed independent practitioner complete the medical assessment, including a medical history and physical examination, within required time frames not to exceed twenty-four hours prior to admission or within seventy-two hours after admission. The medical history and physical completed within thirty days prior to admission or readmission is acceptable for inclusion in the resident's health record and may be requested from the attending physician or licensed independent practitioner. However, the physician must write a summary of the resident's health status and condition, include a plan of care, and the current physical and psychosocial status of the resident for the interim period between the original H&P and seventy-two hours after admission or readmission. State regulations may be more stringent on the time frames for completion of the medical H&P.

For JCAHO subacute program accreditation, the medical assessment is completed either thirty days before admission as outlined above or within forty-eight hours after admission.

The physician should date and sign the history and physical. State regulations and facility policy may dictate cosignature requirements if the documentation is completed by a physician extender.

The health history is vital documentation that supplements many processes within the facility. It provides clear, concise details of the resident's health status and identifies medical problems, issues, concerns, and diagnoses that support assessments, care planning, and reimbursement procedures. It is one of the key documents that indicate physician supervision of the resident's care requirements.

Documentation Required

The resident's health history is a detailed form that triggers the physician to identify facts about the resident's past medical needs and care provisions. It may be dictated but must be completed within specific time frames and be available to clinical staff and HIM coders in a timely manner. The document contains key elements that explain the resident's health condition, status, past medical history, family and social history, and other significant findings.

Because the health history supports the resident's medical reimbursement and medical needs, the quality of the report should be monitored. The quality review of the resident's health history also can support the physician credentialing process.

Quality Requirements

In its health record audit tool, the JCAHO has specific criteria that determine the quality of the assessment of the resident's health history. State regulations and facility policy also provide insight into specific quality requirements for this documentation.

Assessment criteria for the resident's health history may contain the following elements:

- Resident admission history is completed in the required time frames.

- Documentation contains the date and signature and credentials of the professional completing the history.

- Documentation contains the cosignature of the attending physician if the history is documented by a physician extender as required by law or policy.

- Documentation contains all the key elements required by regulation or facility policy (all areas of the form as addressed).

- Handwritten history documentation is legible.

- Annual history is completed as required.

Placement of Documents in the Health Record

The resident's admission or subsequent health history assessments are filed in the designated section of the health record.

Content

The resident's health history (shown in figure 12. 2) may contain the following information:

- Resident's name and health record number

- Resident's age and sex

- Date of assessment

- Name of attending physician

- Allergies

- Diagnosis

- Reason for admission

- History of the present illness

- Past medical and surgical history

- Pertinent family history

- Social history

- ETOH/smoking history

- Diet

- Medications

- Functional status

Figure 12. 2.   Sample history and physical form

XXX Organization
Anytown USA 00000

History and Physical

Resident Name: _____ Health Record Number: _____

Date of Report:_____ Age: _____ Sex: _____ Nursing Stations/Unit: _____

Admission Date:_____ Attending Physician:_____

Reason for Admission: _____

Allergies: _____ PPD Screens:_____

Diagnoses:

History of the present illness:

Past medical and surgical history:

Pertinent family history:

Social history/ETOH/smoking history:

Diet:

Medications:

Functional status:

Review of systems:

Code status as appropriate:

Pertinent laboratory findings:

Impression/plan:

_____   _____
Physician extender's signature and credentials   Date

_____   _____
Physician's signature and credentials   Date

- Review of systems

- Code status, as appropriate

- PPD screens

- Pertinent laboratory findings

- Impression/plan

- Physician extender's signature, date, and credentials (if completing the assessment)

- Physician signature, date, and credentials

Physical Examinations

The physician or physician extender, as allowed by law, completes a physical examination of the resident at the time of the history intake. Usually, the H&P examination is included in one form to simplify the physician documentation process.

The resident's physical examination is a comprehensive review of current health status and functioning ability. The health history captures the resident's past medical requirements; the physical examination provides the assessment of the resident's current health status.

General Requirements

The physical examination provides supporting documentation for the MDS assessment and care-planning process and helps clarify possible areas for interventions, treatments, and services.

General Description/Importance of the Process

The physical examination documentation identifies the following:

- Physician involvement in care

- Current physical status and function

- Possible interventions and treatments

- Deficits and strengths of the resident

- Baseline assessment at admission and ongoing assessment annually

The physical examination is usually the second half of the history assessment or intake. It is similar in format to the history in that it provides triggers or predefined headers for the physician to complete a thorough examination of the resident.

The time frames for the physical examination are as those required for the health history.

Quality Requirements

The physical examination must be comprehensive and thorough to ensure that the assessment and care planning are supported and that medical management of the resident is accurately documented.

The state may require specific components for the physical examination. The JCAHO requires that the H&P be completed according to established time frames as required by facility policy or regulation.

Physical assessment criteria may contain the following:

- Physical examination is comprehensive.

- Physical examination is completed in a timely manner.

- Weight is documented.

- Physical examination includes all components required by regulation and facility policy.

- Physical examination is legible.

Placement of Documents in the Health Record

The documentation of the physical examination is filed in a designated section of the resident's health record.

Content

The content of the physical examination (shown in figure 12.3) may contain the following:

- General
  —Skin
  —Weight
  —Height
  —Vital signs
- Cognitive/mental status
- Head, ears, eyes, nose, throat
- Oral/dental
- Chest
- Breasts
- Heart
- Pulmonary
- Abdomen
- Musculoskeletal
- Neurological
- Pelvic/rectum examination
- Safety issues
- Genitourinary
- Physician extender signature, date, and credentials (if completing the physical examination)
- Physician signature, date, and credentials

Figure 12.3.   Sample physical examination form

XXX Organization
Anytown USA 00000

Physical Examination

General:

Skin:

Weight: _____   Height: _____

Vital signs: Temp _____   Pulse _____   Respirations _____   Blood Pressure _____

Cognitive/mental status:

Head, ears, eyes, nose, throat:

Oral/dental:

Chest:

Breasts:

Heart:

Pulmonary:

Abdomen:

Musculoskeletal:

Neurological:

Pelvic/rectum examination:

Safety issues:

Genitourinary:

_____   _____
Physician extender's signature and credentials   Date

_____   _____
Physician's signature and credentials   Date

Consultation Records

There may be times when the resident requires a consultation by a specialist. The resident's health record will indicate documentation of the consultation with specific recommendations. The specialist also may document in the progress notes to indicate that the consultation is complete. When the resident has to travel outside the facility for consultative services, the following may occur:

- The facility may send its own form for the physician to document on.

- The physician may use a progress note for documentation of the service.

- The physician may have a specialized form or format for documentation of the services.

A consultation is a comprehensive assessment requested by the attending or covering physician to examine a specific body system or identified problem or concern, such as pulmonary, cardiology, genitourinary, or gastrointestinal issues, and so forth. The purpose of the consultation is to provide a focused review of a resident's identified problems or concerns that require consideration for further treatment options, medical interventions, and impressions to complete the resident's care requirements.

A consultation with a specialist is done at the request of the attending or covering physician to further investigate medical issues when the need for a specialist is determined. The request for and completion of the consultation clearly demonstrates physician supervision of the resident's medical needs.

General Requirements

The consultation must be ordered by the physician and, upon completion, must be filed in the resident's health record. No federal requirements specify that consultations are required; however, as identified earlier in this chapter, the physician must oversee the resident's medical care and the consultation provides further supporting documentation of his or her oversight or supervision. State and facility policy may require more specific requirements for a physician consultation.

Consultant or specialist physician orders should be reviewed with the attending physician before being executed except when the attending physician has indicated through an order that the consultant's recommendations are to be implemented.

The consultation provides a physician assessment of specific problems that require further in-depth study and investigation to ensure that the resident's well-being is achieved. The specialist involved provides detailed recommendations to help resolve any problems or issues. Documentation of the consult broadens the assessment, care planning, and treatment options for the resident. The consultation is a communication tool among specialist, attending or covering physician or physician extender, and interdisciplinary team to ensure that the resident receives the best possible care.

The consultation should be done as soon as possible for any emergency situations, but for routine consultations, guidelines suggest that the consultation be completed within fourteen days of the request. Specific requirements of state regulations and facility policy may indicate different time frames for its completion.

The consultation must be written and filed in the resident's health record as supporting documentation of the resident's medical care. The format may differ from facility to facility and may even be documented in the progress note section of the record. The consultation should address the problem(s) identified, provide a focused health history, and offer recommendations and impressions or a plan for continued treatment or follow-up. Finally, it must be dated and signed by the examining physician.

Quality Requirements

Quality concerns for consultation documentation are similar to other required physician documentation. The consultation should address the resident's problem in a timely manner and provide a plan of action to assist the attending or covering physician with medical interventions and recommendations for care planning.

The following criteria can be used to monitor the completeness of the consultation:

- Consult is completed in a timely manner.
- Consult addresses the problem.
- Consult includes a focused health history and pertinent medical information.
- Consult is legible.
- Consult provides an impression or plan of action.

Placement of Documents in the Health Record

The consultation may be placed in the specific specialty consult section, with a generic consultations section, or in another designated section of the record depending on facility policy. If the specialist has written the consultation in the progress notes of the resident's record, it is acceptable to file it in the progress note section. However, care should be taken when thinning the resident's record to ensure that the consult is easily retrievable for clinical staff to refer to as needed.

Other Pertinent Information

Specialists who may provide consultations are limited only by the medical specialty or sub-specialty, but the most often requested consultative specialists are:

- Podiatry
- Dental
- Optometry
- Audiology
- Radiology
- Other specialists, such as:
  —Internists
  —Surgeons
  —Cardiologists
  —Orthopedists
  —Pulmonologists

Content

The consultation form (shown in figure 12.4) should include the following information:

- Resident's name and health record number
- Problem
- Specialist requested
- Date of request
- Health history
- Examination
- Findings/impression
- Recommendations/plan
- Signature of the specialist and credentials
- Date of consult

Figure 12.4.   Sample consult form

XXX Organization
Anytown USA 00000

Consultation Report

Resident Name: _____ Health Record Number: _____

Ordering Physician: _____ Date: _____

Specialty/Physician Requested: _____

Problem: _____

History/pertinent medical information:

Examination:

Findings/impression:

Recommendations/plan:

_____   _____
Physician Signature   Date

Documentation by Nurse Practitioners, Advanced Practice Registered Nurses, and Physician Assistants

Nurse practitioners (NPs), **advanced practice registered nurses** (APRNs), and **physician assistants** (PAs) are used as physician extenders. Federal regulations allow physician extenders to visit the resident in place of the physician where state laws allow their use. They may do so at every other mandated physician visit after the first physician visit in a skilled nursing home. In a nursing facility, a physician extender may fulfill the physician visit requirement if state law allows.

State-specific regulations may dictate the criteria for physician extender services and documentation requirements. Physician extenders must follow all requirements for the progress note as defined in the progress note section of this chapter. A countersignature by the attending physician is not required by federal law; however, many states specify when countersignatures are needed.

"Nurse practitioner is a registered nurse now licensed to practice in the state and who meets the state's requirement governing the qualifications of nurse practitioners. Clinical nurse specialist is a registered professional nurse currently in practice in the state who meets the state's requirements governing the qualifications of clinical nurse specialist. Physician assistant is a person who meets the applicable state requirements governing the qualifications for assistants to the physician" (CMS 2001, PP-154).

The purpose of the physician extenders is to provide a means to provide care to the resident in the event a physician is unavailable. These professionals "extend" the services of the physician to ensure continuity of care as issues or concerns arise in the long-term care setting and the physician cannot be present.

Basically, physician extender documentation requirements mimic physician documentation standards. The HIM professional and facility may follow guidelines for physician reports and progress notes when considering physician extender documentation practices. The only difference may be the countersignature requirements as specified by state and facility policy.

The facility should have a detailed policy outlining the use of physician extenders. It should address the following areas:

- Routine duties

- Nonroutine/emergency duties

- Emergency care

- Collaboration of physician requirements

- Cosignature requirements

- Prescriptive authority

- Quality assurance requirements for the credentialing process

- Coverage requirements for physician in the absence of the physician extender

- Notification of the physician extender practice to the resident and the resident's family or responsible party

- Physician extender expectations for quality of care

- Polypharmacy monitoring
- Scope of practice: Diagnostic and therapeutic procedures the physician extender may order
- Guidelines outlining required consultation with collaborating physician prior to ordering
- Listing of allowable pharmaceutical agents with no consultation requirements
- Listing of pharmaceutical agents that require physician consultation prior to ordering

General Requirements

States provide more specific general requirements for physician extenders.

The physician extender provides a mechanism to ensure that residents have medical oversight in the long-term care setting. He or she works closely with the attending or covering physician to ensure that the resident receives the care needed to maintain or improve functional ability and health status in a timely fashion. The physical extender is usually more accessible to the long-term care staff than is the physician.

These requirements would be driven by physician requirements of documentation.

Quality Requirements

The quality criteria are similar to physician documentation requirements. The criteria for monitoring countersignatures would be added to the physician quality monitors as indicated.

Additional assessment criteria over and above the physician requirements may include:

- Physician consultations are documented as required by medication orders guidelines.
- Physician consultations are documented as required by treatment orders guidelines.

Placement of Documentation in the Health Record

Physician extender documentation is placed in the resident's health record as required for the physician documentation standards.

Content

The content of physician extender documentation would be the same as required for physician documentation.

Summary

Federal requirements make it clear that the physician has medical oversight of the resident's total care. The facility medical staff bylaws provide the foundation for provision of medical services in the facility.

The physician who knows the resident must recommend his or her admission to the long-term care facility and oversee all medical care provided. Documentation stands as the evidence that the physician has oversight of the resident's assessments, care planning, and consultation services, and is knowledgeable about the resident's current health status. The physician's involvement in the interdisciplinary team approach to long-term care must be demonstrated in the resident's health record.

The physician is required to review the total plan of care, including medications and treatments, at each visit to the resident. Each physician visit must be a "face-to-face" visit. Physician documentation discussed in this chapter consists of progress notes, health history, physical examination, and consultations.

If the state allows the use of physician extenders, the physician and facility may utilize their services as outlined in federal and state laws. Documentation standards are similar for the physician extenders. States may provide specific principles and criteria for the documentation practices of physician extenders.

References

American Health Information Management Association. 2001. Long-Term Care Health Information Practice and Documentation Guidelines. Available at www.ahima.org.

Centers for Medicare and Medicaid Services. 2001 (October 31). Guidance to Surveyors—Long-Term Care Facilities, appendix PP in *State Operations Manual*. Available at www.cms.gov.

Joint Commission on Accreditation of Healthcare Organizations. 2004. *Comprehensive Accreditation Manual for Long-term Care*. Oakbrook Terrace, Ill.: JCAHO.

Chapter 13

Physician Orders

The facility must obtain physician orders for each resident's specific needs and provide care and service based on them. (See figure 13.1.) All orders for resident care are obtained from the physician or other authorized individuals as outlined by law, regulation, and professional practice standards before administering care. Physician orders may be verbal or written and may include medication orders. The order must be specific to the resident's needs and must comply with law and regulation (JCAHO 2004, PC-19).

Definitions

A physician order is an instruction or set of instructions that dictates the resident's medical requirements. The orders indicate medications, treatments, services, tests, equipment needed, consultation required, instructions, code status, interventions, and/or nutritional needs to direct the care of the resident.

"Physician orders for immediate care are those written orders facility staff need to provide essential care to the resident, consistent with the resident's mental and physical status upon admission" (CMS 2001, PP-68).

The purpose of physician orders is to direct the medical care of the resident and ensure that the physician has oversight of the resident's medical needs and requirements. The orders provide the medications, nutrition, and routine care that will maintain or improve the resident's functional abilities.

The physician must provide orders on admission to the long-term care facility and as needed to ensure that the resident's care needs and requirements are met. He or she then may stipulate orders at any time during the resident's long-term stay.

All orders are renewed or updated to reflect:

- Changes in the resident's care or needs

- Changes in the resident's health status

- The resident's response to treatment

- The resident's outcomes

- Changes in prognosis, diagnosis, or interventions

- Time frame of review

- Applicable law and regulation

Figure 13.1.   Sample physician order

XXX Organization Anytown USA 00000				
Resident name: _____ Health record number: _____				
Physician Order Sheet				

	Medication	Dose	Frequency No. of Days	Route	
1	T.O. Dr. Healy/B. Careful RN				
2	9/23/2002 at 2:00 a.m.				Medication order
3	Tylenol 650 mg by mouth every 4 hours as needed for pain				
4	B. Careful, RN 9/23/2002				
5					
6	**9/24/2002 Evaluation for physical therapy** *Dr. Healy*				Treatment order
8	**Dressing changes wet to dry 3 times a day**				

Unit & Rm# 1234	Date	Time	Allergic to: NKA	Doctor	

The physician order also indicates the physician's involvement in the interdisciplinary team's care of the resident and signifies physician oversight or supervision and an active role in the resident's care planning.

General Requirements

"At the time each resident is admitted, the facility must have physician orders for the resident's immediate care" (CMS 2001, PP-68). The physician must sign and date all orders. He or she may use a rubber stamp to indicate signature of orders; however, the facility must have a signed statement on file that indicates that the physician with the rubber stamp is the only one who has the stamp and uses it. If the physician uses electronic means to sign computerized orders, a listing of the computer codes and written signatures must be kept available and safeguarded.

For any order or order set discussed in this chapter, the following applies:

- Any existing physician order that is changed would require that the previous order be discontinued and the new order implemented.

- Any physician order that is discontinued must be removed from the resident's care regime.

The Joint Commission on Accreditation of Healthcare Organizations (JCAHO) requires the following:

- PC standards

  —"The attending physician prescribes the medical requirements of care for the residents he or she admits.

    1. Orders, which may be verbal or written, are obtained from the physician or other authorized individuals according to law and regulation and professional practice acts before providing care, treatment, and services.

2. The order is tailored to each resident's needs and includes all elements required by law.

3. All orders are renewed or updated to reflect the following:

   –Changes in care, treatment, or services provided

   –Changes in the resident's physical or psychosocial condition

   –The resident's response to care, treatment, or services

   –The resident's outcome related to care, treatment, or services

   –Changes in diagnosis, treatment, and equipment

   –The minimum review time frame defined by the organization

   –Applicable law and regulation

The organization provides care, treatment, and services according to the most recent order" (JCAHO 2004, PC.5.30).

Physician Oversight of the Resident's Care

The physician must oversee the resident's total plan of care. This is done through participation in the resident's assessments and care planning, reviewing the resident's medical status and providing consultation or treatment or providing orders for such as needed. The attending physician must designate an alternate physician for times when he or she is unavailable. The physician also may delegate and supervise a physician extender to write orders as outlined by federal, state, or accrediting body guidelines.

Physician orders are contained on the physician order sheet. Some facilities may separate medication orders and treatment orders as defined by facility policy and pharmacy practice. The medication form is usually an NCR form, thereby producing multiple copies with the original being retained for the health record.

Written orders are documented at the time of the physician's visit. Verbal orders or telephone orders are documented in the resident's health record at the time of the discussion with the physician with the physician's signature at the physician's next visit or within a time frame required by state law. State regulations determine the timeliness of physician renewal of orders, so the state-specific requirements should be consulted.

Quality Requirements

Legibility is of concern when the physician orders are handwritten. Accuracy and completeness of the order and inappropriate use of abbreviations also may be of concern. Using abbreviations that have been determined to be confusing is a major focus for resident safety. The patient safety issues associated with hospital stays should be reviewed by the long-term care facility, and problematic abbreviations should be eliminated. The Institute of Safe Medical Practice provided a thorough chart in an article describing problematic abbreviations in hospitals (Institute of Safe Medical Practice 2001). The article also provides the long-term care facility with reference material to begin looking at appropriate abbreviations within the organization. The grid of abbreviations included in the article is available in appendix C.

The noting of orders by nursing staff also includes quality issues. Missed orders or orders that contain transcription errors are of concern to the facility as well. The facility should have a policy and procedure as well as a process in place that provides mechanisms to ensure that as few mistakes as possible occur. Both nursing and pharmacy staff must be educated on the noting and transcription of all orders to minimize opportunities for error. The long-term care facility should examine these practices to determine whether there are problem areas that can be improved.

The federal regulation requires that all physician orders be signed and dated. However, the facility may develop specific indicators for physician orders based on organizational policy and procedure or state requirements.

Physician order criteria could include:

- The physician orders all tests and medical requirements.

- Pertinent clinical information is provided when ordering tests, medications, and treatment.

- Physician orders are used to develop the interim care plan for the resident.

- The physician orders food and nutrition needs prior to food being provided.

- Verbal orders for food and nutrition are accepted by appropriate staff per facility policy.

- The physician provides the order for transfer (or discharge).

- Physician orders are timed.

- Medication orders are timed.

- Appropriate abbreviations are used when writing the order.

- Orders are legible.

- Physician extender orders are cosigned as defined by state requirements and facility policy and procedures or bylaws.

- Orders contain specific indications and are complete.

- Orders are renewed as required by regulation and facility policy and procedure.

- All orders are noted by nursing as defined by facility policy and procedure.

- Orders are flagged according to facility policy and procedure.

- Transcription of orders is accurate.

- Verbal/telephone orders are signed appropriately and within the required time frame.

Placement of Documentation in the Health Record

When contained in one format, physician orders are typically filed in the physician order section of the resident's health record. Those facilities that decide to separate medication orders and treatment orders on two separate forms may file them in one section. However, other facilities may decide that when medication orders and treatment orders are written on two distinct forms, the medication orders may be filed in the medication or pharmacy section of the resident's health record and the treatment orders may be filed in the treatment order section. They are filed according to facility policy, in either chronological or reverse chronological order.

Other Pertinent Information

The **interagency transfer form (W-10),** which is sent to the long-term care facility by the referring institution or physician, can be considered a valid set of physician orders for a time period defined by state regulations and facility policy when signed by the attending physician. After the physician has provided written orders at the time of the first visit on admission or readmission as required, the orders on the interagency transfer form are discontinued.

Content of the Order

The content of the order should be accurate and complete. It should reflect the medication and treatment needed, including the reason or diagnosis that justifies the need for the order.

Federal regulations require that the physician provide written, dated, and signed admission orders. State-specific requirements may exist for physician ordering practice and should be incorporated into the facility process for obtaining physician orders. These orders must include diet, drugs (if needed), and routine care to maintain or improve the resident's functional ability.

Incomplete, illegible orders may cause major problems for the long-term facility. Complete, legible orders are imperative for the organization. Medication errors, improper transcription, and extra time spent contacting the physician for clarification are key problems that could develop as a result of improper physician ordering practice.

Medication orders must contain:

- Resident's name and health record number
- Medication
- Diagnoses and reason for medication
- Dose/strength
- Frequency
- Route
- Stop date for certain drugs such as antibiotics
- Parenteral and enteral orders, including fluid amount, flow rate, pump/gravity/bolus use, and stop date
- Date of the order
- Time of the order
- Physician signature and credentials

Treatment orders typically include:

- Resident's name and health record number
- Date of the order
- Treatment ordered
- Reason for the treatment and specific details, if needed
- Date treatment is required
- Date and signature of the ordering physician with credentials

Quality Requirements

Any missing part of the order content can lead to error, miscommunication, and decreased resident outcomes. Clarifying orders can be time-consuming and frustrating for staff and physicians and does interfere with meeting the resident's care requirements. The facility should have a detailed policy and procedure for documentation of physician orders and subsequent transcription and administration processes to ensure that the quality of the resident's care and documentation are consistent. Clinical indications should be included in all orders to help determine need and facilitate interpretation of test results.

The timing and dating of physician orders are extremely important aspects of the physician ordering process. The date defines the exact day of the order, and the time indicates the precise moment the order was documented. These may be important in solving problems related to transcription and medication administration and discontinued, changed, or missed dosages of medications. Faxed orders can be placed in the record in date and time sequence if all orders are dated and timed. Dating and timing all orders will alleviate confusion in situations where faxed orders contradict existing orders or are meant to clarify existing orders.

Criteria for monitoring the content of orders would contain the listing that is included earlier in this chapter. The specific content such as dose, route, frequency, and appropriate abbreviations and legibility should be included as well as clinical indication for the medication, treatment, or test.

Appropriate Abbreviations

As discussed in the previous section on physician orders, proper abbreviations have become a focus for the patient/resident initiative. The following common abbreviations once used for writing orders are no longer considered appropriate according to the Institute of Safe Medical Practice. Long-term care facilities should be made aware of these recommendations because there is a concern in the healthcare sector as to their use. Moreover, the JCAHO is beginning to look at inappropriate abbreviations. These are shown here as a demonstration of current trends in patient safety. It is up to the facility to decide whether it wants to limit the use of these abbreviations. Many are very common throughout the continuum of care.

o.d., or OD	once daily
TIW, or tiw	three times a week
q.d., or QD	every day
qn	nightly or at bedtime
qhs	nightly at bedtime
q6PM, etc.	every evening at 6 PM
q.o.d., or QOD	every other day
U, or u	unit
IU	international unit
x3d	for three days

Some facilities are moving away from approved abbreviation policies and procedures toward providing policies on unacceptable abbreviations to ensure resident safety and quality outcomes. (Appendix C contains an additional list of questionable abbreviations.)

Physician Order Recaps/Renewals

Physician order recaps or renewals are those orders that the resident needs on an going basis to ensure functionality and maintain or improve outcomes. This category of orders includes those state-specific regulations for physician recap or renewal requirements. States may require renewal every thirty to sixty days as outlined in the state public health codes.

Physician recaps or renewals are the reorder of existing resident-required treatments and medications to ensure that resident needs are met. This periodic renewal, driven by state-specific requirements, provides a mechanism for the physician to review and eliminate, change, or discontinue unnecessary or ineffective medications and treatments.

The intent of the renewal of physician orders is to ensure the resident's medical management.

The renewal of physician orders is important to ensure that the overall treatment program and care planning, including medications, are reviewed on a periodic basis. Without this periodic review, usually every thirty to sixty days, the resident would simply continue to receive orders that may no longer be effective or needed.

There are no federal requirements for the renewal of physician orders; federal regulations call only for review of existing orders. When the physician has signed the order renewals, no changes or updates can be made to the signed document. Any changes or additions must come expressly from the physician and can be in the form of a fax, telephone, or handwritten order.

The physician renewal process provides a methodology for continually providing medical management and supervision of each resident within the facility. This process ensures that the physician is a valuable member of the interdisciplinary team actively involved in the resident's care needs and medical management.

State-specific regulations and individual facility policy drive the documentation required for order renewals. However, the same forms and content should be exactly as described in the physician order section of this chapter.

Quality Requirements

These are consistent with the physician orders as described earlier.

Policies and Procedures for Physician Order Expectations

Each facility must develop policies and procedures on physician renewal or orders consistent with state regulations. The process for physician renewal of orders should be detailed to ensure that compliance with the requirements is met. The person or persons responsible for the process should be included in this policy and procedure as well.

Telephone Orders

Telephone orders are physician orders taken over the telephone by authorized clinical staff. Telephone orders are used in situations that may arise in resident care as well. The physician must be contacted prior to writing a telephone order. The order must come from the physician or his or her appointed alternate to ensure the resident's medical management at all times.

The purpose of the telephone order is to ensure continuity of care for each resident. The physician is typically not available to the long-term care setting, and the telephone order allows the physician to meet the resident's changing needs in a timely manner. Although state and federal regulations require that physicians visit and establish face-to-face contact with residents during those visits, the resident may develop health problems or issues and concerns between scheduled visits. The licensed professional staff, as designated by state and facility policy, can provide ongoing medical care to the resident through the use of the telephone order.

The telephone order is a valuable means of ensuring the continuity of care for all residents. The facility should have specific policies and procedures that outline use of the telephone order. It also is important to educate professional staff members on the facility policy and the specific requirements for documenting the telephone order.

General Requirements for Telephone Orders

There are no federal requirements specifically for telephone orders, but physician requirements remain the same as with any order. Federal regulations do call for the availability of physician services twenty-four hours a day in case of emergency. Remember that federal regulations require that all physician orders be dated and signed, so there must be a mechanism in place to have the physician countersign the order. State regulations may define a specific time frame for countersignatures. The telephone order does not take the place of the face-to-face visit requirements spelled out in federal and state regulations.

The telephone order should be written out as soon after receipt as possible to ensure that each component of the order is complete and accurate. It allows the facility some flexibility in providing continuity of care and ensuring that the physician provides and oversees the resident's medical management. Should physician medical services be required when the physician is not scheduled for a face-to-face visit, use of the telephone order provides an easy way to quickly meet resident needs. Use of the telephone order in emergency situations is important because federal regulations do require that a physician be available twenty-four hours a day in the event of emergency situations.

Telephone Order Policy and Procedure

The facility should have a specific policy that outlines use of the telephone order to include:

- Who is authorized to take the order

- How the order is written

- Content of the order

- Time frames for countersignature by the physician

This policy should be based on state-specific requirements, as appropriate.

The documentation required should be spelled out in facility policy. The order will be written in the appropriate section of the record and countersigned as specified.

Quality Requirements

The telephone order can create some unique quality concerns because it is not directly written by the physician. The third party who documents the order must pay close attention to the detail of the transcription of the order not only into the resident's health record, but also into the resident medication or treatment record.

The documentation, or that understanding, of the order is an extremely important step in the process, and the order taken must be written accurately and reflect exactly what the physician ordered. Misunderstanding must be clarified before the order is documented and should be done while talking to the physician on the phone at the time of the request.

The telephone order must contain all the elements of a physician order. It also must contain the name of the person who has taken the order and his or her credentials. Additionally, it should specify the exact time of the order.

The physician must countersign the order in a time frame that is outlined in facility policy. Assessment criteria for the order may contain the following:

- Only qualified professionals take telephone orders.

- Order is timed and dated.

- Person taking the order dates and signs it.

- Order is complete.

- Physician time frames for countersignature are met.

Faxed Orders

The faxed order is an order the physician has sent to the facility via a facsimile machine. Some states do not require that the physician see the resident on a monthly or sixty-day basis; instead, visits are allowed at greater than monthly or sixty-day intervals. However, there are still requirements that the monthly renewal of therapy orders occur. This inconsistency has required facilities to develop alternate methods of obtaining renewal of therapy orders.

Faxing orders also may occur when verbal orders need the physician's signature. Although the physician should sign all telephone orders at the time of the next visit, sometimes an order is overlooked. To ensure compliance with facility policy, the health record department may fax a telephone order to the physician to obtain the necessary signature.

A valid faxed order is any physician order that has been received by fax machine and contains all the elements of a physician order for treatment or medication, if needed. Therefore, it must be signed and dated and should meet the standard for a physician order as outlined in the physician order section of this chapter.

The purpose of the faxed order is to ensure continuity of care. The physician can fax the needed treatments and medication orders form to the facility to allow treatments to start, continue, or be discontinued in a timely manner.

The facility should have a facsimile policy and procedures in place to ensure that the faxing of orders is not abused. The policy should also provide guidelines and checks and balances to ensure that resident identifiable information is protected form unnecessary release. The American Health Information Management Association (AHIMA) provides excellent guidelines for establishing a faxing policy, which includes the guidelines for a fax cover sheet and misdirected fax. (Visit www.ahima.org.)

Physician orders may be faxed to the facility when the following criteria are met:

- Physician orders are signed and kept as an original copy of the order, and the physician can produce the order on request.

- The faxed order should be photocopied to eliminate fading of the copy over time if thermal paper is used to receive the fax.

- Safeguards are in place to eliminate abuse.

- Resigning of the facsimile is not necessary.

- A cover sheet with a confidentiality statement is always used.

- The fax machine is located in a secure location where the public cannot read the content of the fax records

Faxing physician orders can ensure that necessary therapy services continue uninterrupted to meet the resident's needs. It would not be beneficial to the resident to have therapy service interrupted, which could lead to a decline in function.

Documentation Required for Faxed Orders

The faxed physician order must meet federal, state, and accreditation agency rules and requirements. It does not need to be resigned by the physician at the next visit.

The faxed order should be signed and returned on the date of the fax from the facility if the order is generated at the facility site. It should be filed immediately in the resident's health record to ensure that it is placed in proper sequence.

When the fax is generated by the physician's office in response to a telephone call from the clinical staff, the order should be sent as soon as possible and the fax filed immediately after receipt.

Quality Requirements for Faxed Orders

Overuse of fax technology is of concern. The physician should visit the resident face-to-face to establish care requirements. When use of the fax machine becomes excessive, medical management cannot be ensured.

Quality requirements may be established through state regulation or facility policy and procedure and may differ from facility to facility.

Does there appear to be excessive faxing of physician orders? This is easy to monitor because the chart will contain more faxed orders than handwritten ones. Facilities also should include the monitors established for physician orders to check for completeness as well as date and signature requirements.

Placement of Documentation in the Health Record

Faxed orders are placed in the appropriate section of the resident's record as defined by facility policy.

Standing Order Policies

A standing order allows the facility to provide care to residents as a facility standard of care. Standing orders should be used with discretion; in fact, some states do not allow their use at all.

At the time of resident readmission, some facilities may support use of "resume all previous orders" as a standing order set. The attending or covering physician should be contacted prior to the resuming of all previous orders because the resident's condition may have changed and orders may require adjustment. Remember that the physician must oversee the medical management of the resident at all times, and "resume all previous orders" may not be appropriate. Indeed, some states may not allow use of "resume all previous orders."

A standing order is an order or order set that has been determined by the facility to be required in certain circumstances for high-quality resident care. Its intent is to ensure that the resident receives high-quality care in situations when the physician may be unable to provide written orders or when care is of the essence and established protocols define the necessary steps required for specific testing or procedures. The practice allows use of specified protocols to help provide further treatment instructions.

To help the long-term care facility understand the standing order usage, these orders are used in some acute care facilities to ensure that protocols are followed to the letter. Standing order sets for specific tests are generated and placed in the patient's record and later signed by the physician. The order for the specific test that has a clarifying protocol triggers the specific standing order set. Therefore, standing orders may not typically be used in long-term care, although there may be times of an "outbreak" where immediate steps may need to be taken to ensure that all residents receive necessary care and that each resident's health status is protected. If the facility utilizes standing orders, there must be a policy and procedure in place detailing its use and the process by which and for which it is implemented. The policy must be followed when the defined criteria within the policy have been met.

General Requirements for Standing Orders

Facility policy will dictate the use of standing orders. The facility policy for the standing order is extremely important to help clarify and detail the what, when, why, and how of the standing order. Clinical staff must be educated on its use and importance and which residents it affects. When used, the standing order is a legal order that affects the resident's care and treatment. Documentation must support its use and effects on the resident when it is implemented.

When the standing order has been determined to be necessary, it should be documented at the time of implementation.

Placement of Documentation in the Health Record

Placement of the standing order in the health record depends on the type of order and the facility's policy governing placement of orders in the resident's health record.

Other Pertinent Information

Standing orders should be used at a minimum and with great prudence. Prescription, or legend, drugs should never be placed in a standing order set. The policy outlining the use of standing orders must include notification of the attending or covering physician. It is important to keep in mind that specific states may not allow use of a standing order.

There are no federal requirements for the use of standing orders or standing order policies.

Content of the Standing Order

The content of a standing order depends on the order itself. The protocol that may be used to establish specific standing orders must be approved by medical staff and based on acceptable clinical practices for the procedure or test. At a minimum, it should contain all the elements of a physician order and specific procedure or test preparation requirements, as appropriate.

Authentication

Authentication is the signature at the end of the order or entry in the resident's health record. It certifies that the person who completed the order or entry is who he or she says, much like the certification authority in the electronic world. The authentication is the unique identifier of the author of the order.

The signature provides proof that the physician is involved in the care of the resident and has the medical oversight of that resident's care. The physician's signature also demonstrates compliance with federal, state, and regulatory standards, regulations, and guidelines.

General Requirements for Authentication

Federal regulations require that the attending physician sign all physician orders that apply to a particular resident. The signature should include the first initial, last name, and title or credential of the author. The specific requirements for each facility should be outlined in policy, and the policy should be followed. In the event that two individuals have the same first initial and last name, the full name of each would be used to authenticate the document.

The physician's signature demonstrates the legal determination of the author. When signed, the individual signing the document cannot dispute its authenticity. Every physician order must contain a signature as outlined by facility policy and federal and state requirements. Entries in the resident health record should never be signed by anyone other than the author.

Each physician order should be signed at the time of the writing of the order. If the order needs countersignatures such as telephone orders or physician extender orders, the facility policy outlining time frames for procurement of physician signatures should be followed.

Every physician order must have the signature of the attending or covering physician unless specified in facility policy that it is not required, such as physician extender orders.

Quality Requirements for Authentication

The facility should have a policy that outlines the capture of the physician's signature requirement. Health record staff members should monitor countersignatures to ensure that the process is completed according to policy.

Transcription of the Physician Order

The transcription of physician orders takes the order from the resident's health record and places it on the correct form to allow its implementation. The facility defines the process to ensure that each physician order is carried out. It would be time-consuming to leaf though the entire section of physician orders to check orders and determine whether they have been continued or discontinued each time the order had to be carried out. The clinical professional stipulated in facility policy transcribes each order to an appropriate form or format to ensure that the resident receives each specific prescribed order.

Transcription is the act or process of making a written copy of an existing order. Transcription of orders should occur as soon after they are written as possible to ensure that they are implemented for the resident in a timely manner.

The purpose of transcription is to ensure that the order is addressed and implemented. When the physician writes an order, it is placed in the appropriate section of the resident's health record. It would be impossible to have to search for each order in this section every time it had to be provided to the resident. Therefore, the clinical staff develops a process as defined in the facility policy to copy each order to a specific form. This transcription process places all orders in a centralized location per order type to ensure that each is addressed and implemented.

Facility policy defines the transcription process and specifies who is responsible for order transcription. Physician orders may be transcribed to different locations, depending on order type, for ease in implementation of the order. For instance, all medication orders are transcribed to a medication administration record (MAR) or medication Kardex. The physician treatment orders for nonmedications may be placed in a treatment record or directly to the resident's care plan, which centralizes all physician treatment orders and provides a mechanism to ensure that all treatment orders are implemented.

Requests for therapies may be transcribed to a therapy request form, whereas laboratory or X-ray orders are copied to department-specific requisitions for delivery to the ancillary service provider. Usually these orders also are placed on the resident's treatment record to ensure their tracking and completion. This may be particularly true if the order is a recurring order such as a PT and PTT order requesting tests every other day for the monitoring of anticoagulant drug therapy.

General Requirements for Transcription

A check-and-balance system usually is incorporated into the medication order transcription process. When the time comes for medication renewal processing, two nurses or a nurse and pharmacist typically check the medication orders for accuracy.

State-specific regulations may define who would be allowed to transcribe physician orders. A unit secretary or unit coordinator may transcribe them, but a nurse is usually responsible for the accuracy of the transcribed order. If the facility uses unit secretaries to transcribe orders, the process for checking the unit secretary transcription should be outlined.

Depending on facility policy, the documentation format for order transcription differs among facilities. Regardless of the format used, the order must be transcribed accurately and completely. Transcription accuracy eliminates errors in providing care.

Transcription Policy and Procedure

Facility policy may dictate that the transcription of the order would be documented on the order itself. (See figure 13.2.) The person transcribing the order would add the following to the order at the time of transcription:

- "Noted" or "transcribed"

- Date and may include time

- Signature or initials as defined in policy

- Credentials

Quality Requirements for Transcription

The quality concerns inherent in the transcription process focus on the accuracy of the transcription, the capture of each and every physician order, and the accuracy of the transcription process.

Figure 13.2.   Sample transcribed physician order

	XXX Organization Anytown USA 00000				
	Resident name: _____ Health record number: _____				
	Physician Order Sheet				
	Medication	**Dose**	**Frequency No. of Days**		**Route**
1	T.O. Dr. Healy/B. Carre RN				
2	9/23/2002 at 2:00 a.m.				
3	Tylenol 650 mg every 4 hours as needed for pain by mouth				
4	B. Carre, RN 9/23/2002		noted 9/23/02		
5			D. Goodly RN		
6	9/24/2002 Evaluation for physical therapy				
8	Dressing changes wet to dry 3 times a day				
Unit & Rm# 1234	**Date**	**Time**	**Allergic to:** **NKA**		**Doctor**

The following criteria may be used for monitoring order transcription:

- Each order is noted.

- Each order is implemented.

- Each order is transcribed accurately and completely.

Placement of Documentation in the Health Record

After the orders are provided, the forms in which the transcribed orders are captured are filed in the resident's health record in the appropriate section. Permanent treatment records are placed in date order with the medication record or Kardex. Any treatment record that has been a working record—those done in pencil and updated as orders are written—is discarded because the documentation is captured on the original physician order sheet and the transcribed treatment record.

Other Pertinent Information

A nurse is usually identified in facility policy as the person responsible for the overall process of order transcription. As mentioned earlier, some facilities use unit secretaries to supplement the process, but responsibility for order accuracy and implementation falls on the nursing staff.

Physical therapists may be allowed to transcribe orders from a physiatrist, but this stipulation is usually driven by state-specific regulations. In the same manner, respiratory therapists may be allowed to transcribe respiratory orders. It is essential that each facility thoroughly understand any state requirements for the process of order transcription.

There are no federal requirements for the transcription of orders, but state-specific regulations may dictate who may transcribe orders.

Summary

A physician must order the resident's care. Physician orders provide for medical supervision and oversight, and include medications, treatments, and tests. Physician orders on admission to the facility are used to develop the interim care plan for the resident's immediate care needs.

The physician order needs to contain specific information to ensure that proper care requirements are met. The clinical indication for each ordered service should be included in each order. Use of telephone orders and fax orders is acceptable, but should be outlined in facility policy and procedures.

Physicians are required to review orders in specified time frames, which may be driven by either federal or state requirements.

The use of standing orders in long-term care may be limited. The facility would need a policy and procedure for their use.

Authentication is the signature at the end of an order or note that certifies the identity of the author.

The transcription of orders provides a mechanism to place all written orders from the resident's health record on forms that will allow the provision of each order in an efficient manner. The transcription process allows a centralization to ensure that each order is carried out. The facility should have a thorough policy covering the transcription of physician orders.

The Institute of Safe Medical Practice has provided guidelines for the use of appropriate abbreviations for hospitals. The long-term care facility should consider reevaluating the abbreviations used in its organization to enhance resident safety measures.

References

Joint Commission on Accreditation of Healthcare Organizations. 2004. *Comprehensive Accreditation Manual for Long-term Care.* Oakbrook Terrace, Ill.: JCAHO.

Centers for Medicare and Medicaid Services. 2001 (October 31). Guidance to Surveyors—Long-Term Care Policies, appendix PP in *State Operations Manual.* Available at www.cms.gov.

Institute of Safe Medical Practice. 2001 (May 2). Please don't sleep through this wake-up call. Available at www.ismp.org.

Chapter 14

Medication and Treatment Records

Medication and treatment records are forms that provide a mechanism to track that all medications and treatments were provided to the resident. Medication records are logs that provide detailed listings of medications, dosage, time, date, and name of the person who administered the medication. They also contain the listing of any resident allergies as well as the resident's name, medical record number, and room number, for ease in administration. The information required to complete the medication record is entered as soon after the medication dosage is given as practical. Medication records are kept for those residents whose needs require the administration of medication by nursing staff. Treatment records provide the same mechanism for documentation of treatments that the resident requires. A medication record also is kept for those residents who self-administer drugs and contains the same medication information but will not contain nursing documentation of the dosage, time, or date of administration.

Medication Records

Medication records are transcribed from the physician's orders. The form is used for document capture and to support the delivery of each medication or treatment ordered by a physician. (See figures 14.1 and 14.2.)

Medication administration records (MARs) are tools used to capture the delivery of each drug to the resident. The MAR identifies medications a resident is scheduled to take, how often they should be administered, and at what dose they are to be administered.

The purpose of the MAR is to provide a means to confirm that each drug was provided as indicated in the order. The medication record also captures the nurses' initials when providing the drug. The tool provides an easy way to organize the resident's medication orders and to ensure that each medication is given as ordered.

There may be two types of medication records: one for regular medications and one for prn medications, or medications administered as needed. Each type of record is similar in content, and some facilities use one form for both regular and prn medication orders.

The documentation tool is an extremely important tool to capture each drug and its dose, route, and interval as well as its original order date, renewal date, and expiration date. The MAR stays on the medication cart that is wheeled to the resident's room where the delivery of the medications can be given in a logical and efficient manner by following the scheduled medication administration.

Figure 14.1.   Sample medication administration record

Medication Administration Record

XYZ Organization
Anytown USA 00000

Month	Year	Resident name	Med Rec #	Room #	Allergies		Page
Physician					Diagnosis		

Nurse Alert

Code Status

			Time	Exp Date	1	2	3	4	5	6	7	8	9	10	12	14	16	18	20	22	24	26	28	30
Org Date Ordered	Renew date	Drug Dose Route Interval			1	2	3	4	5	6	7	8	9	10	1 12	1 14	1 16	1 18	1 20	2 22	2 24	2 26	2 28	2 30	3
Org Date Ordered	Renew date	Drug Dose Route Interval	Time	Exp Date	1	2	3	4	5	6	7	8	9	10	1 12	1 14	1 16	1 18	1 20	2 22	2 24	2 26	2 28	2 30	3
Org Date Ordered	Renew date	Drug Dose Route Interval	Time	Exp Date	1	2	3	4	5	6	7	8	9	10	1 12	1 14	1 16	1 18	1 20	2 22	2 24	2 26	2 28	2 30	3

One-time Dose and STAT Medication Administration

Date	Time	Drug/dose/route/	Nurse	Date	Time	Drug route	Nurse

PRN Medication Administration and Refusals and Holds of Scheduled Medications

Date	Time	Medication	Reason	Effect				See Nursing note	Nurse
				None	Fair	Good			

Figure 14.2.   Sample treatment administration record

Treatment Administration Record

XYZ Organization
Anytown USA 00000

Month	Year	Resident name	Med Rec #	Room #	Allergies		Page
Physician		Nurse Alert		Code Status	Diagnosis		

Org Date Ordered	Renew date	Drug Dose Route Interval	Exp Date	Time	1	2	3	4	5	6	7	8	9	10	1	12	1	14	1	16	1	18	1	20	2	22	2	24	2	26	2	28	2	30	3
Org Date Ordered	Renew date	Drug Dose Route Interval	Exp Date	Time	1	2	3	4	5	6	7	8	9	10	1	12	1	14	1	16	1	18	1	20	2	22	2	24	2	26	2	28	2	30	3
Org Date Ordered	Renew date	Drug Dose Route Interval	Exp Date	Time	1	2	3	4	5	6	7	8	9	10	1	12	1	14	1	16	1	18	1	20	2	22	2	24	2	26	2	28	2	30	3

Nursing Treatment Notes

Instructions   1. If the treatment is a medication, the nurse must initial.
2. If the treatment is a PRN Medication, there must be an explanation in the nursing notes.

Date	Time	Treatment	Initial	Reason	Result

227

Physician Orders and Transcription

A physician must order each medication. The nursing staff then transcribes each medication to the medication administration record to ensure that the resident receives those ordered drugs. States may have specific requirements for the administration of medications. The Joint Commission on Accreditation of Healthcare Organizations (JCAHO) requires that documentation of each medication given be included in the resident's health record.

The facility should have a policy and procedure on the MAR that would coincide with the transcription of orders policy and procedure. It is important to establish a check-and-balance system for monitoring the physician order and its transcription to the MAR. Errors can occur in the transcription process, and the facility needs to ensure that steps are taken to minimize any error in the process.

Upon admission to the facility, the physician writes the medication and treatment orders for the resident. The nurse or appointed person then transcribes the medications to the MAR while the order is sent to the pharmacy for processing. Should the resident's stay be interrupted, a new MAR should be initiated based on new orders written by the physician. This eliminates the possibility of errors occurring in medication administration. The new orders provided by the physician may include changes in the medication regime. Therefore, starting a new medication administration record can more accurately capture the correct drug orders. If medications are discontinued or adjusted, the new MAR would contain only what the physician has ordered at the time of readmission.

Trying to discontinue and reenter new or readjusted medications can make the MAR cumbersome to manage because of multiple pages and discounted items. The possibility of medication errors increases when pages are inadvertently disregarded at medication administration.

The MAR is a detailed form that captures the necessary information that is required to administer drugs to the resident. Because it contains information for an entire month, the form is sturdier than regular documents in the resident's record. The MAR details the drug usage for a thirty- to thirty-one-day cycle and is renewed at the beginning of each calendar month.

The MAR should be completed at the time of administration of the medication to the resident. This provides assurance that the medication was given at the specified time.

Quality Requirements

Completeness of the medication administration record is always of concern. Should areas be left blank, it would appear that the required medication was not given to the patient. The process for completion of the MAR should be a quality concern for the facility.

Transcription of the medication to the MAR also is a quality concern as discussed in chapter 13.

The facility should not sanction the process of simply filling blank areas on any documentation captured in the health record. The practice is determined to be deliberate falsification and is illegal.

Facilities should use concurrent monitoring or a self-monitoring, shift-to-shift approach to ensure that the MAR is complete. This process could be conducted at the time of the narcotic check and count, which may be required by law.

Assessment criteria may contain the following elements:

- Each medication is contained on the resident's MAR.
- The MAR indicates that all medications were administered.
- Effects of prn medications are captured on the MAR.

Placement of Documents in the Health Record

The MAR documents are filed according to facility policy. Some facilities may choose to create a separate section for these records called the medication and treatment section. However, due to volume, other facilities may decide to move them to a miscellaneous section or file them directly into overflow files. Overflow files are storage files maintained for each resident as the volume of the health record mandates. They contain the depleted health record documents filed according to health information management policy. (Refer to chapter 1 for HIM practices.) Treatment records are filed in the same manner.

Other Pertinent Information

Use of the prn MAR allows the capture of only those medications that are needed on an as-needed basis and helps keep the MAR more organized and efficient. This document also captures the effects of the drug administered.

Content

The content of the MAR may contain the following information:

- Facility name
- Resident name, health record number, and room
- Month and year
- Allergies
- Code status
- Diagnoses
- Original date ordered
- Renewal date
- Drug, dose, route, and interval
- Expiration date
- Days of the month for initials of the nurse administrating the drug
- Effect of the medication as required

The medication records must be kept up-to-date, and a mechanism to show discontinued medications must be established. This mechanism should be outlined in facility policy and procedures. Typically, the medications that are discontinued are highlighted in a manner to indicate that they are no longer to be given. Some institutions may choose to highlight in a particular color to demonstrate that the medication is no longer applicable. Figure 14.3 shows a highlighted administration record indicating that the medication was discontinued. The shading across the document (which normally would be highlighting) indicates that the medication is no longer to be given to the resident.

The medication record also must indicate when the resident is not in the facility, such as during acute care stays. When a resident is transferred to an acute care facility, documentation that the resident is on leave of absence (LOA) may be indicated. The nurse would write either "LOA" or "Leave of Absence" in the days and times in which the resident is not present in the facility to take the medications.

Figure 14.3. Discontinued medication

XYZ Organization
Anytown USA 00000

Medication Administration Record

Month	Year	Resident name	Med Rec #	Room #	Allergies	Page
Physician		Nurse Alert		Code Status	Diagnosis	

Org Date Ordered	Renew date	Drug Dose Route Interval / Medication Discontinued	Exp Date	Time	1 2 3 4 5 6 7 8 9 10 12 14 16 18 20 22 24 26 28 30 3
Org Date Ordered	Renew date	Drug Dose Route Interval	Exp Date	Time	1 2 3 4 5 6 7 8 9 10 12 14 16 18 20 22 24 26 28 30 3
Org Date Ordered	Renew date	Drug Dose Route Interval	Exp Date	Time	1 2 3 4 5 6 7 8 9 10 12 14 16 18 20 22 24 26 28 30 3

Treatment Records

The resident's treatment record contains the treatments the resident is ordered to receive. As discussed in the MAR section of this chapter, treatments must be ordered by the physician or may be prescribed interventions based on accepted protocols established to be necessary by the facility to provide proper and effective care. These protocols must have had documented physician approval prior to use.

The treatment record is the transcribed set of treatment orders prescribed by a physician to attend the resident's needs. The purpose of the treatment record is to provide one location for the capture of the resident's treatment regime so that it is easy to determine what, when, how, and where treatments are to be given.

The treatment record provides a detailed list of all treatments that are necessary for the care of the resident. These may include dressings and dressing changes, lotions, ointments, or creams to be applied, care of decubitus ulcers, special shampoos, sun block, bowel regimes, diet supplements, special equipment requirements, ventilator settings, and the like. The treatment record makes it easier for the nurse caring for the resident to see all required treatments in one document that specifies the treatment and time it must be provided. It also tracks the actual provision of the treatment by requiring the nurse to initial the appropriate space on the treatment record.

General Requirements for Treatment Records

Centralization of all treatment on one treatment record gives the nurse the ability to better ensure that all treatments are provided in a timely manner to each resident. Documenting the provision of care is extremely important to demonstrate that the care-planning process and care provision have been accurately completed.

Transcribing the treatments onto the treatment record is an important step in the process of providing care to the resident. The accurate transcription of each treatment ordered is vital to the process of healthcare provision. Each treatment must be transcribed properly and accurately to ensure that the resident receives the care ordered by the physician.

Documenting the treatment provided also is a key component in care provision. The treatment record provides a means to quickly and easily determine that all required care was provided as scheduled. Empty spaces on the treatment record would indicate that care was not given. The documentation of treatments should be done at the time the treatment is provided. As care is given, the nurse initials the form to indicate completion of the treatment.

Similar in format to the MAR, the treatment record is a form that captures all of the information for providing each resident's full regime of treatments.

Quality Requirements for Treatment Records

The treatment record must be accurate and complete. Areas that are inadvertently left blank are quality concerns.

Assessment criteria for monitoring the treatment record may include the following:

- Resident identification is present.

- Allergies are documented on the treatment record.

- All treatments are included in the form.

- Treatments that have been discontinued have been removed according to policy.
- Each treatment is provided.
- The form is complete.

Content

The content of the treatment record may contain the following information:

- Facility name
- Resident name, health record number, and room
- Month and year
- Allergies
- Code status
- Diagnoses
- Original date ordered
- Renewal date
- Treatment required (if an ointment or possible medication, the form will contain drug, dose, route, and interval)
- Expiration date
- Days of the month for initials of the nurse administrating the drug
- Reason for the treatment
- Effect or result of the treatment as required

Summary

Medication records are used to capture the delivery of each drug to the resident. The MAR provides a mechanism to capture each drug given to the resident and to ensure that doses are not missed. Nursing initials in the appropriate space on the MAR indicate that each drug was given.

Treatment records are a mechanism to capture the delivery of any ordered treatment required by the resident. This form provides a centralized location for all treatments ordered by the physician.

Both the MAR and the treatment record provide an easy, centralized location to ensure that all drugs and treatments are provided to the resident as required.

References

Joint Commission on Accreditation of Healthcare Organizations. 2004. *Comprehensive Accreditation Manual for Long-term Care.* Oakbrook Terrace, Ill.: JCAHO.

Centers for Medicare and Medicaid Services. 2001 (October 31). Guidance to Surveyors—Long-Term Care Facilities, appendix PP in *State Operations Manual.* Available at www.cms.gov.

Chapter 15

Flow Sheets

Flow sheets are used in various ways in the long-term care setting. Nursing flow sheets track the health status of each resident on a day-to-day basis and support care planning and assessment. **Nursing assessment records** (NARs), or activities of daily living (ADL) flow sheets, track residents' functional status and support the Minimum Data Set (MDS) process. Service delivery records track the provision of rehabilitative services such as nursing restorative care, occupational therapy, physical therapy, and speech–language therapy, and document residents' responses to these services. Clinical flow sheets track delivery of many kinds of specific clinical services to long-term care facility residents. The common purpose of all of these flow sheets is to document that required services were delivered to the facility's residents and to provide a means of communication among healthcare workers.

Nursing Flow Sheets

The nursing flow sheet is used to capture the daily care and monitoring of each resident and provides supporting documentation for resident care. A comprehensive shift-to-shift assessment of the resident's status, the nursing flow sheet helps communicate resident health status to all care providers, especially the nursing staff. Additionally, the nursing flow sheet documents the nursing staff's clinical observations and provides detailed information on the resident's general daily health condition.

Description

Nursing flow sheets are comprehensive tools used to collect the daily documentation of the resident's health status and to support the care-planning and reassessment process. The purpose of the nursing flow sheet is to provide a mechanism to reassess the resident's overall health status and body systems daily, shift by shift.

The ability to document clinical observations on a shift-by-shift basis supports the care-planning and assessment process throughout the clinical units of the facility. The nursing flow sheet also may capture the response to care over time and clarifies the resident's nursing care needs.

General Requirements

The daily nursing flow sheet must be dated and signed by the nurse overseeing the care of the resident on a shift-by-shift basis. Facility policy should define the process for nursing flow sheet documentation and content as well as the timeliness of the documentation process.

There are no federal requirements for nursing flow sheets. However, state regulations may include specific nursing requirements that can be included on the nursing flow sheet.

Nursing Daily Assessments

Nursing flow sheet documentation provides a thorough reassessment of the resident on a shift-to-shift basis and tracks body system functions and health status. As stated earlier, documenting an accurate reflection of the resident's health status helps support the assessment and care-planning process. Nursing flow sheets provide a methodology to determine resident problems on a regular basis. They should be completed at the time care is provided and the resident is assessed.

A daily documentation tool, the nursing flow sheet contains columns for documenting the resident's care needs every eight hours.

Quality Requirements

Documentation completeness is of the utmost importance. Also at issue is that the flow sheet must be documented at the time of care and reassessment. It goes without saying that a nursing flow sheet should never be completed before the nurse sees the resident, nor should it simply be considered an exercise to check off the boxes, as has sometimes been the case in the past.

Assessment criteria for the nursing flow sheet may contain the following:

- The nursing flow sheet contains the resident name and health record number.
- The nursing flow sheet is accurate.
- The nursing flow sheet is complete.
- An appropriate person as defined by policy signs the nursing flow sheet.

Placement of Documentation in the Health Record

The nursing flow sheet is placed in a designated section of the resident's record upon completion.

Content

The nursing flow sheet may contain the following data points:

- Facility name
- Resident name and health record number
- Date
- Neurological sensory assessment
- Motor functions
- Cardiovascular assessment
- Vascular assessment
- Pulmonary assessment
- Gastrointestinal assessment

- Genitourinary assessment

- Comfort

- Nutrition

- Psychosocial

- Skin integrity

- Pain assessment

- Care plan update check

- Initials and signature of the nurse

The flow sheet may contain individual boxes for each factor of the assessment (figure 15.1) or may simply require a check mark for function within normal limits and exceptions, which would require a nursing note (figure 15.2).

Figure 15.1.   Sample nursing flow sheet indicating individual factors

XYZ Organization Anytown USA 00000 **Nursing Flow Sheet** Date			
Assessment	**11–7**	**7–3**	**3–11**

Neurological	___Alert
	___Oriented
	___Awake
	___Follows commands
	___Speech clear
	___Pupils equal/
	    reactive to light
		___Alert
		___Oriented
		___Awake
		___Follows commands
		___Speech clear
		___Pupils equal/
		    reactive to light
			___Alert
			___Oriented
			___Awake
			___Follows commands
			___Speech clear
			___Pupils equal/
			    reactive to light

Figure 15.2.   Sample nursing flow sheet indicating normal and exception assessments

XYZ Organization Anytown USA 00000		**Instructions:** Check WNL for normal assessments. Check "exceptions" that vary from normal. (All "exceptions" checked must have a nursing note.)				
Date		**Nursing Flow Sheet**				
Assessment	**Time**	**11–7**	**Time**	**7–3**	**Time**	**3–11**
Neurological Alert and oriented to person, place, time. Follows commands. Speech is clear.		___WNL ___Exception		___WNL ___Exception		___WNL ___Exception
Pupils Equal/reactive to light		___WNL ___Exception		___WNL ___Exception		___WNL ___Exception

Nursing Assessment Record or ADL Flow Sheet

There is no federal requirement for documentation to be entered in either an NAR or an ADL flow sheet. However, state-specific regulations may require documentation of this type. The facility will require ADL charting as outlined in policy. Many times, facilities do allow the nursing assistant to provide ADL or nursing assistant charting. The ADL flow sheet or NAR tools should be included in the facility policy.

The purpose of the ADL flow sheet is to document the day-to-day functional status of the resident. (See figure 15.3.) The form captures activities of daily living—those normal human functions that we complete on a daily routine such as bathing, dressing, eating, and the like.

When a facility determines that the nursing assistant documents on a flow sheet, it is reflective of the comprehensive assessment process and often the ADL flow sheet will contain the MDS ADL requirements and scoring techniques to ensure a means to capture those required data elements.

Some facilities may require that the nurse document on the actual ADL flow sheet after discussing the resident's care with the nursing assistant. Regardless of whether the nurse or the nursing assistant completes the flow sheet, the completeness of the documentation should be checked at the end of each shift to provide concurrent monitoring of the form.

General Requirements

The nursing assistant flow sheet or ADL flow sheet supports the MDS assessment process, and scoring on the flow sheet should mimic MDS scoring to ensure data consistency between the documents.

Figure 15.3.   Sample activities of daily living flow sheet

XYZ Organization
Anytown USA 00000

ADL Flow Sheet

Resident name: _____   Health record number: _____

Month and year: _____

ADL scoring:	**Self-performance**		**Support needed**	
	0 = independence	3 = extensive assistance	0 = none	3 = 2 or more people
	1 = supervision/cueing	4 = total assistance	1 = setup	8 = did not occur
	2 = limited assist	8 = did not occur	2 = one person	

ADLs		**Sun**			**Mon**			**Tues**			**Wed**			**Thur**			**Fri**			**Sat**		
		N	D	E	N	D	E	N	D	E	N	D	E	N	D	E	N	D	E	N	D	E
Bed mobility	Self-support																						
Transfer	Self-support																						
Walk in room	Self-support																						
Walk in corridor	Self-support																						

Documentation of resident ADLs provides another means to support the accurate reflection of the resident's current health status. Recording activities of daily living demonstrates the resident's functioning ability on a shift-by-shift basis and can be used over time to show decline or improvement for the comprehensive assessment and care-planning process. The documentation contained on the ADL flow sheet is valuable and important for the interdisciplinary team. Documentation done on the ADL flow sheet should be completed as close to the time of care as possible.

There are no federal requirements for an ADL flow sheet; however, the resident's health record must contain documentation that supports the MDS comprehensive assessment process.

The ADL flow sheet is a comprehensive tool that captures the elements required on the MDS for charting activities of daily living. It may contain information for the entire week so that decline or improvement can be seen during the seven-day time frame.

Quality Requirements

Once again, completeness of the ADL flow sheet is essential. Accurately documenting the resident's function provides a means to further support the entire care process.

Assessment criteria for the ADL flow sheet are similar to the nursing flow sheet criteria previously discussed.

Placement of Documentation in the Health Record

The ADL flow sheet is placed in a designated section of the resident's health record.

Content

The ADL may contain the following elements:

- Facility name
- Resident name and health record number
- Date of the flow sheet
- Shift performing the documentation
- Temperature
- Diet and supplements
- Cognition
- Mood
- Behavior
- Mobility
- Ambulation
- Elimination: Bladder
- Elimination: Bowel
- Sleep pattern
- ADLs
  —Bed mobility
  —Transfer

- —Walking in room
- —Walking in corridor
- —Locomotion on unit
- —Locomotion off unit
- —Dressing
- —Eating
- —Toilet use
- —Personal hygiene
- —Bathing
- Nail care
- Range of motion
- Safety
- CNA initials and signature (if appropriate to facility policy)
- Nurse initials and signature

Each item is coded according to the MDS scoring guidelines, as appropriate.

Service Delivery Records

Service delivery records are various forms that are developed to capture data concerning the rehabilitation services provided to the resident. These forms are used for nursing restorative care (figure 15.4), occupational therapy (figure 15.5), physical therapy, and speech–language therapy.

Service delivery records or flow sheets are those documents used to record rehabilitation or nursing restorative care charting.

The purpose of the service delivery record is to document services and record treatment time for the specific discipline provided. These forms support the comprehensive assessment, billing, and reimbursement processes by capturing the time spent to provide the particular service.

The service delivery record is specific to the discipline providing the particular service required. Each form contains a section, usually on the back of the form, for progress notes as well. Each discipline-specific form contains the data elements required to provide the treatments and interventions that have been ordered by the resident's physician.

The facility should have a policy and procedure for documentation of the service delivery record. The policy should outline when service delivery records are used and by which disciplines within the facility. Further, it should contain the forms that are required to ensure that the process is completed properly.

General Requirements for Service Delivery Records

There are no federal requirements for service delivery records, but there are requirements for the provision of care by nursing and therapy departments. State regulations may require specific elements to be documented in the resident's record. The service delivery record is a mechanism to accomplish this process.

Figure 15.4. Sample nursing restorative care service delivery record

XYZ Organization
Anytown USA 00000

Nursing Restorative Care Service Delivery Record

Resident name: _____   Health record number: _____

Month and year: _____

	1	2	3	4	5	6	7	8	9	10	11	12	13	14	15	16	17	18	19	20	21	22	23	24	25	26	27	28	29	30	31
Ambulation																															
Assistance																															
Distance																															
Range of motion																															
Toleration																															
Good																															
Fair																															
Poor																															

Monthly review only—specify treatments

Comments

Signature _____   Date _____

239

Figure 15.5.   Sample occupational therapy service delivery record

XYZ Organization
Anytown USA 00000

Resident name: _____

Month and year: _____

Last Evaluation Date: _____

Occupational Therapy Service Delivery Record

	NAME	TITLE	INITIAL

HCPC/CPT code	Description	1	2	3	4	5	6	7	8	9	10	11	12	13	14	15	16	17	18	19	20	21	22	23	24	25	26	27	28	29	30	31
97003	Initial evaluation																																
97004	Reevaluation																																
97530	Therapeutic activities																																
97535	ADL training																																
97703	Orthotic/prosthetic check																																
97504	Orthotic fitting and training																																
Total																																	
Initials																																	

There must be a current order signed by a physician for the delivery of therapy. (See chapter 13 for further information on the process of physician orders for therapies.) The service delivery record must be dated and signed by the person responsible for providing the care and treatment to the resident. Accuracy of the data is vital to the overall assessment and billing processes within the facility. The service delivery record allows each discipline to capture treatments and interventions as well as the length of time spent providing the services. It is a concise method for demonstrating the documentation of the actual delivery of care for these required services. The service delivery record should be completed as soon after the delivery of care as possible to ensure documentation accuracy.

Quality Requirements

Accuracy of the documentation of the times on these service delivery forms is a quality concern because the total time can impact billing and reimbursement processing.

The following assessment criteria may be used to monitor the service delivery record:

- Treatments are identified.

- Times are indicated for each treatment.

- Signatures and date are recorded.

- The current plan of care for therapy is signed by a physician.

- Progress notes are captured according to facility policy.

Placement of Documentation in the Health Record

Each specific rehab discipline files its service delivery record in the discipline-specific section of the resident's health record. This places all documentation for the specific discipline together for easy access and monitoring.

Nursing restorative service delivery records are filed with related nursing restorative documentation in a designated section of the resident's health record.

Content

The service delivery forms may contain the following information:

- Facility name

- Discipline

- Resident name and health record number

- Month and year

- Last evaluation date

- Signature, title, and initial of each professional providing care

- CPT/HCPCS code

- Description of the treatment or intervention, such as initial evaluation, reevaluation, therapeutic activities, ADL training, and the like

- Grid for minutes

- Total treatment minutes of the day

- Initials for the individual completing the document

- Progress notes on the back as defined by facility policy

Clinical Flow Sheets

Long-term facilities have developed many different types of flow sheets to capture important service delivery health information on each resident. These clinical flow sheets may consist of the following, although this is not an all-inclusive listing:

- Abnormal involuntary movement scale

- Antipsychotic drug use monitoring

- Bowel and bladder flow sheet

- Diabetic flow sheet

- Education flow sheet

- Injection site rotation

- Intake and output

- Interim blood pressure sheets

- IV therapy

- Monthly blood pressure sheets

- Pain flow sheet

- Pressure ulcer flow sheets

- Urinary flow sheet

- Vital signs

- Weight sheets

Federal regulations do not require specific flow sheets, but state or facility-specific requirements or policies drive the use of these types of documents. The format differs between each flow sheet and has different time frame requirements such as every seven days, fourteen days, daily, or just on a monthly basis.

Clinical flow sheets are filed in the nursing section of the resident's health record.

The purpose of these types of clinical flow sheets is to capture the delivery of services provided to each resident. Each flow sheet represents a means to document that the required service was given.

Federal and state requirements mandate that each resident receive the care the physician has ordered. In an attempt to show that the services requested are given, long-term care facilities have created clinical flow sheets to capture the delivery of each type of service required by the resident to maintain or improve functional well-being. These documents are valuable tools that help to communicate the care given to the resident. Not every resident will have each of the previously listed flow sheets in his or her health record because each resident requires a medical regime designed specifically for his or her needs.

These documents become significant pieces of the entire resident's health record. They help demonstrate that the care the resident required as determined by the assessment and care-planning process has been provided and provided in the detail needed. These documents support the overall care of the resident, help clarify specific delivery of care methods, and contribute to the assessment and care-planning process for each resident.

Clinical service delivery flow sheets should be completed as soon as possible after care is provided.

Quality Requirements

As with any document contained in the resident's health record, these forms, when used, must be completed in their entirety to provide the full and accurate detail of the services provided to the resident. Assessment criteria are as outlined in the previous flow sheet discussions.

Placement of Documentation in the Health Record

Placement of clinical flow sheets in the resident's health record is determined by the type of service delivered, the discipline involved in recording the service delivery, and facility policy. However, for the most part they are located in the nursing section of the resident's health record.

Content

The content of each flow sheet differs depending on the service delivery required.

Summary

Flow sheets are comprehensive tools used to collect daily documentation of the resident's health status. They support the care-planning and reassessment process within the facility. Each facility has policies and procedures describing the particular flow sheets used to document the care provided.

Nursing flow sheets provide a mechanism for capturing clinical observations. ADL flow sheets provide a means of tracking the day-to-day status of each resident. Service delivery records allow specific disciplines to document services provided and treatment times. Clinical flow sheets contain various ways to document other necessary services provided to the resident, such as education, intake and output, blood pressure, pressure ulcers, and vital signs.

The documentation captured on each flow sheet supports the MDS process in long-term care and is a very important aspect of recording the care and service provided. Flow sheets are an important addition to the resident's health record and ensure that the resident's health status is completely and accurately illustrated. They facilitate communication to all clinical staff to ensure a clear understanding of the resident's condition, needs, and requirements.

References

Centers for Medicare and Medicaid Services. 2001 (October 31). Guidance to Surveyors—Long-Term Care Facilities, appendix PP in *State Operations Manual*. Available from www.cms.gov.

Chapter 16

Laboratory and Special Reports

Physicians depend on information gathered from many kinds of laboratory and diagnostic test results to help them establish the correct diagnosis and treatment plan for each patient and to assess changes in residents' health conditions. Laboratory test reports and special diagnostic test reports form an important part of the resident's health information in long-term care settings.

Laboratory Reports

Laboratory reports contain the results of tests on the resident's body fluids such as blood, sputum, and urine. They also indicate whether microorganisms are present in those specimens. The physician must order all laboratory tests. Test results are key documentation containing further information on, and clarification of, the resident's medical condition.

Laboratory results are diagnostic testing outcomes made by a chemical, microscopic, microbiologic, immunologic, or pathologic study of secretions, discharges, blood, or tissue. They must be included in the resident's health record. The reports are used to help clarify resident symptoms and provide clinically pertinent information for diagnosis determination. The laboratory performs tests, experiments, and investigative procedures for diagnostic study.

The purpose of the laboratory testing is to assist physicians in determining the resident's diagnoses. The printed reports provide the documentation that shows evidence of the testing outcomes.

The printed laboratory reports provide the outcomes of testing procedures and are valuable documentation that the interdisciplinary team can use to care for the patient. Based on the results of laboratory testing, treatments and interventions are planned to manage the resident's identified needs.

Laboratory reports should be included in the admission information sent with each resident upon admission to the facility. If these results do not accompany the resident at the time of admission, health record staff usually requests them from the referring facility or the physician's office. Receipt of these test results eliminates the need to retest the resident on admission to the long-term care setting.

During the resident's long-term care stay, laboratory tests must be done as required by state law and as symptoms and conditions warrant. Many long-term care facilities do not have on-site laboratories and, instead, depend on outsourced services for laboratory testing and results. The long-term care facility may use different techniques to ensure that test results are received for filing into the resident's health record. Results may be telephoned into the facility and taken by licensed staff, usually nursing staff, for immediate reporting to the physician for medical management and orders as needed. They may be faxed to a designated secure location for distribution to the particular nursing stations or units for notification and filing into the resident's health record. Some facilities also use a courier service to deliver printed reports or have the reports printed directly to a dedicated printer in the facility.

General Requirements

State-specific laws and regulations may require certain laboratory studies be done on each resident at specified time frames. Certain tests may be required on an annual basis; other testing requirements may stipulate longer time frames between tests. Check with all applicable state requirements to develop specific policies on laboratory testing procedures that will be needed for each resident.

Federal regulations require that the attending or covering physician order all laboratory, radiology, and diagnostic services. They also require that the physician be notified immediately of laboratory findings and findings from radiology or other diagnostic services.

State-specific requirements may exist for certain laboratory testing. These may include, but are not limited to:

- Fasting blood sugar (FBS)
- Complete blood count (CBC)
- Blood urea nitrogen (BUN)
- Urine routine and microscopic (R & M)
- Stool for occult blood

Laboratory Testing

Usually the long-term care setting depends on other entities or outsourced services to provide laboratory testing and/or results for its constituency. Utilization of appropriate services and resources becomes a major concern not only to the facility, but also to the resident due to the unavailability of recent laboratory results. The cost of care rises not only for the institution and the resident, but also for the nation as testing is redone to satisfy regulatory requirements. The necessity for further testing when results are unavailable and the appropriateness of retesting and invasive testing regimes on the resident due to unavailable testing results does not provide residents with effective and efficient continuity of care, nor does it provide an "efficacy" of healthcare services. The acute care facility and the long-term care facility must communicate resident needs and health conditions, including pertinent resident diagnostic testing results, to ensure continuity of care and to provide a true continuum of care for the customer—the resident.

One of the great concerns in the long-term care environment is that of getting the necessary documentation to support the resident's condition on admission, readmission, or after transfer and return to an acute care facility. In the hectic routine in the acute care facility and the heavily regulated long-term care environment, there is a "disconnect" in communication of resident medical conditions, diagnostic results, surgical procedures, outcomes, and care requirements.

Long-term care is driven in reality by the resident's healthcare needs. Federal regulations are clear in stating that the facility must "provide the necessary care and services to attain or maintain the highest practicable physical, mental, and psychosocial well-being, in accordance with the comprehensive assessment and plan of care" (CMS 2001, PP-83). To more effectively provide the necessary care to each resident, the interdisciplinary team must have the documentation, including laboratory reports, from other institutions that have provided care to the resident prior to the long-term care stay.

The actual laboratory reports containing preliminary and final diagnostic test results must be kept in the resident's health record. These reports are typically computer generated. After reports are final, the preliminary reports may be destroyed to ensure that the resident's health records are up-to-date and accurately reflect his or her condition.

Laboratory test results should be filed into the resident's health record upon receipt so that the interdisciplinary team can begin planning care.

Quality Requirements

Physician notification must be completed as required by federal requirements.

There are quality concerns inherent in receiving the laboratory reports for the resident's continued care. The documents are necessary to ensure proper care.

Preliminary reports should be removed after they have been finalized.

Laboratory test requests should be tracked to ensure that they are completed. This checklist of requested tests should be compared to laboratory reports received to ensure that results are reported and tests are actually completed.

Mechanisms for tracking receipt of admission laboratory reports should be established to minimize the need to retest residents for state- or facility-specific required laboratory tests.

The resident care plan should be updated, as appropriate, after receipt of preliminary and final laboratory test results.

The following assessment criteria may be used for quality purposes:

- Resident laboratory reports are received on admission, readmission, or after transfer and return to the facility.

- Resident laboratory results are requested and received if they did not accompany the resident to the facility.

- Preliminary reports are removed when final reports are received.

- A laboratory test request list is maintained.

- Laboratory tests received are matched to the request list upon receipt to ensure that all tests are completed.

- Resident care plans are updated, as appropriate, upon receipt of preliminary and final laboratory reports.

- Physician is notified of results.

Placement of Documentation in the Health Record

Depending on facility policy and guidelines, laboratory reports may be filed in the following manner:

1. Laboratory reports are filed in the laboratory section of the resident's record.

2. Laboratory reports are filed only in the laboratory section of the resident's record after review and signature requirements have been met.

3. New laboratory reports are placed at the front of the physician order section until signature requirements are met and then are permanently filed in the laboratory section of the resident's record.

Other Pertinent Information

The facility should have a policy and procedure on the options used for reporting laboratory results. For example, the policy might include the following kinds of information:

- Laboratory policy
    - —Admission testing requirements (laboratory reports accompanying the resident on admission and after transfer and readmission)
    - —Annual testing requirements
    - —Other required testing (six months, three months or quarterly, every month, and so on)
    - —Testing requirements for specified drug analysis (for example, electrolytes for diuretic usage)
- Telephone reporting of laboratory results
    - —Further reporting to physician offices
    - —STAT or "please call" results reporting
    - —Critical results reporting
    - —Positive microbiology and serology reporting
- Laboratory reports
    - —Delivery methods and location
    - —Laboratory review
    - —Notification to physician of abnormal levels
    - —Notification of tracking mechanisms
    - —Signature requirements
    - —Distribution to specific units or stations
    - —Placement in the resident's health record
    - —Laboratory request and receipt tracking mechanisms and checks
    - —Facsimile processing mechanisms

Content

In general, laboratory reports contain the following elements:

- Resident's name and health record number
- Unit or station and room
- Date of test
- Date of report

- Designation "preliminary" or "final"
- Category of test, chemistry, microbiology, and the like
- Name of test or tests
- Results of test
- Normal ranges
- Abnormal results

Special Reports

Special reports include the results of imaging and pathology testing, among other procedures. Imaging may include a full range of radiological service diagnostic test results, including the more common X-ray, EKG, Holter Monitor, MRI, CT scan, and respiratory therapy reports such as pulmonary function testing and pulse oximetry results. X-ray reports are the most common test result found in the resident's health record.

Special reports include imaging, pathology reports, and respiratory therapy testing results completed for diagnostic purposes. However, there may be instances where other special reports are included in the resident's health record.

Purpose of Special Reports

The purpose of special reports is to further define and determine diagnostic testing results for residents. The reports help clarify and detect resident problems. From these special tests, the physician can determine the cause of problems or conditions that the resident may develop. The reports are used to assist in planning the complete care of each resident.

Diagnostic testing, and the resulting special reports, is an extremely valuable tool used to detect causes of diseases and resulting deterioration from those diseases. These special reports assist in detecting, establishing, or confirming a diagnosis. Special diagnostic testing helps determine the nature of a disease, injury, or congenital defect, and the testing procedures can aid in monitoring the progression of disease.

Requirements

The request for and receipt of special reports for the resident's diagnostic services cannot be overlooked by the facility. As with laboratory diagnostic reporting, the facility should clearly define the process in policy and procedure and ensure that the policy is implemented and follow-through is complete. Reporting to the physician is also a step in the process that should be defined and follow-through monitored for compliance.

The physician must order all special testing procedures. When the special testing reports are received, the physician must be notified and orders written for management of identified issues. The interdisciplinary team must implement a care-planning process to ensure that the test results and physician orders are incorporated into the resident interventions and services. The tracking of a request for and receipt of special testing is essential to ensure that each resident's needs are met.

Each test that is ordered must have a correlating resulting report to file in the resident's health record. The results of diagnostic special reports should be filed in the resident's health record upon receipt of the reports.

Quality Requirements

Management of special test requests, results reporting, physician notification, and incorporation of care requirements into the resident's care plan are vital from a quality standpoint. The facility should ensure that these processes are in place and working efficiently to make certain that proper resident care needs are being served.

Assessment criteria may include the following:

- Special test requests are tracked.
- Special test results are received and compared to the test request checklist to ensure completion of the test.
- The physician is notified of special test results.
- The resident care plan is updated as indicated.
- Special test results are filed in a timely manner.
- Nursing notes reflect test results and actions taken if required by facility policy.

Placement of Documentation in the Health Record

Special reports are usually filed in the laboratory section of the resident's health record or contained in a separate section—"Special Reports" or "Radiology"—as defined by facility policy.

Reports found in this section may include:

- Chemistry
- Hematology
- Urinalysis
- Stool testing results
- EKG/ECG
- EEG
- Radiology reports
- Holter monitors
- Pulse oximetry

Other Pertinent Information

The facility should develop a policy and procedure for tracking and managing special results reporting documentation. The policy may contain the following criteria:

- Diagnostic reports
  - —Admission testing requirements (special diagnostic reports that accompany the resident on admission and after transfer and readmission)
  - —Annual testing requirements
  - —Other required testing (six months, three months or quarterly, every month, and so on)

- Telephone reporting of special diagnostic results

    —Further reporting to physician offices

    —STAT or "please call" results reporting

- Special diagnostic reports

    —Delivery methods and location

    —Review

    —Notification to physician

    —Notification to tracking mechanisms

    —Signature requirements

    —Distribution to specific units or stations

    —Placement in the resident's health record

    —Special diagnostic request and receipt tracking mechanisms and checks

    —Facsimile processing mechanisms

Content

Depending on the special diagnostic test, the contents may differ slightly, but at a minimum should contain the following criteria:

- Resident's name and health record number
- Unit or station and room
- Date of test
- Date of report
- Designation "preliminary" or "final"
- Name of test
- Results of test
- Impression
- Physician signature and date

Summary

Laboratory and special reports such as X rays, EKGs, Holter Monitor, MRI, CT scan, and respiratory tests must be included in the resident's health record. These reports contain the outcomes of testing procedures and provide valuable information on the resident's current health condition. Physician notification of test results must be completed according to federal and state requirements.

The facility should devise efficient systems to ensure that all ordered laboratory and special tests are completed, results reported, and reports filed in the resident's health record. There must be a process to ensure that resident care plans are updated as determined by test results.

Laboratory and special tests are ordered in response to resident symptoms and conditions. The results are extremely important to the provision of care to the resident. The test results may indicate resident improvement or decline and thus may trigger care plan review and revision. Test reports provide further diagnostic determinations to support the assessment and care-planning processes in long-term care.

Reference

Centers for Medicare and Medicaid Services. 2001 (October 31). Guidance to Surveyors—Long-Term Care Facilities, appendix PP in *State Operations Manual.* Available at www.cms.gov.

Chapter 17

Discharge Documentation

Before discussing discharge documentation, it is important to discuss and understand the federal requirements for transfer and discharge from a facility.

Federal Requirements Specific to the Facility for Transfer or Discharge of Residents

Federal regulations severely limit the facility's capability to transfer or discharge a resident after he or she has been admitted to the facility. This is to protect the rights to receive care. The resident may not be transferred or discharged unless:

1. Transfer or discharge is required to ensure the resident's welfare because his or her condition cannot be managed in the facility.

2. Transfer or discharge is required because the resident's health status has improved and no further services are necessary.

3. Transfer or discharge is required for reasons of safety.

4. Transfer or discharge is required to protect the health of other residents.

5. Transfer or discharge is necessary because the resident has failed to pay for the required stay after reasonable notice was provided. (The resident cannot be transferred or discharged from the facility for nonpayment if the bill has been submitted to a third-party payer.)

6. Transfer or discharge is required because the facility is closing.

Federal requirements mandate that should any of the first five scenarios occur, the resident's health record must reflect the events. For scenarios 1 and 2, the resident's attending or covering physician must document the reason for transfer or discharge in the resident's health record. Should scenario 4 occur, documentation by any physician must be completed in the resident's health record. "To demonstrate that any of the events specified in 1–5 have occurred, the law requires documentation in the resident's clinical record. To demonstrate situations 1 and 2, the resident's physician must provide the documentation. In situation 4, the documentation must be provided by any physician (See §483.12(a)(2))" (CMS 2001, PP-32).

The facility also must arrange adequate preparation and orientation for residents to ensure a careful discharge or transfer from the facility. In addition, federal regulations require the facility to notify the resident or resident's family or legal representative of the reasons for the transfer and to provide documentation of those reasons in the resident's health record. Notification must occur at least thirty days prior to transfer or discharge except when the transfer or discharge is necessary for one of the following reasons:

- Transfer or discharge is necessary to ensure the safety of others.

- Transfer or discharge is necessary because the resident's health has improved.

- Transfer or discharge is necessary medically because the resident's health has deteriorated.

When the resident's stay is less than thirty days, notification must be provided to the resident or the resident's legal representative as soon as possible.

The notice of transfer or discharge must contain information on the resident's right to appeal the facility's decision and the name, address, and telephone number of the state long-term care ombudsman. If the resident has a developmental disability, the notice also must contain the name, address, and telephone number of the advocate agency for the mentally ill.

Content of the notice before transfer must include the following components:

- Statement of advance notice (either thirty days or as soon as practicable, depending on the reason for transfer/discharge)

- Reason for transfer/discharge

- Effective date of transfer/discharge

- Location to which the resident was transferred/discharged

- Right of appeal

- How to notify the ombudsman (name, address, and telephone number)

- How to notify the appropriate protection and advocacy agency for residents with mental illness or mental retardation (mailing address and telephone numbers) and whether the facility notified a family member or legal representative of the proposed transfer or discharge (CMS 2001, PP-35).

Federal regulations also require that Medicaid-eligible residents be provided with a notice of the facility's bed-hold policy and readmission policies before transfer to an acute care hospital or for therapeutic leave. The resident, family member, or responsible party must be provided with a written notice that discusses the length of time for a bed hold within the facility. Additionally, the facility is required to have a policy that allows the resident eligible for Medicaid services who was transferred but did not return in the allotted bed-hold time frame to return to the facility in the first available bed.

The facility may want to consider adding to these policies the fact that the notice was indeed provided the resident upon transfer out of the facility by documenting it in the resident's health record for proof of compliance with these regulations.

Other Pertinent Information

The facility should have a detailed policy and procedure for transfer and discharge of a resident to ensure that federal regulations are followed in the institution. Moreover, it should have policies for bed hold and return after bed hold has expired.

Quality Requirements

Facilities should ensure that the notice of transfer contains all federal requirements. It also should be monitored to ensure that any state-specific regulations are included.

Assessment criteria that may be monitored to ensure that the transfer and discharge process is completed according to regulations are as follows:

- Accommodations of needs have been met.

- Reason for the transfer/discharge is documented by appropriate professionals as required by regulations.

- When the discharge is for safety reasons, documentation reflects the process by which the facility made the determination.

- Did the transfer or discharge occur after the payment source change?

- Are there reasons why the resident's need could not be met or documented?

Discharge Documentation

Federal regulations require that the reason or need for the transfer or discharge be documented in the resident's health record. In addition, each resident must be notified in writing of the reasons for the transfer or discharge and the facility bed-hold policy. For purposes of this discussion, discharge documentation refers to those records that must be completed at the time the resident is transferred to another facility or discharged from the facility. These documents include:

- Medication education and drug discharge documentation

- Clinical discharge summaries or recap of the stay

- Comprehensive assessment

- Discharge plan of care

- Transfer form

- Physician discharge summary

"Transfer and discharge includes movement of a resident to a bed outside of the certified facility whether that bed is in the same physical plant or not. Transfer and discharge does not refer to movement of a resident to a bed within the same certified facility" (CMS 2001, PP-32). The documentation discussed in this chapter is required for these occasions.

The purpose of discharge documentation is to record the summary of the resident's stay in the facility. This type of documentation provides a concise recapitulation of the resident's stay and health status at discharge or transfer.

General Requirements

Although there are no federal regulations for disciplines to recap the resident's stay, it is considered good practice for each discipline that has cared for the resident to complete a form of discharge summary documentation. Nursing may be required by state or facility policy to do a discharge note instead of a formal summary. State regulations and facility practice also may mandate that therapists, dietitians, and physicians complete a "recap" of the resident's stay and include it in the resident's record upon discharge. Upon an emergent transfer to an acute care facility, therapists and dietitians may not write formal summaries but, rather, a final progress note that discharges them from service. State regulations may dictate when to specifically document discharge summaries or transfer summaries.

Documentation at transfer or discharge captures the resident's stay and provides a condensed, thorough synopsis of the resident's health status and overall care, including any procedures done during that visit.

Documentation of discharges made **against medical advice** (AMA) should contain a release of responsibility. The facility should have a policy on the AMA discharge to include pertinent discussions with the resident.

Education provided the resident at the time of discharge also should be documented, such as therapy education and education concerning dietary need and requirements.

Discharge Instructions

Discharge instructions are directions given the resident that explain the necessary care requirements he or she is to follow after being discharged from the facility. These include medications, therapy, dietary and nursing instructions, and/or scheduled appointments for follow-up in the community. Moreover, the discharge instructions may include community services that the resident can use.

Purpose of Discharge Instructions

The purpose of discharge instructions is to ensure that the resident receives the care he or she needs after being released from the facility. They are written in simple terms to ensure that the resident (1) has the required information, (2) understands the information, and (3) has contact information, if necessary.

General Requirements

State regulations may mandate the need for discharge instructions. Federal requirements call for a postdischarge plan of care.

The facility should have a policy for completion of the discharge documentation that is required. Check state regulations to determine if discharge instructions are needed in the specific state and determine when the instructions are necessary to ensure compliance.

A nurse, case manager, or discharge planner usually completes the discharge instructions. Therapy, dietary, and social services instructions may be completed by appropriate personnel and signed and dated. State requirements also may dictate who must sign discharge instructions.

Discharge instructions must be completed prior to the resident's discharge and be given to the resident at discharge.

Discharge Instructions Provided to the Resident

The discharge instructions or postdischarge plan of care provides a comprehensive means of providing the resident or continued care providers with a set of directions for continued treatment, home programs, or community services. When discharge instructions are provided directly to the resident, it is extremely important to ensure that the discharge instruction sheet contains only language that the resident will understand. Abbreviations are not acceptable because many abbreviations can mean more than one thing. Common language makes the documentation easy to understand and leaves fewer needs for clarification. Figure 17.1 offers a comparison of acceptable and unacceptable language for use in discharge instructions.

The resident always should receive the original discharge instructions. A photocopy or **no-carbon-required** (NCR) copy of the form should be placed in the resident's health record.

Quality Requirements

The issue of layman's terms is the most important quality issue for discharge instructions. Another area of concern is that of ensuring that the document is complete. If areas of the form are not applicable, the form should be so noted with "not applicable" rather than the abbreviation N/A, which is not necessarily a layman's term.

The following assessment criteria may be used to monitor discharge instructions:

- Discharge instructions are written in plain language.

- The discharge instructions contain no inappropriate abbreviations.

- Discharge instructions are included in the resident's health record.

Placement of Documentation in the Health Record

Discharge instructions are placed in the discharge section of the resident's health record.

Content

The discharge instruction may contain the following information:

- Resident name and health record number

- Therapy instructions

Figure 17.1.   **Unacceptable and acceptable language**

Unacceptable Language	Acceptable Language
$\uparrow$ movement as instructed	Be sure to walk short distances every 2 hours.
$\downarrow$ concentrate sweets	Do not eat sweet foods such as cakes or brownies.
NAS diet	Do not add salt to your food.
Shift $\leftarrow$ to $\rightarrow$ in bed	Remember to change bed positions often.
Use O_2 as needed.	Use your oxygen as you need to.
Use assistive devices PRN.	Be sure to use your cane as you need it.
If C/O SOB call your physician.	If you get short of breath, call your doctor.
$\uparrow$ ® leg	Elevate your right leg when sitting.
$\varnothing$ bending > 90°	Do not bend more than 90 degrees.

- Social services information

- Diet and specific instructions

- Special instructions or activities

- Discharge plan

- Mode of transportation

- Follow-up services

- Destination

- Reason for the discharge

- Discharge date and time

- Resident or representative signature and date

- Other required signatures and dates

Comprehensive Assessment

The comprehensive assessment requirement for discharge contains a minimum amount of required data for the submission. The information is captured on the discharge tracking form.

The purpose of the discharge tracking form is to ensure that there is a mechanism to track each resident's location. The form was established by the Centers for Medicare and Medicaid Services (CMS) to identify the resident's location. It is an extremely modified form with minimum data to be submitted to the state as outlined in the MDS submission guidelines. The professional staff who are required to complete the form must be sure that the data are reported accurately.

The Comprehensive Assessment Discharge Process

The discharge tracking form is required when a resident is discharged from the institution except for brief home visits, other temporary leaves of absence, or when he or she is seen in an acute care facility observation unit. If the resident is admitted to the acute care facility from the observation unit, the discharge tracking form is required. It is the only form that is required at the time of discharge from the facility.

General Requirements

The correct reason for the discharge must be documented on the discharge tracking form in section AA8a. There are three choices:

- Section AA8a, number 6: The resident was discharged with no anticipated return.

- Section AA8a, number 7: The resident was discharged with an anticipated return.

- Section AA8a, number 8: The resident was discharged before the initial assessment was completed.

The MDS discharge tracking form must be completed within seven days of the date of R4. The form must be submitted to the state within thirty-one days of the date of R4. Accuracy of the data is important because it ensures data quality, which reflects the resident's current health condition.

Placement of Documentation in the Health Record

The discharge tracking form may be placed in the comprehensive assessment and care-planning section of the chart as the last MDS assessment form or at the front of the chart upon discharge.

Content

The discharge tracking form contains the following information:

- Section AA, items 1 through 9 (Item 8 content requires only one of the three discharge codes.)

- Section AB, items 1 and 2

- Section A, item A6

- Section R, items 3 and 4

Postdischarge Plan of Care

Federal regulations require a **postdischarge plan of care** that is documented in conjunction with the resident or the resident's family or responsible party. This care plan must be as comprehensive as the plans used for treatments, interventions, and services provided in the nursing facility.

A post-discharge plan of care for an anticipated discharge applies to a resident whom the facility discharges to a private residence, to another NF or SNF, or to another type of residential facility such as a board and care home or an intermediate care facility for individuals with mental retardation. A 'post-discharge plan of care' means the discharge planning process which includes: assessing continuing care needs and developing a plan designed to ensure the individual's needs will be met after discharge from the facility into the community (CMS 2001, PP-82.6).

The purpose of the postdischarge plan of care is to assist the resident in adapting to his or her new living arrangement.

Postdischarge Plan Components

The postdischarge plan of care must be comprehensive just as the plan of care was while the resident received care in the facility. It should include details on how to gain the care needed and where to gain the services identified. This plan is important to ensure that the resident continues to attain or maintain the highest practicable level of physical and psychosocial well-being.

The postdischarge plan of care should contain the following information:

- Resident's and family's preferences for care

- Description of how to access the services needed

- Coordination of care when there are identified needs for multiple caregivers

- Specific needs such as personal care, dressing requirements, therapy needs, educational requirements, and the means to obtain the care identified

When the resident leaves the security of the facility and the care provided by the interdisciplinary team, he or she needs to feel confident that the discharge plan will continue to provide the services and treatment needed to continue to make gains or hold gains that have been achieved. The resident and resident's family should feel confident that they have the ability and understanding to continue to gain or to provide the necessary needs of the resident. The comprehensive postdischarge plan provides that security to the resident even after leaving the facility.

Discharge Process

The discharge process should begin before admission or at least at admission to the facility. Discharge planning will be documented as outlined by facility policy. The policy should identify the person responsible for discharge planning in the facility. The policy on discharge planning will outline the necessary documentation required for the process.

The postdischarge plan should be completed and necessary education provided to the patient prior to discharge.

State regulations also may contain criteria for discharge planning and a specific postdischarge plan. These state-specific requirements also will be contained in any discharge planning policies and procedures to ensure that the facility has a thorough process in place.

Quality Requirements

The postdischarge plan and the planning process must be completed as described by facility policy and procedure, which incorporates federal and state requirements for the process. To ensure quality outcomes, the process must be complete and accurately documented.

Assessment criteria for the postdischarge plan of care may include the following:

- Postdischarge planning is complete.
- Postdischarge plans include needed care requirements.
- Community services required by the resident have been identified.
- Postdischarge education was provided to the resident.

Placement of Documentation in the Health Record

The postdischarge plan is contained in the care plan section of the resident's health record. The discharge instructions may be a piece of the postdischarge plan and are filed as indicated earlier in the chapter.

Federally Required Discharge Summary

When discharges are planned for those residents being sent home or to another facility, federal regulations require completion of a summary of the resident's stay based on the comprehensive assessment in addition to the postdischarge plan of care and the comprehensive assessment discharge tracking form.

This **discharge summary** is not the physical discharge summary but, rather, a discharge summary based on the comprehensive assessment. It is a recapitulation of the resident's visit.

The purpose of the discharge summary is to provide a summary of the resident's stay at the facility, which is used in conjunction with the postdischarge plan of care to provide continuity of care for the resident upon discharge from the facility.

The discharge summary is used with the postdischarge plan of care to ensure individualized discharge planning and notification of essential health-related information to the continuing care provider.

Discharge Charge Summary Requirements

The discharge summary must include a recapitulation of the resident's stay and descriptions of any significant changes in the resident's physical or mental condition, including declines and improvements, such as major:

- Changes in the resident's activities of daily living (ADLs)

- Changes in the number of behavioral symptoms

- Changes in decision-making ability

- Changes in incontinence patterns

- Changes in mood

- Weight loss or gain

- Changes in the use of trunk restraints

- Changes in the incidence of pressure ulcers

- Improvement or deterioration of resident's condition

The federal government mandates this discharge summary.

The discharge summary must be "available for release to authorized persons and agencies" and thus must be completed at the time of discharge (CMS 2001, PP-82.5).

Quality Requirements

Assessment criteria for the discharge summary are similar to those required for completion of the comprehensive assessment.

Placement of Documentation in the Health Record

The discharge summary is placed in a designated section of the health record.

Interagency Transfer Form

The interagency transfer form (W-10) must be completed for each resident who is discharged from the facility. Its form may be driven by state requirements. It provides a detailed account of the resident's conditions, medications, treatments, diet, and possible medical equipment required.

The interagency transfer form consists of fundamental medical facts about the resident to ensure that continued care is provided. The purpose of the interagency transfer form is to provide continuity of care to the resident upon discharge from the facility.

Interagency Transfer Form Process

Nursing facilities must receive the interagency transfer form, also known as a W-10, from the resident's physician at admission, which certifies that nursing home care is appropriate for him or her. The interagency transfer form is used on discharge to house all of the resident's healthcare needs in one form that is easily accessible and identifiable to the professional who will continue to provide care to the resident. It is used for all discharges except deaths.

Completion of the interagency transfer form provides the healthcare providers with important health data concerning the resident. A physician must sign the interagency transfer form, which may be used as the initial physician order for continued resident care after the resident is discharged from the long-term care environment.

The interagency transfer form should be completed for all resident discharges as defined by facility policy with the exception of deaths or AMA discharges. Moreover, it must be completed at the time of discharge and accompany the resident when he or she leaves the facility.

The form is a permanent part of the resident's health record. The original interagency transfer form is sent to the clinical establishment providing the required care, a copy is kept for permanent filing in the resident's health record, and a second copy is typically provided to the transport services for billing, if necessary. For those instances where the resident provides his or her own transportation, this copy is not needed.

Clinical establishments providing the required care may include:

- Acute care hospitals
- Other nursing or skilled nursing homes
- Physician offices
- Home health agencies
- Visiting Nurse Association (VNA)
- Therapy clinics
- Hospices
- Other healthcare providers

Quality Requirements

Because the interagency transfer form provides extensive health information about the resident, completion of the form in its entirety is necessary. As stated earlier, the health information on the form should reflect the resident's current health status, medications, special requirements, or equipment required and dietary needs.

The assessment criteria for the interagency transfer form may include the components of the form itself such as:

- Insurance information is included.
- All special needs are contained on the form.
- Diet is included.
- Diagnoses accurately reflect the resident's condition.
- Physician has signed the form.
- Form is complete with all data elements addressed even if "NA."

Placement of Documentation in the Health Record

The discharge interagency transfer form is usually placed in with other discharge records in a designated section of the resident's record.

Content

The transfer form is extensive and can be easily adapted for each long-term care facility as long as the required elements are included. The form typically includes the following elements:

- Resident's name, address, and telephone number
- Gender
- Date of birth
- Admission date
- Discharge date
- Martial status
- Religion
- Responsible party, relationship, and telephone number
- Referred by facility name, contact person/unit, and telephone number
- Referred to facility name, contact person/unit, and telephone number
- Follow-up by name and address of the physician or clinic, telephone number, and date of appointment
- Health record number
- Medicare number
- Social Security number
- Department of income maintenance number or social services number, as appropriate
- Other insurance numbers
- Pertinent history, diagnoses, and reason for transfer
- Skin condition
- Advance directives
- Organ donor
- Medications, frequency, last given
- Allergies
- Diagnosis given and prognosis
- Clinician's name to whom an explanation has been provided
- Therapeutic goals
- Resident service start date
- Services required (nursing, occupational therapy, speech therapy, physical therapy, home health aid, other)

- Treatment for condition for which the resident was hospitalized

- Resident homebound

- Certification for listed services provided by acute care, chronic hospital, SNF, ICF, home health agency, rehab center

- Physician signature and date

Other data that may be added by the facility include the following:

- Behavioral status

- Vital signs

- Diet

- Cognitive status

- Personal needs, such as bathing, dressing, transfer, toileting, feeding, meal preparation, administration of medication (identified as independent [I], supervision [S], physical assistance [PA], total dependence [TD], and/or tube feed [TF])

- Purified protein derivative (of tuberculin) (PPD) testing results

- Lab/X rays

- Speech (not impaired versus impaired)

- Sight (not impaired versus impaired)

- Restraints

- Height and weight

- Bladder control

- Bowel control

- Glasses

- Cane or walker

- Prosthetics

- Dentures

- Ostomy appliance

- Hearing aid

- Responsible party notified

- Previous hospitalization dates

Physician Discharge Summary

There is no federal requirement for a physician to complete a discharge summary at the time of the resident's discharge from the facility. However, the physician discharge summary may be mandated by state-specific regulations.

A physician discharge summary is a complete medical synopsis of the resident's stay at the long-term care facility. The purpose of the physician discharge summary is to consolidate the resident's stay into one document for easy review and to help further the continuing care of the resident.

Discharge planning starts at the time of admission and includes the entire interdisciplinary team, including the physician. The postdischarge plan, the nonphysician discharge summary, and the physician discharge summary all address the particular needs of the resident and include postdischarge instructions and plans for follow-up care as indicated by specific resident needs. These three separate, yet interrelated, documents help convey the facts of the resident's visit and current health condition to those clinical professionals who will become responsible for the continued care of the resident.

Discharge Summary Process

The resident's discharge summary should completely and accurately describe his or her condition at the time of discharge. Each diagnosis that has been established during the resident's long-term care stay should be listed, using no abbreviations for clarity.

The facility should have a policy and procedure that outlines the process for capturing the physician discharge summary and pertinent components that are required by state-specific requirements. In addition, the facility may choose to create a form or have a format for dictation readily available for the physician to use for each discharge summary documented.

State-specific requirements, accrediting agencies, and facility policy will drive the timeliness of the documentation of a physician discharge summary. The Joint Commission on Accreditation of Healthcare Organizations (JCAHO) requires that all physician discharge summaries be completed within thirty days of discharge.

Quality Requirements

The physician discharge summary is a vital document that can support the physician's involvement in the resident's care and care-planning process. Incorporated within the physician's discharge summary are those medical treatments that are required to ensure that the resident receives continued care and interventions. Also discussed in the document are the medical interventions and services the resident utilized during his or her stay at the facility. The quality of the documentation is a key component of physician quality assurance programs and can be used to facilitate the physician credentialing process.

States may have specific criteria that must be included in the physician discharge summary. These criteria should be included in the assessment criteria that are examined through the quality process.

Assessment criteria for the physician discharge summary may include the following:

- Diagnoses are documented without abbreviations.

- Physician discharge summary is completed within the specified time frame as required by regulations and facility policy.

- Procedures performed during the stay are present.

- Test results are present.

- Condition on discharge is documented.

- Physician signature and date are present.

Placement of Documentation in the Health Record

The physician discharge summary may be placed with other discharge records in a designated section of the resident's health record.

Other Pertinent Information

A brief narrative progress note should be entered into the resident's health record at the time of discharge. The information contained in the note may include:

- Date and time of discharge
- Disposition
- Condition at discharge
- Discharged destination
- Individual taking responsibility for the resident

Content

The physician discharge summary may contain the following information:

- Resident name and health record number
- Admission date
- Discharge date
- Reason for admission
- Weight loss (if yes, interventions)
- Disposition
- Complications
- Discharge diagnosis to include principal and all secondary pertinent diagnoses with no abbreviations
- Discharge recommendations
- History of the resident stay
- Laboratory/radiology findings
- Functional level at discharge
- Physician signature and date
- Physician extender signature, if applicable, and date

Summary

Federal regulations limit the ability of long-term care facilities to transfer or discharge residents after they have been admitted. The facility must prepare residents for discharge and provide documentation of the reasons for the move in the resident's health record.

Discharge documentation stipulations may be found within federal, state, and accrediting agency requirements. Discharge documentation may encompass a number of elements and reports. For example, the facility must give discharge instructions to the resident at discharge. These instructions must be written in simple terms and explain the care requirements the resident must follow after discharge from the facility. Medication education and drug discharge documentation demonstrate that the resident has been educated on each drug in his or her regime at discharge. Clinical discharge summaries or recaps of the resident's stay are documents that provide a means for the clinician to give a concise recap of the resident's stay at the facility. The comprehensive assessment form captures the discharge information for MDS submission. The discharge plan of care is a report that provides the plan of care for the resident's discharge.

The interagency transfer form provides detailed data about the resident's health status and current health condition. This report contains detailed, concise information to help facilitate the care at the receiving facility. It must accompany each resident at discharge or transfer. State-specific requirements may drive the content of this form. The physician discharge summary (if required) is usually a detailed recap of the stay from the physician's perspective. It provides the medical summary of the resident's stay at the facility.

References

Centers for Medicare and Medicaid Services. 2001 (October 31). Guidance to Surveyors—Long-Term Care Facilities, appendix PP in *State Operations Manual*. Available at www.cms.gov.

Joint Commission on Accreditation of Healthcare Organizations. 2004. *Comprehensive Accreditation Manual for Long-term Care*. Oakbrook Terrace, Ill.: JCAHO.

Chapter 18

Accident and Incident Reports

Accidents or incidents occasionally occur in the long-term care setting as they do in other settings. When they happen, they must be reported and the facts of the event must be documented in the resident's health record. An example of an accident or incident may be a fall, a minor injury, a broken bone, a cut, or the like. Facility staff may make an error that also would require reporting, such as the right medication given with an adverse effect or a dose of medication that was not given.

Bumps, falls, and mistakes do happen. When they occur, the facility should have a policy and procedure in place to report them. The incident report (or, as it is coming to be known, the occurrence report) is completed as outlined and sent to the risk manager or appointed personnel for follow-up and investigation. The actual report of the occurrence is never documented in the resident's health record.

Categories of Accidents and Incidents

Accidents and **incidents** are those mishaps, misfortunes, mistakes, events, or occurrences that may happen during the normal daily routines and activities in the long-term care setting. However, regardless of how minor an accident or incident is, it must be reported to the designated personnel.

The purpose of the accident and incident report is to identify the event and investigate its cause and possible solutions so that it does not occur again.

Accidents and incidents may be classified into different categories, as follows:

- Events that have caused a death or may present an immediate danger of death or serious injury

- Outbreaks of disease or outbreaks of food-borne disease

- Abuse of a resident

- An event such as loss of power, heat, water, or so on that may necessitate evacuating one or more residents to a safe inside location or another outside location

- Fires

- A serious injury or significant change in a resident's condition

- A medication error of clinical significance

- An adverse drug reaction of clinical significance

- Minor injuries, distress, or discomfort to a resident, such as minor falls, bruises, and cuts

General Requirements

There are no federal requirements for accident or incident reports. States may have specific regulations or requirements as may accrediting agencies.

State law drives some of the reporting requirements to state public health agencies and or public safety agencies.

The facility should have a policy in place that discusses these categories of accidents and incidents and fully outlines what is expected of staff when these events occur within the facility.

The facility policy should cover the following areas:

- Purpose

- Policy statement

- Procedure

- Reporting the accident or incident

- Assisting accident and incident victims

- Burn reporting

- Department of Mental Retardation notification

- Medical device reporting

    —Malfunction of medical device

    —User error

- Reportable events for each accident or incident

- When report is required for each accident or incident

- Timeliness of reporting for each accident or incident

- What forms to use for each accident or incident

- Where to file reports for each accident or incident

- Responsibility for reports and documentation for each accident or incident

- Responsibility for investigation for each accident or incident

- Responsibility for follow-up for each accident or incident

- Responsibility for review for each accident or incident

- When to use cause-and-effect analysis

- Sentinel event reporting specifics

- Categories of accident and incidents

- What events get reported to outside authorities with time frames

- Filing systems/techniques for report retention (each is numbered, each is classified, and so on)

When an incident occurs, the facts of the occurrence should be documented as outlined by facility policy. However, documentation does not indicate that an incident report has been filed nor does it refer to the report in the documentation. However, the resident's health record must reflect the facts of the injury and how it was received. Facilities should not document what is unknown, only the facts as presented at the time of the accident or injury. The policy the facility has developed for the management of accidents and incidents should be followed.

The following two examples illustrate appropriate and inappropriate reporting of an injury:

- *Incorrect:* Resident fell and complains of broken bone in leg. Occurrence report filed.

- *Correct:* Resident fell and complains of pain in leg. No swelling, area is red. Called physician. Physician ordered X rays of leg. Results are pending.

Care Planning after the Incident or Occurrence

Accidents and injuries affect the resident's condition, even when they are minor. Assessing the resident after an accident or incident ensures that he or she receives appropriate care and that care planning is accurately reflected.

Care provisions are the important aspect of accident and incident reporting, followed by investigative techniques to ensure that problems are identified, issues are resolved, and/or solutions are found. Just documenting an accident or incident does nothing to ensure proper care provisions, investigations, solutions, or resolutions to possible problems or process faults.

Documentation of follow-up notes should be continued in the resident's health record until the injury is resolved. The resident's care plan must be updated as well.

Documentation of the Event

Documentation of the facts provides a means to capture the resident's current condition and provides a legal record of the facts as they occurred.

The report of the accident or incident allows the facility the opportunity to provide in-depth investigation into possible cause and effect. Further examination may provide the opportunity to make improvements in processes, equipment, behavior, or the facility, if needed.

Quality Requirements

The quality of documentation is a crucial factor in health record charting. Accidents and incidents that must be reported to public health agencies may require investigation by state authorities. When documentation is inadequate, the finding may not be favorable for the facility. Following facility policy for accident and incident reporting is an extremely vital component of the entire process.

Documentation includes not only charting the facts in the resident's record, but also ensuring that the incident or occurrence report is complete and accurate as well. Each area on the report must be addressed completely.

Timeliness of documentation should be outlined in the facility policy on accidents and incidents, and the policy must be followed as outlined.

The quality indicator (QI) reports do provide the capability for reporting the identified sentinel event triggers that are reported to the state through the Minimum Data Set (MDS) submission. Patient safety initiatives are under way in hospital settings to ensure that patients receive high-quality care. States are now introducing legislation to mandate adverse event reporting by hospitals. Although this specific initiative is not yet a requirement of the long-term care industry, facilities should be vigilant in tracking, investigating, and reporting adverse events not considered sentinel events to oversight agencies.

Quality Requirements

Quality assessment criteria may include the following:

- The resident's health record reflects the facts of the accident or incident.
- The resident assessment is completed in a timely manner.
- Documentation is done in a timely manner according to policy.
- The incident or occurrence report is complete.
- The incident or occurrence report is filed in a timely manner.
- Investigation is completed in a timely manner with appropriate follow-up provided.
- Accidents and incidents that must be reported to public health agencies are reported in a timely manner.
- The resident's care plan is updated as appropriate and necessary.

Placement of Documentation in the Health Record

Placement of the documentation of the accident or incident should be charted as outlined in facility policy. Some facilities may require the documentation to be placed on progress notes; others may require it to be charted in the nursing narrative notes. Placement of the assessment must be followed as outlined.

The actual report of the accident or incident does not get filed in the resident's health record. Facility policy should specify where these reports are filed. Moreover, facility policy should reflect retention schedules for keeping such accident and incident or occurrence reports.

Content

The content of a typical incident or occurrence report may contain the following:

- Classification of the incident or occurrence
- Facility license number
- Year
- Level of care
- Bed capacity
- Original report
- Subsequent report
- Licensure classification of facility
- Institution
- Address

- Date
- Name of persons involved (employees and residents, if applicable)
- Address
- Age
- Sex
- Resident information

  —Name

  —Date of admission

  —Diagnosis

  —Condition before occurrence (mental/physical)

  —Condition after occurrence (mental/physical)

- Employee

  —Name

  —Department

  —Title

  —Returned to work with little or no treatment

  —Sent home

  —Sent to hospital

  —Name of hospital

- Visitor or other identified person
- Date of occurrence
- Time of occurrence
- Exact location
- Witnesses (names and titles)
- Part of body injured
- Restraint used (describe)
- Exact description of occurrence
- Name of attending physician and address
- Physician notified, date, and time
- Date and time physician completed the examination
- Physician's finding and orders
- Notification of family (name of person notified, date, and time)
- Insurance company (name of company, date, time, and how notified)

- Administration (name, signature, date, and time)
- Name of person making report (signature, title, date, and time)

Specific reports to report medical device and burns may differ from state to state. Please refer to the facility-specific policy for details on correct form use.

Summary

Accidents and incidents do occur. The facility should be fully prepared to manage these types of occurrences. The facility should outline in policy the person within the institution responsible for overseeing and carrying out the incident or occurrence reporting process. Each accident or incident should be reported and tracked to ensure that problems are identified and that solutions to the problem are developed and implemented.

Facility policy should classify categories of incidents and initiate processes to manage each grouping. These categories would typically range from minor occurrences to major, life-threatening events.

Incident or occurrence reports are completed for any type of accident or injury regardless of severity or simplicity. Incident or occurrence reports concerning resident accidents or incidents are never filed in the resident's health record. However, the resident's health record documentation should contain the detailed objective facts surrounding the incident, which include a description of the accident, any injuries involved, the medical treatment or interventions initiated, and outcomes of the immediate care provided. Follow-up notes should be documented, as needed, until the injury is resolved.

Reporting to external agencies also must be completed on a timely basis as outlined in the facility policy on accidents and incidents. Managing accidents and incidents is an important aspect of care for each long-term care facility. Effective management of accidents and incidents will help control adverse outcomes and provide a healthful environment for every resident.

References

American Health Information Management Association. 2001. Long-Term Care Health Information Practice and Documentation Guidelines. Available at www.ahima.org.

State of Connecticut. 2002. *An Act Creating a Program for Quality in Health Care.* Available at http://www.cga.state.ct.us.

Chapter 19

Data Quality and Coding Issues

"The services provided or arranged by the facility must meet professional standards of quality and be provided by qualified persons in accordance with each resident's written plan of care" (CMS 2001, PP-82.3–82.5).

Data quality and coding are pertinent issues in the long-term care environment. Data quality hinges on complete documentation and accurate coding practice. It influences the Minimum Data Set (MDS) submission process and subsequent quality indicators (QIs) and ORYX outcomes as well as the coding process, which is an integral part of the reimbursement process in long-term care.

The Joint Commission on Accreditation of Healthcare Organizations (JCAHO) performance initiative ORYX uses outcome data as part of the accreditation process and to monitor the performance of organizations on a quarterly basis. The JCAHO intends to use this continuous monitoring process to supplant the three-year accreditation format it currently uses. Facilities that do not comply with ORYX risk loss of accreditation. ORYX indicators are used to continuously assess key performance processes and present an ongoing picture of skilled nursing performance.

Data quality and accuracy is crucial to documentation and reimbursement practices because it provides the level of detail needed for high-quality resident outcomes, resident care planning and assessment processes, appropriate coding practices, and final reimbursement. Ultimately, data quality and accuracy supports decision making, not only in the resident care areas, but also at the administrative level.

Because data quality and accuracy is crucial in coding and reimbursement practices, the facility should provide education to staff concerning work flow processes, data collection and abstraction, and data integrity. The long-term care facility should have both a quality improvement program and a compliance plan that includes correct coding practices and the importance of data quality throughout the organization.

Qualitative and Quantitative Monitoring Processes

The facility may consider implementing qualitative and quantitative monitoring processes. The quality improvement program would define reporting and follow-up mechanisms, the quality improvement committee, auditing and monitoring systems (including focus audits for identified problem areas or concerns), and QI and survey or licensure issues.

Communication must also be a priority because many problems can be avoided if cooperation and information-sharing is an established standard among HIM, coding and billing staff, physicians and other care providers, and other departments. Although specific coding problems vary in each facility, reviewing and evaluating coding, payment, and compliance practices tend to reveal the same three weaknesses. These are:

- Lack of information
- Inadequate or faulty documentation
- Poor communication between physicians and coders (Hapner 2001)

The compliance plan should incorporate all of the following departmental compliances:

- **Chargemaster** review

- Coding and documentation practices

- Coding validation audit

- Review of the health record documentation to determine the extent that documentation supports the bill

- Denial review to determine potential problems

Health record compliance plans should include the following components:

- Mission statement

- Code of ethics

- AHIMA Standards of Ethical Coding

- Oversight for the program

- Organizational chart

- Coding structure

- Coder qualifications

- Job descriptions

- Policies pertinent to coding/billing for the department

- Documentation practice policies

- Retention policy

- Education

- Committee descriptions, as appropriate

Also for consideration of long-term care facilities is the **Nursing Home Quality Initiative.** The Centers for Medicare and Medicaid Services (CMS) has performed a pilot project in six states that identifies quality measures that reflect the quality of care in nursing homes. "The

6-state pilot is the first step in the Nursing Home Quality Initiative, a campaign to improve the quality of care in Nursing Homes. This new initiative will hold nursing homes more accountable for the quality of care they give" (CMS 2003). The quality initiative intends to provide consumers with the ability to compare nursing homes and to make decisions about the care they may receive in the long-term care setting. The Nursing Home Quality Initiative was implemented in November 2002.

Ten approved measures have been identified for monitoring the quality of care in a nursing home. (See figure 19.1.)

The following criteria were used to guide our decisions:

1. The measures must be both valid and reliable.
2. To the extent possible, the measures used for the national rollout should be consistent with those in the pilot.
3. Changes to the measures should be based on clear and obvious lessons learned from the pilot, from the validation, and from comments received from our partners.
4. Where a possible change is open to much debate, we left the measure for now, and will let the debate occur via the National Quality Forum (NQF) process (CMS 2002, p. 1).

The CMS is committed to the public reporting of quality measures and guarantees to their beneficiaries and their families that information will be shared in a "timely fashion." This initiative was developed to allow individuals to have the information to make an informed decision about the selection of an appropriate nursing facility should they ever need to consider placement for themselves or a family member.

The MDS 3.0 is scheduled to be released for use in nursing homes beginning in 2004.

Data Quality

Data quality encompasses the accuracy, conformity, completeness, consistency, integrity, and validity of the data that are gathered and reported for the MDS process, health record documentation practice, and coding and reimbursement, as well as quality initiatives within the facility and at the state and federal levels. If the data submitted for MDS assessments and coding for reimbursement are not accurate, complete, consistent, or valid, or do not conform to the

Figure 19.1.   Measures for monitoring quality of care

The quality measures (without facility admission profile [FAP] unless otherwise designated) that will be reported are as follows:

*   Residents with a loss of ability in basic daily tasks
*   Residents with pressure ulcers
*   Residents with pressure ulcers (with FAP)
*   Residents with pain
*   Residents in physical restraints
*   Residents with infections
*   Short-stay residents with delirium
*   Short-stay residents with delirium (with FAP)
*   Short-stay residents with pain
*   Short-stay residents who walk or walk better (with FAP)

requirements and do not ensure integrity, they are a serious risk to the facility. The MDS data will produce inaccurate QI and quality measure reports, bills will not be paid, and the health record will not substantiate the facility's legal business.

Obviously, the purpose of data quality is to ensure that the resident's health information is precise. The resident's health information contains not only his or her health record, but also the billing information that is gathered to generate bills and obtain reimbursement for services. Without data quality, the resident's health information is unreliable.

In figure 19.2, a section of a form is provided and contains many fields that require data entry. The figure demonstrates poor data quality because many areas of the form remain blank.

Figure 19.3 shows a form with complete data fields, but contradictions are present within the form. This, again, is poor data quality and will lead to poor facility outcomes.

Data quality is important in the long-term care environment and an integral part of each of the following:

- The admission process and placing the resident in the appropriate setting

- Documentation practice and the final health record

- The assessment and reassessment process and subsequent care planning

- The MDS process, which triggers the QI, QM, and ORYX reporting, and RUGs assignment

- Coding and subsequent reimbursement practices

- Optimal resident care

- Resident safety

Figure 19.2.   Sample of poor data quality due to incomplete data

XXX Organization
Anytown, USA 00000

Resident Name: Jane Doe   Health Record Number: 77-66-55

Nursing Flow Sheet

Date	11 to 7	7 to 3	3 to 11		11 to 7	7 to 3	3 to 11
Hygiene				**Bowel**			
Bed bath	ej		cp	Continent	ej	nj	cp
Shower	NA		cp	Incontinent			
Oral care		nj	cp	Enema			
Peri care			cp	Suppository			
Bladder				**Activity**			
Continent	ej	nj		Awake		nj	cp
Incontinent	NA	NA	NA	Napping	ej	nj	NA
Catheter	NA		NA	Turned	ej	nj	cp
Last void	NA	8a	10p	Bed transfer		nj	cp

Figure 19.3. Sample of poor data quality due to contradictory data

XXX Organization
Anytown, USA 00000

Resident Name: Jane Doe

Health Record Number: 77-66-55

Nursing Flow Sheet

Date	11 to 7	7 to 3	3 to 11		11 to 7	7 to 3	3 to 11
Hygiene				**Bowel**			
Bed bath	ej	NA	cp	Continent	ej	nj	cp
Shower	NA	nj	cp	Incontinent	NA	NA	NA
Oral care	ej	nj	cp	Enema	NA	NA	NA
Peri care	ej	nj	cp	Suppository	NA	NA	NA
Bladder				**Activity**			
Continent	ej	nj	cp	Awake	NA	nj	cp
Incontinent	NA	NA	NA	Napping	ej	nj	NA
Catheter	NA	NA	NA	Turned	ej	nj	cp
Last void	NA	8a	10p	Bed transfer	NA	nj	cp

- Continuity of care
- High-quality resident care
- State, federal, and accreditation process

The lack of quality of documentation impacts each of these areas and, of course, translates to poor data quality. The accurate, timely, and complete documentation of key processes in the long-term care setting has a major influence on the outcomes of the facility operations but, more important, ensures higher-quality resident outcomes as well. The visionary concept of data quality in long-term care enhances information flow, communication, complete documentation practice, high quality, accurate care planning, and outcomes that provide the resident with the best possible care and quality of life, which directly reflect on the organization's success and image.

General Requirements

General documentation requirements support data quality. The specific documentation requirements for long-term care are discussed in each chapter of this book. It is imperative that these guidelines be followed and all health record forms be completed thoroughly and accurately. Remember, if it is not documented, it did not happen. The Long Term Care and Subacute Medical Record Review Form for Open and Closed Medical Records is available from the Joint Commission on Accreditation of Healthcare Organizations (JCAHO) Web site (www.jcaho.org) and is a valuable tool for monitoring documentation practice and completeness of health records. Both open and closed health records should be monitored for completeness. Completing the audit on open charts provides the opportunity to correct problem areas using proper documentation guidelines while the audit of closed records provides a mechanism for monitoring discharge documentation practice. It encompasses the following criteria:

- Assessments and reassessments

- Physician visits

- Subacute criteria

- Demographic data

Coding Guidelines

Official coding guidelines must be followed when coding resident diagnoses (available at www.cdc.gov/nchs/data/icdguide.pdf.) These guidelines provide the foundation for proper coding assignment and are a valuable source of information for those employees with coding responsibility.

Also, the American Health Information Management Association (AHIMA) publishes an excellent reference book, *ICD-9-CM Coding for Long-Term Care,* that provides important information to further define and explain proper coding practice for the long-term care setting. In addition, coding professionals should be familiar with the CPT procedural coding classification system, which is used for billing and reimbursement, and the HCPCS codes, which are used for supplies and equipment the resident may require.

The physician query process described in chapter 1 can assist facilities when clarification is needed on correct coding assignment questions. However, this process should be used at a minimum for coding questions.

Documentation of Data Quality

Documentation of data quality should be reflected in the facility's policies and procedures, as appropriate. Staff training in proper documentation practices ensures data quality and integrity. Each form in the resident's health record is designed to capture the important aspects of care that feed into data quality and provide an accurate reflection of the resident's treatment. Each form should be completed in its entirety and signed to signify data accuracy and integrity.

High-quality documentation drives data quality influencing coding assignments and provides clear, concise, accurate details of the resident's health status and care-planning needs. Documentation that should be included in the resident's health record and reflects data quality and accuracy includes:

- Resident's demographics

- Legal status

- Prior care provided

- Resident assessments, ongoing and significant change status, comprehensive assessments and reassessments

- Medical assessments and reassessments

- Pertinent diagnoses and diagnostic impressions

- Reason for admission and treatment

- Care plan and goals

- Advance directives

- Informed consent

- Orders for care, treatment, or resuscitative services, and medications, including every dose and adverse effect

- Diagnostic and therapeutic procedures and tests

- Progress notes

- Clinical observations

- Consultations

- Relevant diagnoses and final diagnoses

- Discharge plans

- Discharge summaries

- The provision of care, including nursing, nutrition, activities, medical, rehabilitative, and social services

- Care provided by outside services

Coding Basics

The facility should have competent, credentialed coders to perform the coding function. It also should provide ongoing training and resources to ensure compliance with correct coding practice. Moreover, it should have updated coding references to ensure accurate and complete coding practice. At minimum, a credentialed health information management (HIM) professional should oversee the coding process. If the facility hires nurses or billers to perform diagnoses code assignments, they must be trained in correct coding practice and use of the coding guidelines, official coding rules, standards, and standards of ethical coding practice. The AHIMA Standards of Ethical Coding is available from www.ahima.org.

The Health Information Portability and Accountability Act (HIPAA) of 1996 requires the use of ICD-9-CM and CPT codes for its transaction standard code sets for electronic billing.

The facility also should have a policy in place that discusses coding standards to ensure that acceptable coding procedures and references are used when coding patient diagnoses. This policy should outline the number of resources needed and the responsible party for ensuring that the resources are updated and current. Moreover, the policy should outline who is responsible for coding practices and those individuals who will complete the actual coding assignments. This includes written and system references. It is important to remember computerized coding resource updates.

CPT and HCPCS codes are utilized for consolidated billing for Medicare. These code sets are used to indicate services and supplies provided to the resident. All long-term care coders should have training in all aspects of coding classifications including ICD-9-CM, CPT, and HCPCS code sets.

Coding ICD-9-CM Diagnosis Codes on Admission

Admission coding provides the MDS coordinators or nurses the ability to place the proper diagnoses codes on the first MDS submission. It provides the baseline assessment of problems identified by the physician at admission and is a foundation for the billing process. However, coding should not stop at admission or readmission. It is extremely important to use concurrent coding methods to ensure proper compliance with the billing and claim submission process. Concurrent coding practices ensure that services rendered are captured for proper billing.

The facility should have a detailed process for assigning ICD-9-CM codes and coding standards required for the organization. At a minimum, diagnosis code assignment should be done as follows:

- At admission and readmission

  —Documents used should include physician history and physical, physician orders, interagency transfer forms signed by the physician, and hospital referral information, as appropriate (discharge summary, history and physician, consultations, and so on)

  —Documentation should be done as soon after admission or readmission as feasibly possible and as documentation allows. It should be completed and placed in the resident's record as defined by MDS completion requirements.

- Quarterly, as indicated by the MDS schedule, but may be needed more often to ensure that diagnoses are captured for billing purposes

  —Documents used should include physician progress notes, orders, referral information, and consultation. This process will capture the following diagnoses:

  –Pneumonia

  –Respiratory infections

  –Septicemia

  –Urinary tract infections

  –Viral hepatitis

  –Wound infections

  –Fevers

  –Recurrent lung aspiration

  –Other problems as indicated

- At discharge

  —All physician documentation as well as the facility discharge summary, if available

Diagnosis/Problem Sheet

The resident assessment process, resident care planning, comprehensive assessment process, and QI/QA results reporting give the facility the ability to demonstrate resident outcomes. Data quality drives the ultimate outcomes of the residents and the facility's ability to demonstrate to the public how good the institution is in providing care and treatment. Poor data quality produces poor data outcomes, poor care planning, and poor facility results, whereas high-quality data can help establish more referral, financial viability, a steady workforce, and quality applicants to ensure high-quality care for each resident served. Figure 19. 4 illustrates the importance of data quality to the facility.

Diagnosis codes are typically placed on a diagnoses sheet of the problem list. (See figure 19.5.) The problem list may be maintained by nursing and contains all nursing diagnoses and pertinent problems. (See figure 19.6.) The diagnoses sheet, if used, is begun by the coding professional upon assignment of resident diagnosis codes at admission. Addenda or additional diagnosis codes should be added to the diagnosois sheet by nursing staff. Actual ICD-9-CM coding assignment should be completed by the coding professional. These forms are updated according to facility policy but should be done at a minimum on an annual basis at the time of the annual history and physical to ensure data quality of diagnoses and code assignment. Those diagnoses that are not pertinent should be not be carried over to the new diagnoses sheet.

Updating/Monitoring Diagnoses

A diagnoses sheet makes updating and monitoring diagnoses easier for the coding professional. All pertinent diagnoses are placed in one area of the health record for easy assess not only for the coding professional, but also for the nursing staff and the physician. The sheet allows the physician a reference point for the annual history and physical, and it provides a simple format for nurses to record any new or exacerbated diagnoses. The coding professional can update and monitor this sheet and place diagnoses assignments for ready access for the MDS assessments as well.

Figure 19.4.   Data quality and high-quality outcomes

Resident's admission
- Correct placement
- Correct demographics/contacts
- Correct insurance information
- Insurance authorization

Resident's assessments
- Accurate, complete documentation
- Timely medical attention
- Correct and accurate referral data
- Interdisciplinary team approach

Resident's care planning
- Each resident need is addressed in the care-planning process
- Problems and interventions identified
- Medical needs planned for

Resident's MDS submission
- Accurate, correct, complete comprehensive assessment

QI/QM reports
- QI: Deviations and declines can be easily explained from documentation
- QM provides additional data for consumers to see facility quality

Resident outcomes

Resident outcomes achieved even if resident has deviation or decline because documentation backs treatment and care plan and resident progress toward defined goals

Facility outcomes
- More referrals
- Financial viability
- Steady workforce
- Quality applicants

Figure 19.5.   Sample diagnoses sheet

XXX Organization
Anytown, USA 00000

Diagnoses/Diagnoses Addendum Sheet

Resident Name: _____   Date: _____

Health Record Number: _____   Room: _____

Diagnoses	ICD-9-CM Assignment	Diagnoses Addendum	Date	ICD-9-CM Assignment
Rehabilitation	V57.89			
Late effect of stroke	438.20			
With aphasis	438.11			
And dysphasia	438.12			
COPD	496			
Hypertensions	4019			

Figure 19.6.   Sample problem list

XXX Organization
Anytown, USA 00000

PROBLEM LIST

Resident Name: _____ Health Record Number: _____ Room:_____

Physician: _____

Diagnosis: _____

Allergies and symptoms:_____

Problem Number	Date Identified	Problem	Date Resolved	Signature

_____   _____   _____   _____
MD's SIGNATURE   DATE   RN's SIGNATURE   DATE

Only diagnoses that are affecting care or are being treated should be reported for claims submission and reimbursement. The updating and monitoring process ensures that compliance with proper coding, billing, and reimbursement procedures is simplified and that only pertinent diagnoses are reported. This process centralizes the diagnoses assignment practice and provides a simple, easy location to refer to for the resident's current diagnoses codes.

The diagnoses sheet should be replaced annually to reflect only those diagnoses that are pertinent to the resident's current treatment and care-planning process. The used sheet is removed to the overflow files where it can be easily retrieved for clinical staff.

Concurrent Coding

Concurrent coding is an important aspect of data quality. This process ensures that the resident's current diagnoses are accurately reported. Those diagnoses that are no longer pertinent should be eliminated, and any new diagnoses that have developed or been treated should have proper code assignment.

Coding Resources

Essential coding resources include:

- Up-to-date ICD-9-CM, CPT, and HCPCS codebooks

  —ICD-9-CM is updated annually on October 1.

  —CPT and HCPCS references are updated annually on January 1.

- Current medical dictionary

- Anatomy and physiology textbook or equivalent software

- Physician's desk reference

- Current subscription to American Hospital Association's *Coding Clinic for ICD-9-CM*

- Current subscription to American Medical Association's *CPT Assistant*

Data Quality and the Survey Process

The quality indicators (QIs) and subsequent quality measures (QMs) developed for CMS support the facility's survey process. The QIs identify resident care problems through MDS data submission. They provide a snapshot of the quality of care within the facility. Surveyors have the information prior to the survey process. The facility must use the QI report to examine problem areas, implement improvement plans, and monitor progress for improvement. *Quality Indicators: A Practical Guide to Assessment and Documentation* (2000, Opus Communications) is a useful reference that can help the facility prepare for the survey process, improve reimbursement, plan care, and ultimately provided better outcomes.

The facility is only as good as the data that support its business practices. Data quality is reflected in all documentation and drives reimbursement and the survey process.

Quality Requirements

Audits performed for documentation practices can be both qualitative and quantitative. *Qualitative audits* are more subjective because they focus on whether documentation demonstrates that resident care was provided appropriately. *Quantitative audits* are more objective because they focus on determining that documentation is complete, signed, and done in a timely fashion. Audits also verify that each form is completed in its entirety with each data field filled.

The facility should conduct ongoing quantitative monitoring to ensure that records are completed and done in a timely manner. Audits should be completed on a sample of admission and discharge records as well as concurrent review. The purpose of audits is to identify problems or concerns and implement improvement plans as indicated. Periodic, ongoing audits ensure that documentation practice is followed and charts are complete. Concurrent auditing helps identify areas of documentation that may have been omitted or may be inaccurately reflected. If the audit determines that data are either omitted or inaccurate, the information can be completed following proper documentation guidelines, ensuring that resident care needs are accurately captured and subsequently delivered. Audits help facilitate documentation accuracy and completeness and improve data quality and outcomes.

Quality audits for documentation may include:

- Consistency in documentation

- Replication or redundancy

- Inconsistency or contradiction in documentation

- Omissions of documentation

- Use of practice guidelines, standards, regulations, and clinical protocols

These areas of documentation should be completed on a continuing basis as defined by the facility's quality improvement program and individual departmental quality reviews. The JCAHO has established criteria to help with documentation monitoring and can be located at www.jcaho.org. It helps clarify key areas within the health record to monitor. The audit tool shown in table 19.1 can be used to further develop both qualitative and quantitative monitoring criteria. It provides a thorough reference to the actual standards that apply to each indicator.

Coding assignment drives the reimbursement of healthcare services rendered. Coding assignment accuracy should be monitored on a regular basis. It is essential that a qualified credentialed health information management professional (HIM) perform these audits. (See figure 19.7.)

Coding and Billing Association

The coding and billing association is an important aspect of compliance. The relationship between the financial and HIM staff is key in providing quality reimbursement practices. Both billers and coders need to understand the importance of each role and to determine proper and ethical practices that will ensure that the billing process is completed accurately and in a timely manner in order to improve reimbursement for the facility. Working together as a team to ensure that compliance with coding and billing regulations and requirements is met will facilitate quality practices, improve outcomes, and help ensure the organization's financial viability.

Table 19.1. **Modified version of the JCAHO open and closed health record audit**

Open and Closed Medical Record Review					
Month/Year					
	Standard	**Process Standards**	**Yes**	**No**	**Comment**
Resident Names					
Identification data	IM.7.2.a	PE.1			
Resident's legal status, as appropriate	IM.7.2.b	PE.1			
Resident's assessment	IM.7.2.d	PE.1			
The initial medical assessment conclusion of impressions on history and physical examination. (24 hrs before or 72 hrs after admission, 48 hrs for **subacute**)	IM.7.2.e	PE.1.2.1			
The physician visits at a minimum once in the first 30 days, and at a minimum once prior to discharge for planned lengths of stay of 30 days or less.		TX.1.4.3			
Covering physician is identified, as appropriate.		TX.1.4.4			
The diagnosis	IM.7.2.f	TX.1.4			
The reason(s) for admission	IM.7.2.g	PE.2.1 PE.2.1.1			
Neuropsychiatric status, mental, affective, cognitive status, sleep, memory, recall, decision-making ability		PE.2.1.2			
Communication status, hearing, speech, language, voice and modes of expressions		PE.2.1.3			
Rehab status and needs		PE.2.1.4			
Psychosocial status, cultural ethnic factors, emotional status, and social skills		PE.2.1.5			

(Continued on next page)

Table 19.1. (continued)

	Standard	Process Standards	Yes	No	Comment
Spiritual status and needs		PE.2.1.5.1			
Musculoskeletal, GI, CV, foot care needs		PE.2.1.6			
Activities status and needs		PE.2.1.7			
Nutrition & hydration status, needs, risks, deficiencies, cultural, ethnic, religious food preferences, special dietary requirements, nutrient intake patterns		PE.2.1.8			
Dental status & oral health		PE.2.1.9			
Pain: Origin, location, severity, alleviating & exacerbating factors, current treatment & response		PE.2.1.10			
Response to stress		PE.2.1.11			
Assessment indicates means to enhance activity and recreational skills		PE.2.1.12			
Assessment of resident's and family's educational needs, preferences, abilities, and readiness to learn		PE.2.1.13			
Initial assessments completed within established time frame		PE.1.2			
Entries are dated, author identified and authenticated		IM.7.8			
Reassessments	IM.7.2.0	PE.3			
Orders for care and treatment as required by law and regulation	IM.7.2.1	TX.1.4			
The care plan and goals	IM.7.2.h	TX.1			
Interim plan of care		TX.1.1			
Interdisciplinary care plan developed according to time frames		TX.1.1.1			
Care planning is individualized to resident.		TX.1.2			

Table 19.1. **(continued)**

	Standard	**Process Standards**	**Yes**	**No**	**Comment**
Goals are reasonable, measurable, and have time frames.		TX.1.2.1			
Care is planned and coordinated by interdisciplinary team.		TX.1.3			
Resident and family participate in care-planning activities.		TX.1.4.1			
Care plan is reviewed and revised, as indicated.	TX.3.1	TX.3.1			
Care plan is reviewed according to time frames.		TX.3.1			
Indication of known advance directives	IM.7.2.i	TX.1.3.1			
Informed consent per policy	IM.7.2.j	RI.2.1.8			
All orders, renewal of orders, for resuscitative services that are to be withheld or life-sustaining treatment that is withdrawn	IM.7.2.k	TX.1.3.1			
Verbal orders dated and signed	IM.7.7	TX.1.4			
Entries dated, author identified and signed	IM.7.8	TX.1.4			
All diagnostic/therapeutic procedures/tests done as well as results reported	IM.7.2.m	TX.2.1			
Progress notes done by authorized staff	IM.7.2.n	TX.2.1			
Clinical observations	IM.7.2.p	TX.3			
Consultation reports	IM.7.2.q	TX.3			
Every medication ordered or prescribed	IM.7.2.r	TX.4			
Every dose of medication administered and any adverse drug reaction	IM.7.2.s	TX.4			
All relevant diagnoses established during the course of care	IM.7.2.u	TX.1.4			
Effects of medications	IM.7.4	TX.4			

(Continued on next page)

Table 19.1.   **(continued)**

	Standard	Process Standards	Yes	No	Comment
Needs/alternatives and orders for restraints	TX.8.1	TX.8.1			
Care provided to prevent & treat health-related complications		TX.2.5			
Provision and response to:					
Activities program	IM.7.3.1	TX.3			
Nutrition care services	IM.7.3.2	TX.3			
Nursing services	IM.7.3.3	TX.3			
Medical treatment	IM.7.3.4	TX.3			
Rehabilitation services	IM.7.3.5	TX.3 TX.6.5			
Social service interventions	IM.7.3.6	TX.3			
Education based on assessed needs	IM.7.3.7	PF.3 PF.3.5			
Education about pain and managing pain	IM.7.3.7	PF.3 PF.3.5			
Significant changes in resident's condition	IM.7.3.8	PE.3			
Discharge records					
Discharged records completed within 30 days	IM.7.6.1				
Discharge plan, or reason for lack of an ongoing plan when discharge potential does not exist	IM.7.2.v	PE.2.3			
Every medication dispensed/prescribed on discharge	IM.7.2.t	CC.5			
Referrals/communication to external or internal caregivers and community agencies	IM.7.2.w	CC.4.1.2			
Physician's summary/final diagnosis when the resident is admitted.	IM.7.2.x	CC.5			
Discharge information given to resident/ organization	IM.7.5	CC.5			

Source: www.jcaho.org

Figure 19.7.   Sample audit tool

XXX Organization Anytown, USA 00000 **Coding Quality Monitor** Date: _____						
Resident	**Principal Dx correct**	**Secondary Dx correct**	**Sequence of Dx correct**	**Pertinent Dx are captured**	**4th and 5th digits are present**	**Comments**

Compliance

"The creation of compliance program guidance is a major initiative of the OIG in its efforts to engage the private health care community in combating fraud and abuse" (DHHS 2000, p. 14289). The program was begun to provide facilities with guidance on initiating internal controls to monitor and improve compliance with statues, regulations, and program stipulations. The compliance program guidance is available at http://www.hhs.gov/oig. The program content includes the following seven elements:

- Implementation of written policies, procedures, and standards of conduct (This includes the code of conduct for the organization and other policies and procedures to prevent fraud and abuse, including a quality of care philosophy.)

- Designation of a compliance officer and committee

- Education and training

- Communication mechanisms

- Implementation of "well-published disciplinary guidelines"

- Completion of internal monitors and audits

- Detection response and corrective action planning

The effort of the program reduces fraud and abuse and helps ensure that the resident receives high-quality care. The checks and balances inherent in the compliance program ensure this quality of care through the seven defined elements with the program.

The benefits of a compliance program may include:

- Internal controls to monitor adherence with statues, regulations, and rules

- Duty to accountable corporate behavior

- Determination of employee and contractor conduct

- Ability to prevent unlawful and unethical conduct

- Effective responses to employee's compliance issues

- Improved quality, effectiveness, and consistency of services provided

- Open atmosphere for employees to report potential concerns allowing the ability to complete internal examinations

- Centralized distribution of information concerning statues, regulations, and program directives

- Improved internal communication

- Investigative process of suspected misconduct and reporting and cost reduction

- Early detection through self-monitoring

The program was designed to considerably decrease the risk of illegal or improper behavior. It is meant to be tailorable to the facility size and scope of practice and should have a top-down approach. The potential risk areas identified for nursing facilities by the Office of the Inspector General (OIG) include:

- Quality of care

- Resident rights

- Employee screening

- Vendor relationships

- Billing and cost reporting

- Record keeping and documentation

Quality of Care

Inherent in the compliance program are the data quality concerns that include the following:

- Comprehensive, accurate assessments with measurable objectives and time frames

- Improper or inadequate treatment and services

- Failure to satisfy each resident's needs and preferences (lack of documentation to prove needs and preferences were considered)

- Insufficient staffing levels, which leads to poor documentation practice

- Lack of documented therapy services

- Lack of documented activities of daily living

- Lack of documented activity programs

Billing, Coding, and Cost Reporting

The facility must constantly assess its billing practices. The risk areas for billing and cost reporting are the most commonly investigated by the OIG; thus, the facility must develop policies and procedures for these risk areas. When developed, staff must be continually educated on proper practice. Monitors should be implemented when problems arise so that quality improvement activities can be started.

Billing, coding, and cost-reporting concerns include:

- Billing for items of services not provided
- Sending claims for equipment, supplies, and services that are not medically necessary
- Sending claims to Medicare Part A when residents are ineligible for coverage
- Duplicate billing
- Not identifying and refunding credit balances
- Sending claims for services not ordered
- Intentionally billing for insufficient care
- Inaccurate information about the resident's medical condition on the MDS
- Upcoding RUGs
- Upcoding level of service
- Billing for items or services included in per diem rates
- Billing for items already covered by a third-party payer
- Altering documentation or not acquiring a physician's signature
- Failing to maintain proper documentation to support diagnoses, treatment, and the like
- Improper ICD-9-CM code assignments
- False cost reports

These risk areas can be linked to the quality of documentation practice and data quality concerns as well. "A key component of ensuring accurate information is the proper and ongoing training and evaluation of the staff responsible for coding diagnoses and regular internal audits of coding policy and procedures" (DHHS 2000, p. 14296). Under the compliance program, it is important to hire knowledgeable professionals for diagnoses code assignments.

The facility needs to implement periodic compliance audits. "These assessments should focus both on nursing facility's day to day operations, as well as its adherence to the rules governing claims development, billing and cost reports and . . . the nursing facility's compliance with Medicare requirements" (DHHS 2000, p. 14302). Quality monitoring is an important aspect of the compliance program and data quality and integrity.

The compliance program provides a foundation for monitoring and improving data quality and coding assignments, thus improving organizational performance and radiant outcomes as well as reimbursement. Tying it all together with a thorough quality program ensures that data quality and integrity are enhanced and organization performance is improved so that the resident receives the benefit of high-quality care and improved outcomes.

Chargemaster

The chargemaster that supports the facility from a coding, billing, and reimbursement standpoint must be reviewed from a compliance perspective. If the facility chargemaster is not kept up-to-date, billing rejections, incorrect reimbursement, and Medicare compliance issues may affect the facility's financial stability. At a minimum, the chargemaster should be reviewed annually or as the need arises. The integrity of the facility's chargemaster files helps ensure organizational compliance.

Chargemaster file errors can affect the organization's revenue, reduce biller productivity, and impact the accuracy of cost-reporting data. Improper chargemaster data, along with an incorrect charge structure, can lead to implications of Medicare/Medicaid program fraud or abuse.

The facility should have a policy and procedure for chargemaster compliance. This policy should outline the following information:

- Chargemaster file content

- Assessment of revenue codes

- Assessment and mapping of CPT codes and HCPCS codes

- Billing descriptions for clarity

- Charge structure

- Duplicated CPT codes

- Assessment chargemaster functionality

- Coordination with financial services, health record or health information management, and compliance to identify billing problems and identified denial issues

Summary

Data quality is the cornerstone of data integrity and accurate documentation in any business. The quality of the data gathered and assessed for healthcare and business needs is imperative. Without constant diligence to ensure that the information captured and documented is of the utmost accuracy and completeness, there is no guarantee that the resident will receive the necessary interventions and treatments to achieve the highest practicable well-being.

Proper diagnoses code assignment is crucial to reimbursement practices. Continual education must be provided to coding staff to ensure proper diagnoses code assignment. Updated reference material must be maintained to ensure that code assignment is done accurately, efficiently, and effectively.

Every long-term care facility that participates in Medicare and Medicaid reimbursement must have an organizational compliance plan in place. Federal government regulations detail the exact requirements for the organization's compliance program.

Review of the facility chargemaster is a must for compliance. The facility should have a policy and procedure that outlines its chargemaster monitoring process.

References

American Health Information Management Association. 1999. Standards of Ethical Coding. Available at www.ahima.org.

Centers for Medicare and Medicaid Services. 2001 (October 31). Guidance to Surveyors—Long-Term Care Facilities, appendix PP in *State Operations Manual*. Available at www.cms.gov.

Centers for Medicare and Medicaid Services. 2003. Nursing Home Compare. Available at http://www.medicare.gov/NHCompare/home.asp.

Centers for Medicare and Medicaid Services. 2002 (October 24). Quality Measure Criteria and Selection. Available at http://www.cms.hhs.gov/providers/nursinghomes/nhi/final_qm.pdf.

Commeret, Karen, and Julia Hopp. 2000. *The Quality Indicators: A Practical Guide to Assessment and Documentation.* Marblehead, Mass.: Opus Communications.

Department of Health and Human Services. 2000. *Federal Register* 65, no. 52. Available at http://www.cms.hhs.gov.

Final Compliance Program Guidance for Nursing Facilities. 2000. 65 FR 14289, March 16. Available at http://www.hhs.gov/oig.

Hapner, Peggy. 2001. Covering the bases of coding compliance. *Journal of AHIMA* 72(5): 69–71. Available at www.ahima.org.

Health Insurance Portability and Accountability Act of 1996. Available at http://aspe.os.dhhs.gov/admnsimp.

Joint Commission on Accreditation of Healthcare Organizations. 2004. *Comprehensive Accreditation Manual for Long-term Care.* Oakbrook Terrace, Ill.: JCAHO.

Chapter 20

Reimbursement for Long-Term Care Services

Reimbursement is payment for services and supplies rendered. In the long-term care environment, reimbursement is based in part on the prospective payment system (PPS) for Medicare. Managed care, private pay, private insurance coverage, Veterans Administration (VA), and Medicaid payments also are reimbursement methods in the long-term care arena.

Medicare and Medicaid may be the largest payers of long-term care services due to the nature of illness and characteristics of residents in the industry. To receive reimbursement from Medicare, the facility must meet the *Conditions of Participation* requirements for long-term care.

State regulations and requirements drive Medicaid payments. In most instances, state regulations supersede federal regulations based on state Medicaid laws. Because each state may regulate its Medicaid program differently, each facility should determine appropriate policy and procedure for Medicaid reimbursement processing.

Services provided under PPS, and for that matter for other insurance payers, must be medically necessary. For Medicare reimbursement, the facility must demonstrate through accurate, concise, timely documentation and physician certification and recertification that care is medically necessary to receive reimbursement payments.

Medicare has established guidelines for compliance plans to decrease fraud and abuse of reimbursement for all healthcare providers that participate in the Medicare program. These plans are designed to ensure that the correct services are provided and billed properly. Medicare claims typically are denied when documentation does not prove that the services rendered were medically necessary. Correct coding and billing processes are key components of facility compliance plans.

Reimbursement Methodologies

The following are reimbursement methodologies that may be used in the long-term care industry:

- Medicare PPS system
  - RUGs classification determines the reimbursement allotment. (See discussion of RUGs in chapter 10 and refer to the revised April 1, 2001, Payment Rates: PDF File, and the Nursing & Therapy Minutes [used in calculating preliminary rates: April 10, 2000, *Federal Register* PPS Update] PDF File, available from http://www.cms.hhs.gov/providers/snfpps/default.asp.)
  - Proper diagnosis code assignments are required.

- Medicaid or state payment system: May be paid in predetermined schedules as specified by the particular state

- Managed care contracts where payment levels may be predetermined: Based on contracted predetermined payment schedules

- Managed care contract with carve-outs: May pay more or less for carve-out of services and supplies

- Private pay from private insurance

  —Based on published total charges

  —Only pay room and board to the facility

  —Resident pays ancillary services directly to vendors.

- Veterans Administration: Preestablished per diem rate that is updated annually

- Private pay: Payment in full (out of pocket) for services rendered

The purpose of payment systems—whether Medicare, Medicaid, VA, managed care, or private pay—is to ensure that only appropriate, necessary services and supplies are provided to the resident for accurate reimbursement.

Medicaid is a state-run and -regulated program; therefore, facilities must check state-specific rules and requirements. Each state may mandate different guidelines for claims reimbursement. Residents also may be required to follow strict regulations for placement in the long-term care facility in order to be eligible for Medicaid services and programs.

Managed care contracts, regardless of type, may be individualized by category of the resident's medical condition. It is important to be familiar with each managed care contract benefit assignment prior to resident admission to the facility. These contracts may be very specific as to payment resources for services delivered.

In October 1996, Congress passed Public Law 104-262, the Veterans' Health Care Eligibility Reform Act of 1996. This legislation paved the way for the creation of a Medical Benefits Package—a standard enhanced health benefits plan generally available to all enrolled veterans. Like other standard health care plans, the Medical Benefits Package emphasizes preventive and primary care, offering a full range of outpatient and inpatient services (Department of Veterans Affairs, 2003.

Medicare Part B coverage is elective insurance in which the resident chooses to participate. It is simply a coinsurance that the resident has paid money into for additional coverage options. It provides payment for ancillary services such as laboratory tests, therapy, and radiology, among other services. Medicare Part B billing is included in the consolidated billing processing and requires the same stringent documentation guidelines as Medicare Part A.

It is extremely important to follow proper facility policies and procedures for billing and coding for all insurance payers. The rest of this chapter primarily discusses Medicare Part A coverage—not because it is more important than other payment systems but, rather, because it is regulated by the federal government and has strict guidelines that must be followed by all long-term care facilities.

The Medicare PPS became effective with the start of the first cost-reporting period on or after July 1, 1998. "The PPS payment rate is adjusted for case mix and geographic variation in ages and covers all costs for furnishing covered SNF services (routine, ancillary, and capital-related costs" (CMS 2002). The payment rates are increased each federal fiscal year.

As discussed earlier in this book, the health information coding professional should be competent and involved in the coding and monitoring process for assignment of resident diagnoses codes for billing. He or she must thoroughly understand the need for accurate code assignment and its importance to the billing cycle. Those professionals responsible for billing also must recognize the need for accurate and complete code assignment, including ICD-9-CM, CPT, and HCPCS codes, to ensure that proper billing is accomplished. The Health Insurance Portability and Accountability Act (HIPAA) of 1996 requires the appropriate use of these code sets for electronic data interchange.

ICD-9-CM diagnosis code assignment on a billing claim form furnishes the information to help establish that services are medically necessary. Each code number provided on the claim form represents a specific disease or condition for the resident that has been abstracted from physician documentation. Improper diagnosis code assignment placed on the bill to account for services billed could potentially be considered fraudulent if the resident's health record does not support that diagnosis.

> CPT and HCPCS codes represent services or supplies. When a CPT or HCPCS code is reported on a claim form, the facility is indicating that the specific service or supply represented by the code was provided and medically necessary. It is important that all services and supplies represented by the CPT or HCPCS codes be supported by documentation in the medical record regardless of whether it is a Medicare part A claim (where all services are lumped together under one revenue code) or a Medicare part B claim (where each item is line item billed per service and per day) (AHIMA 2001).

Under HIPAA, if facilities electronically bill healthcare claims, appropriate ICD-9-CM, CPT, and HCPCS code sets must accompany all claims. Professional coders must be accurate and thorough in assigning all diagnosis codes for reimbursement purposes. Therefore, although some reimbursement methodologies may not currently place much emphasis on ICD-9-CM, CPT, or HCPCS code sets, they must be assigned properly on all claims submitted electronically in the future.

Coding professionals must never assume from documentation that diagnoses are present. The physician documentation is of the utmost importance for proper coding practice. It is critical that the physician document exactly what is happening with the resident on admission. There must be thorough documentation of the physician's thought process in order to capture proper code set assignment for each diagnosis the resident may have to ensure that the highest reimbursement is received for care.

The admission process as outlined in chapter 1 must be clearly defined and efficient. Resident demographic and insurance information must be documented accurately at the time of admission to ensure that the billing process is completed correctly and accurately. Preauthorization for resident care must be received prior to or at admission to ensure that proper reimbursement is received. This preauthorization, precertification, or preapproval is required regardless of payer. A well-defined registration process helps capture proper resident demographic and insurance information for billing purposes and decreases the chances of incorrect billing processes.

It is important to remember that precertification for specific tests, procedures, or interventions may be required as well. Facility policy and procedure should outline which individual is responsible for obtaining the precertification for these resident treatment requirements.

General Requirements

Residents with Medicare benefits in skilled nursing facilities (SNFs) are limited to one hundred days of coverage, usually after a qualifying hospital stay. Residents whose stay will be reimbursed by Medicare have a slightly different completion schedule than non-Medicare residents do.

The physician must certify that the long-term care stay is medically necessary. (See chapter 10 for a discussion of physician certification and recertification.)

"Certain services are excluded from the SNF PPS only when furnished on an outpatient basis by a hospital or a CAH [critical access hospital]:

- Cardiac catheterization services
- Computerized axial tomography (CT scans)
- Magnetic resonance imaging (MRI)
- Radiation therapy
- Ambulatory surgery involving hospital operating rooms
- Emergency services
- Angiography services
- Lymphatic and venous procedures" (CMS 2002)
- Ambulance services that take the resident to these listed tests

"The SNF PPS incorporates adjustments to account for facility case mix, using the system for classifying residents based on resource utilization known as Resource Utilization Groups, Version III (RUG-III)" (CMS 2002). Information taken from the most recent Minimum Data Set (MDS) is used to categorize each resident into a RUG-III group. (See chapter 7 for discussion of RAIs, RAPs, MDS, and RUGs.)

Each of the forty-four RUGs categories has a specific payment code associated with it. Reimbursement is affected when required MDS submission schedules are not met. The first twenty-six RUGs categories are the highest-paying RUGs categories. Facilities must take special care to ensure that they have accurate data and meet required time frames for therapy services to capture reimbursement at these higher levels.

Accurate therapy documentation is a key component in placing residents in the appropriate RUGs category. Discrepancies in actual time spent in therapies on the MDS and the resident's health record must be resolved prior to submission of the MDS data and the claims request.

Those residents whose care requirements fall into the following categories will be placed in one of the top twenty-six RUGs assignments:

- Rehabilitation
- Extensive care
- Special care
- Clinically complex

Those residents who may fall into the lower eighteen RUGs categories may not necessarily meet SNF level of care definitions, such as those residents in the preceding list of categories.

The payment rates under the Medicare PPS system are published in the "*Federal Register* before August 1 of the year preceding the affected fiscal year" (CMS 2002).

HIPAA has set transaction and code set standards for healthcare. The law stipulates that healthcare providers, payers, and clearinghouses use specified code sets and follow the official coding guidelines instituted for each code set when submitting electronic claim transactions. Fiscal intermediaries and other payers must understand the official coding guidelines and can no longer set their own rules for reporting diagnoses that may conflict with these official specifications.

HIPAA standards mandate one claim form for all electronic claim submissions regardless of payer type. Prior to HIPAA transaction standards implementation, it was estimated that there were more than 400 different claim forms for submission of healthcare bills. HIPAA transaction standards will simplify claims processing by eliminating the many different forms. (See chapter 22 for more information on HIPAA transaction standards.)

The accuracy of all MDS assessment dates may affect reimbursement as follows:

- Assessment reference (ARD) on section A3a
- Date of entry on section AB1
- Face sheet signatures on section AD
- Signature dates for certification of accuracy
- Date RN assessment coordinator signed section R2b
- Completion date for prospective payment and quarterly MDS assessments, section VB2 is the completion date

Consolidated Billing

"Under consolidated billing (both Medicare part A and part B), health information and billing staff must be concerned with the accuracy of the vendor invoices received and billed under the facility's provider number. When a vendor bills the facility for services provided to a Medicare resident, they should provide the CPT/HCPCS code and date of service. To assure accuracy, the facility should have a process to review vendor invoices prior to billing Medicare. The goal of the review process is to assure that the service or supply was provided (based on medical record documentation), physician ordered, and medically necessary" (AHIMA 2001, p. 70).

Consolidated billing excludes the following services:

- Physician's professional services
- Certain dialysis-related services
- All ambulance services except when a medically necessary transport from one SNF to another SNF and covered ambulance transportation to obtain dialysis
- Erythropoietin for certain dialysis patients
- Chemotherapy
- Chemotherapy administration services
- Radioisotope services
- Customized prosthetic devices

Under consolidated billing, CPT and HCPCS codes are used to demonstrate services and supplies. The long-term care facility should consider employing health information management (HIM) staff with basic training in, and understanding of, the CPT and HCPCS coding systems to ensure accurate capture of code assignment for these services and supplies.

Reimbursement

Reimbursement, regardless of the methodology, must be completed accurately and with proper diagnosis code assignments to ensure adherence with established compliance guidelines within the facility. When established, the compliance plan covers the entire facility's activities, not simply the Medicare billing practice. (See chapter 19 for compliance program information.)

Medicare reimbursement is derived from the MDS assessment criteria. The MDS assessment that triggers the RUGs category assignment also must be accurate and complete. As discussed throughout this book, poor documentation produces poor reimbursement processes.

Documentation ultimately drives the reimbursement process. It is extremely important that the documentation practices discussed at length in this book be adhered to and monitored to ensure that:

- Care is medially necessary.

- Certification and recertification are completed.

- Care planning reflects required care needs and services.

- Data quality and accuracy are paramount.

- Diagnoses code assignment is accurate, and documentation that supports code assignment is present and complete.

- Documents are dated and signed to prove services were provided.

- MDS assessments are accurate.

- Physician has oversight of the resident's medical care.

- Physician orders are renewed as required.

- Resident care needs and services are provided consistently.

- Supporting documentation backs up the MDS assessment.

Documentation Required

The health record must reflect the care and services provided to the resident. The documentation in the resident's health record must be accurate and complete to ensure that there is evidence that care was medically necessary.

Quality Requirements

Claim rejection and denials due to coding, incorrect submissions, or documentation errors are critical quality concerns. Processes should be in place to review that chargemasters are appropriate and mechanisms have been established to ensure proper reference material for coding professionals.

Billing and coding professionals must attend educational sessions to ensure compliance with standards. Monitoring Medicare transmittals also is a necessity.

Incorrect resident identifiers on the MDS may not place the resident in the common working file. This may cause a denial of the claim. The following identifiers or numbers must be accurate:

- Name

- Gender

- Date of birth

- Social Security number

- Medicare number

The facility should develop an ongoing audit to monitor the accuracy of MDS codes not only for reimbursement and compliance, but also for accurate and complete documentation. This audit ensures that the highest allowable reimbursement is achieved and guarantees the highest-quality resident outcomes. High-quality resident outcomes are what should drive the facility in all aspects of service; reimbursement is secondary to resident outcomes.

The billing and HIM staff must continually communicate in all aspects of the billing process. When billing claims are denied, systems and processes must be in place to ensure that problems are identified and solutions implemented. Proper sequencing of diagnosis codes also is important. It is never appropriate for the billing staff or any staff member to change diagnosis codes in order to have claims paid. Denials and rejections of claims should be examined immediately upon notification of those denials, and the resident's health record should be reviewed prior to resubmission of claims information. It may be necessary to consult with the fiscal intermediary (FI) to determine problems and solutions.

When consulting with FIs on coding assignment, always request any coding advice in writing and keep a written log of all discussions and advice. Should the FI refuse to provide advice in writing, request the staff person's name and immediately document the conversation. This summary should be sent back to the FI for an official record. File a copy of this document with billing and claims policies.

Should individual payer policies conflict with official coding rules and guidelines, the policies should be received in writing as well. Reasonable efforts should be made to educate the payer on proper coding practice. This effort should be documented as well.

The following may be included in assessment criteria:

- Claims forms are correct.

- Documentation supports diagnoses codes.

- Therapy documentation supports reported time spent in therapy.

- Denials due to coding are monitored.

- Incorrect submissions are monitored

- Documentation errors are monitored.

- Chargemaster review is complete.

- Reference material for coding professionals is up-to-date.

Assessment criteria for monitoring compliance with transaction standards may include the following:

- Data fields are correctly designed.

- Data in the fields are correct.

- References are up-to-date.

- Diagnosis assignment ensures fourth- and fifth-digit assignment.

- Code assignments reflect Official Coding Guidelines and *Coding Clinic* requirements.

- Quality checks on ICD-9-CM and CPT assignments are completed as outlined by the facility.

- Billers have complied with submission policy.

- Data fields are complete.

- Coding and billing staff are updated on HIPAA requirements as policy changes occur.

- Denial of claims is monitored.

The following information must be accurate on MDS submissions:

- Name

- Gender

- Date of birth

- Social Security number

- Medicare number

- Therapy times accurately reflected for appropriate RUGs assignment

- Therapy time documented in the health record not in conflict with MDS or billing data

Accuracy of all MDS assessment dates is as follows:

- Assessment reference (ARD) on section A3a

- Date of entry on section AB1

- Face sheet signatures on section AD

- Signature dates for certification of accuracy

- Date RN assessment coordinator signed on section R2b

- Completion date for prospective payment and quarterly MDS assessments on section VB2

Timeliness of Documentation

Diagnosis codes should be documented at admission and discharge, and a mechanism should be established through policies and procedure for the need for concurrent coding requirements. The facility should attempt to centralize concurrent coding processes with the coding professional to minimize coding professional efforts to review each resident's chart daily. Alerting the coding professional to infections, test orders, antibiotic drug use, and the like allows him or her to limit record review to the records of residents who are receiving new services for accurate diagnosis code assignment.

Other Pertinent Information

Medicare reimbursement is not the only reimbursement methodology in long-term care, but it is a specific system that requires much attention. The PPS requires attention to detail not only in the claims processing and submission, but also in the data quality of the MDS assessment. The data gathered and submitted in the MDS assessment triggers the RUGs payment category.

With other payment systems such as DRGs for acute care hospitals, the accurate assignment of diagnosis codes triggers the payment category based on physician documentation. Although accurate documentation of diagnosis codes is extremely important in the acute care world, an automated clinical data-gathering system (the MDS) does not trigger the payment category. Therefore, long-term care has two different problems in which to focus for compliance. Not only must the MDS assessment done by interdisciplinary clinical staff be scrutinized and monitored consistently to capture the accurate and complete data, the coding assignments based on physician documentation must be accurate and timely as well.

These differences between the long-term care PPS and the acute care payment system is in the requirement for documentation of supporting information for proper payment category. DRGs require coding assignment from physician documentation, whereas nonphysician clinical staff documentation triggers RUGs categories. Both systems require that trained coding professionals assign accurate diagnosis codes for claims submission.

Issues

Healthcare claims submission for other reimbursement methodologies have typically fewer regulatory requirements to follow when submitting healthcare claims. This is not to say that there is less attention to detail when submitting these claims; rather, because Medicare standards are so high, other claims processing is accomplished on the same set of high standards. Compliance plans should cover the entire organization's billing, claims, and coding processing, not just the Medicare system.

Staff must be educated, and reference materials must be updated and available to ensure that MDS assessments are accurate. All staff completing the MDS assessment should have available the following references:

- MDS questions and answers issued by CMS since 1996 as well as all appropriate corrections issued to questions and answers
- Medicare memos relating to SNFs
- Medicare Program Integrity Manual
- Medicare Provider Reimbursement Manual
- Medicare Skilled Nursing Facility Manual
- Medicare transmittals relating to skilled nursing facilities
- Resident assessment instrument (RAI) manual

Staff may obtain education from the following:

- American Association of Nurse Assessment Coordinators
- Fiscal intermediary for the facility
- National Subacute Association
- Private seminars
- State healthcare associations
- Train-the-trainer and in-house programs

Fraud and Abuse

The federal government has issued model compliance plans for long-term care facilities that must be implemented. (See chapter 19 for the requirements of a compliance plan to prevent fraud and abuse.)

Policies and Procedures

Both billing and HIM or health records departments will have to have policies and procedures in place to manage reimbursement in long-term care. The fiscal intermediary and the HIM professional must work closely to ensure that proper billing and coding functions are complete.

Types of policies that the facility may include as it complies with HIPAA transaction standards include:

- Access to electronic systems and processing requirements
- Admission processing
- Auditing process for quality and accuracy in each area, as needed
- Charge entry procedures
- Chargemaster monitoring
- Claims processing and submission
- Code set accuracy
- Coding assignment processing
- Coding time frames
- Complaint management
- Compliance plan
- Data submission criteria
- Denial processing and monitoring
- Documentation required to code accurately
- EDI processes detailed for each payer
- Managing resident's request for claims-processing information
- Oversight of claims-processing function
- Oversight of coding function
- Partnership with HIM for code assignment
- Reference material required for code assignment
- Vendor listing for healthcare claims processing for tracking purposes

Summary

Several reimbursement methodologies are used in the long-term care environment for payment, but the Medicare PPS is a large portion of the process. If the facility does use the

Medicare system for payments, the Medicare *Conditions of Participation* must be met. This requirement provides detailed specifics that must be achieved to continue to receive Medicare reimbursement.

HIPAA requires that proper code sets be included in all claims to all payers. The importance of proper ICD-9-CM, CPT, and HCPCS code assignment must be emphasized in long-term care facilities. Properly trained health information professionals should be the individuals given responsibility for proper coding practices. Physician documentation should be accurately and concisely recorded to ensure proper diagnosis assignment.

The clinical data and time spent in therapy placed on the MDS trigger the RUGs reimbursement category. Proper documentation practices are critical to the reimbursement process. Improper assignment of the RUGs category through poor documentation practices will result in loss of reimbursement.

Consolidated billing practices should be well documented and correctly followed for proper reimbursement of services provided. Quality review of the process is recommended.

The facility must develop a compliance plan for participation in the Medicare program that encompasses all facility activities and billing and coding practices for all payers, not just the Medicare program. The compliance plan ensures that fraud and abuse are eliminated throughout the facility.

Reimbursement is an important aspect of any facility's business and financial viability, but it should be a secondary activity that results from high-quality resident care and outcomes. Reimbursement is not the purpose of the business but, rather, the result of ensuring that the resident achieves the highest practicable physical, mental, and psychosocial well-being.

References

American Health Information Management Association. 2001. Long-Term Care Health Information Practice and Documentation Guidelines. Available from www.ahima.org.

Centers for Medicare and Medicaid Services. 2002 (March 27). *Medicare Skilled Nursing Facility Manual.* Transmittal 372. Available at www.cms.hhs.gov.

Centers for Medicare and Medicaid Services. 2003. Skilled Nursing Facility Prospective Payment System. Available at http://www.cms.gov/providers/snfpps/.

Consolidated billing for SNF resident claims. Available at http://www.snfinfo.com/ppsrc/index.cfm#Consolidated.

Department of Veterans Affairs. Available at http://www.va.gov/health_benefits/.

Chapter 21

Automation of Health Information

The **electronic health record** (EHR) is an evolving software system that has been slower to become fully developed than the healthcare industry had originally anticipated. Efforts to minimize medical errors and increase patient safety have been influential in promoting an electronic physician order-entry system and clinical record. The onus is on many institutions in the healthcare industry to implement such products.

The healthcare industry as a whole also looks to provide faster, more effective executive information through electronic software systems. Case management, quality assurance, and risk management directors look to address concerns or problems through the use of electronic software systems that are interfaced with EHR systems to provide total quality management of resident care needs. The long-term care industry will use computerized systems to translate skilled nursing services and documentation practices to provide similar software systems for their environment.

The long-term care industry already has a sound foundation for an EHR in its Minimum Data Set (MDS) assessment software systems. These comprehensive assessment software products provide extensive and integrated systems to gather clinical data, provide electronic transfer to the state, and interface with billing systems to produce **electronic data interchange** (EDI) for faster reimbursement. Many of these systems also support the care-planning process to create the actual care plan directly through the comprehensive assessment data entered into the software system. These are the beginnings of the long-term healthcare EHR. Further development of databases and data repositories will allow the long-term care facility to better analyze the clinical data captured in the existing electronic systems before receiving their quality indicator (QI) reports. In a sense, the long-term care industry is ahead of the healthcare industry with its comprehensive assessment mandated to be electronic. Some hospitals do not yet have electronic clinical data available in their institutions.

Issues Unique to the Computerization of Medical Data

"Medical data are a collection of observations about a [resident]. These observations can be objective measurements, such as blood pressure reading, or the subjective assessment of a [resident's] level of pain or anxiety. This is the primary difference between medical data and the business data collected by most corporations. In fact, since these data are used in medical decision making, which impacts the quality of life (or death), they become even more important" (Priest 2000, p. 28).

Although information systems used to gather medical data and data in corporations or other organizations will have similar hardware components, the software used to capture resident care data is different. "The delivery of health services is an information-intensive process. High-quality resident care relies upon careful documentation of each resident's medical history, health status, current medical conditions, and treatment plans" (Austin and Boxerman 1998, p. 3). The very nature of health information—the private, detailed medical facts about an individual—also greatly adds to the complexity of medical data over that of corporations or other organizations. Although other corporations may have an individual's demographic and specific financial information, the healthcare industry collects and utilizes personal, private health-related information.

Concerns regarding the nature of medical data also have resulted in passage of federal legislation for the protection of those data. The Health Insurance Portability and Accountability Act (HIPAA) of 1996, further clarified in the transaction, privacy, and security standards promulgated by the Secretary of Health and Human Services, provides standards for the protection of those data.

"The nature of medical data has a tremendous impact on the methodologies used in system design, implementation, and evaluation. Integrated hospital information systems, medical records, home care, and physician office systems impact everyone working in the health care environment. Security and privacy issues, and the use of the Internet, can make them a key barrier to proliferation of the electronic medical record" (Priest 2000, p. 28). (See figure 21.1 for categories of health information systems.)

The detailed clinical data, clinical laboratory, radiology, vital signs, and history and physical elements of the resident's care are characteristics that make medical data difficult to computerize. Those objective and subjective data elements about a resident require many different formats to capture the data to the extent necessary.

Options among Software Systems

Many products currently on the market provide a means to gather clinical data required in the comprehensive assessment process. They range in functionality from the CMS RAVEN product that provides a basic software system to allow submission to the state for reporting the MDS to more comprehensive systems that create both preprogrammed and query-reporting capabilities.

Figure 21.1.   Categories of health information systems used in the healthcare industry

Clinical	Strategic decision support	Electronic networking
Computerized patient records	Planning and marketing	Insurance billing and claims processing
Medical decision support	Financial forecasting	Regional/national databases
Automated instrumentation	Resource allocation	Online purchasing
Clinical research and education	Performance assessment	Provider networks
Administrative	Outcomes measurement	
Financial		
Scheduling		
Human resources		
Materials management		
Office automation		

Source: Austin and Boxerman 1998, p. 6.

They differ greatly in price as well. Although the CMS RAVEN system is free, it does not have the sophistication and sufficient reporting capability that a more costly system includes.

Many products available on the market include software that is integrated for registration, billing for all payers, accounts receivable, general ledger, admission, discharge and transfer, and resident trust funds. These systems typically interface with the facility's existing MDS software product or provide an MDS option within their system for seamless data sharing. In the comprehensive MDS software products available, data can be exported to facilitate development of online care plans and to provide assistance in monitoring QI triggers. These integrated modules inherent in the comprehensive software systems allow information needed for Medicare PPS billing to be exported, including RUG scores, modifiers, and assessment reference dates.

Best-of-breed information systems, those systems deemed the best in an area of expertise, also may be purchased. Using this approach may require interface programming so that the systems can communicate with each other. In the best-of-breed approach to software solutions, the facility buys those systems that are considered top of the line; thus, each information software system may be purchased from a different vendor. The end result provides the facility with the best financial system, the best MDS system, the best clinical documentation system, the best physician order-entry system, and so on.

The right information technology (IT) solutions will provide a competitive advantage to the facility through enhancement of effective business strategies and real-time data-reporting capabilities. The use of information systems can provide a competitive advantage for the facility not only in capturing the data effectively, but also in reproducing them appropriately to enhance resident and facility outcomes.

Advantages of Computerized Environments

"Effective healthcare information systems can provide up-to-the minute information on clinical and administrative matters, and they can process that information to allow a healthcare executive to make effective strategic decisions" (Austin and Boxerman 1998, p. 3). Having to extrapolate data manually, handle paper resident records, and hand-tabulate multiple-page audit tools is time-consuming and fraught with error. Computerized information systems would be able to manage an information-intensive environment in a much more organized, systematic, and productive manner. A computer software and data management system:

- Automatically extrapolates information
- Saves hours of manual data auditing and hand tabulation
- Produces efficient and effective information for executive decision support

According to an Institute of Medicine report, there are many reasons for supporting an electronic medical record. Electronic medical records:

"1. Support [resident] care and improve its quality.

2. Enhance productivity of healthcare professional.

3. Reduce administrative costs associated with healthcare delivery and financing.

4. Support clinical and health services research.

5. Accommodate future developments in healthcare technology, policy, management, and finance.

6. Protect [resident] date confidentiality" (Austin and Boxerman 1998, p. 14).

Computerizing the health record system has certain advantages when it comes to managing information. Austin and Boxerman (1998, p. 35) identified the following characteristics of useful management information:

"• Information—not data

• Relevant

• Sensitive

• Unbiased

• Comprehensive

• Timely

• Action-oriented

• Uniform (for comparative purposes)

• Performance-targeted

• Cost-effective"

Computerization ensures that these characteristics are available. Properly designed systems can provide information, not just data. The data in a well-designed system are relevant, sensitive, and particularly unbiased. Moreover, they can be more comprehensive, timely, and uniform. A computerized system is more performance targeted and cost-effective than one in which data are gathered manually. Speed and accuracy are two key advantages to a computerized system.

Information systems support resident care and improve its quality in numerous ways. They:

• Enhance the productivity of healthcare professionals

• Improve communication among residents, clinicians, and physicians

• Reduce the administrative costs associated with healthcare delivery and financing by providing better utilization of resident care treatments, faster claims submission and payment, and ease of access to information

• Support clinical and health services research and track outcomes

• Accommodate future developments in healthcare technology, policy, management, and finance allowing better strategic planning and management

• Protect resident data confidentiality, provide security and technical mechanisms, and allow for privacy of resident information

Well-designed systems support outcomes management, which is the current focus in the healthcare environment and an initiative that the Joint Commission on Accreditation of Healthcare Organizations (JCAHO) incorporated into its ORYX performance measures. Computerized systems enhance data gathering for MDS submission, thus allowing state reviewers and the Centers for Medicare and Medicaid Services (CMS) to monitor and respond to outliers of resident care. These same computerized data systems provide the same information to the organization for better understanding of issues and problematic areas of resident care prior to regulatory oversight inspections.

Data from the information system are used to generate a number of performance reports, including resident satisfaction, ratios of residents to staff, and other key indicators of cost and quality. Outcome reports are generated on the cost-effectiveness of alternative treatment modalities, with data from these assessments used to create practice guidelines of the clinics (Austin and Boxerman 1998, p. 15).

The computerized environment can provide information for strategic decision support systems as well.

Until recently, very little priority was assigned to the use of information for strategic planning and management in healthcare facilities. Managed care and market-driven reform have quickly changed this situation. Organizations that wish to survive in the current environment must be able to:

1. access the health risks of the population they serve or plan to serve in the future;
2. forecast the costs and revenues anticipated from contracts with HMOs and exclusive provider arrangements; and
3. measure the clinical outcomes of services provided and continuously improve service quality in order to compete successfully for business in the medical marketplace (Austin and Boxerman 1998, p. 16).

Computerized systems give organizations the ability to have information at their fingertip. Further, they have the potential to create a paperless environment. Moreover, computerization allows for a timely, current, accurate, relevant, complete, and detailed presentation. One-time data capture eliminates the need to have several clinicians repeatedly ask residents for the same information. Finally, it is good for the documentation of resident care. The capture of data from individual visits can be compiled to indicate episodes of care. Properly designed information systems can benefit resident, care provider, and organization alike.

Disadvantages

"Unfortunately, it's impossible to put an exact dollar figure on the value of information" (Haag, Cummings, and Dawkins 2000, p. 21). One of the greatest disadvantages to computerized systems is cost. Information system solutions require many hours of clinical, information technology, and professional expertise to prepare the system for implementation, not to mention upgrade costs. Clinical staff training and actual implementation of the EHR requires much time and effort that are taken directly from resident care.

A computerized system is only as good as the person inputting the data. That is the "garbage in, garbage out" adage. "The intelligent use of information in health services management does not just happen. Rather, the administrator must ensure that it occurs in a systematic, formally planned way" (Austin and Boxerman 1998, p. 4). Without attention to detail, data integrity and data criticality are affected. Even table-driven systems can suffer from inattention to detailed data selection.

computers are only tools to aid in the accomplishment of a wider set of goals. . . . Information technology by itself is not the answer to management problems; technology must be a broader restructuring of the organization, including reengineering of business processes. Alignment of information systems strategy with business goals of the health care organization is essential (Austin and Boxerman 1998, p. 5).

If computerized systems are not designed correctly, organizations cannot obtain the information derived from the data.

Another disadvantage is in the realm of employee acceptance of the new system. "The application of information technology in health services organizations inevitably involves change, often major change, in the way business is done. Change is threatening to organizational stakeholders, particularly employees" (Austin and Boxerman 1998, p. 37). Employees can feel threatened by a computerized environment—particularly worrying about job elimination and job redesign—because they may not have the required computer skills. "You have to realize that the success of IT as a set of tools in your organization depends on the careful planning for, development, management, and use of IT with the two other key business resources—people and information" (Haag, Cummings, and Dawkins 2000, p. 5).

Acceptance is limited due to the cost of hardware, software, and work hours to implement. A demonstration of a computerized software package can look easy to use, but in reality it takes many long hours to implement the system in the manner most effective for a particular organization.

Selection Process

Implementation of a computerized system requires buy-in and commitment from the facility's board of directors and senior management. It also relies on clinical input and feedback on desired systems and system approaches. Thus, clinicians have to be committed to the project as well. Moreover, the organization must have a well-defined strategic plan, and the information system's goals, objectives, and priorities must match it. Information requirements and priorities must be clearly defined, and the information architecture and infrastructure must be available to support the organization's strategic direction. Finally, an adequate budget must be firmly established to support the move to a computer-stored resident record.

Integration among existing systems that will be used with the computer-stored resident record also must be in place. Likewise, policies and procedures for data security, physical and technical safeguards, disaster planning, contingency planning, access controls, virus protection, training, and sanctions must be in place.

Before selecting the appropriate software system, the organization must have an understanding of the hardware (physical devices) and infrastructure (blueprint of information technology) required to implement it. This involves consideration of a number of elements, including:

- Client/server network architecture
- Storage and data warehouses
- Interface engines
- Wide-area networks
- Database requirements
- Workstations
- Compliant with HL7 standards

The organization also must consider the following:

- Goals and objectives for the facility
- Goals and objective of the system

- Management information requirements

- Crucial success factors

- Information preferences

- Priority applications

  —Clinical

  —Administrative

  —Decision support

- Specifications

  —Centralized approach versus decentralized approach

  —Network architecture

  —Location of data and data owners

  —Security and controls

- Software plan

  —Vendor packages

  —Homegrown solutions

  —Contracted tailoring

  —Combination

- Information technology plan

  —Staffing

  —Outsourcing

  —Combination

- Resource requirements

- Capital budget (hardware, software, network, communication devices)

- Operating budget (staff, supplies, consultants, training, help line support, licensing, and annual fees) (Austin and Boxerman 1998, p. 175).

To assist in the selection process, the organization must recognize the competitive environment and strategically examine its internal need and requirements. The scope of the project, system requirements, and system design implementation and support must be defined as well. Figure 21.2 depicts the systems process planning that should be used.

Examining existing systems and processes for data gathering and streamlining and simplifying administrative processes also should be done prior to implementing a computer-stored resident record. Moreover, preparing or integrating systems such as eligibility and benefits verification, automated payment processing, electronic claims submission, centralized resident scheduling, enrollment, and master resident index must be accomplished. The organization should prepare for a paperless environment.

Figure 21.2. The systems planning process

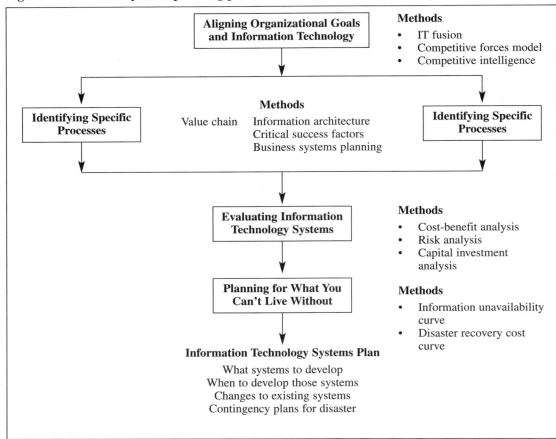

The requirements for connectivity and seamless interfaces hinder the need to link health-care providers. The lack of standards and a standardized vocabulary hampers the facility's ability to provide connectivity and seamless interfaces. Moreover, vendor buy-out by other vendors also plays a role. The facility may find itself with products that are no longer supported and with the need to purchase and implement new systems. Finally, the cost of system purchases, implementation, and training is prohibitive.

No two systems are similar enough to interface smoothly. There are even interface problems among a single vendor's products. The many vendor products and choices make it difficult to link systems to systems. And, as mentioned earlier, implementation and training requirements take away valuable clinical and physician treatment time from residents, which creates cost-effectiveness issues.

However, an integrated delivery system does enhance communication among clinicians, physicians, and residents. It allows diagnoses and diseases to be stored and tracked, enabling all problems to be accessed by appropriate clinical staff and providing more timely and higher-quality care. Repeat testing is decreased because test results are readily available for clinical care. "Web sites provide network access to centralize an individual's personal and demographic information, healthcare contracts, immunizations, office visits, tests, treatments, health histories and a personal health journal" (Priest 2000, p. 31). Continuity of care is better served because resident data are available in real time. Duplication of effort is reduced, and utilization review and case management are more successful.

Selection Team

The selection team depends on the system required but should include representation from those areas that will have hands-on application use. For a clinical system, the team must be interdisciplinary to ensure buy-in and support of the system after it is implemented. Nurses and physicians are extremely important members of the team selecting a clinical solution for the facility. The line staff, including nursing, therapy, and ancillary staff, should have input in the selection process because they will ultimately have to use the product. They understand the current work flow and can provide valuable insight into information system software selection. The facility must remember that the installation of a clinical system is not an IT project but, rather, a facility project that should include key end users. Health record personnel should be included in the selection process because they understand records processing and can help determine if the system will meet federal and state requirements for documentation practice. After the clinical system is implemented, they will have to use it to accomplish their many and varied tasks in record management, coding, indexing, filing, and retrieval. System success depends largely on user buy-in and proper selection to meet the organization's goals and objectives.

Implementation

Implementation of the information system is a multifaceted process that requires thoughtful planning. Successful software installations require a detailed and systematic approach to ensure that goals and objectives are met.

The following steps must be completed when implementing an information system:

1. Perform a thorough analysis of the functionality needed.
2. Design an approach for functionality (in-house development, vendor selection, output, input, database, data flow specifications, and so on).
3. Determine the systems required to meet the functionality.
4. Purchase or develop the system.
5. Install the system (customize).
6. Test the system.
7. Operate the system (actual use).
8. Maintain the system (update).
9. Evaluate the system (goals achieved).
10. Improve the system.

Depending on the system's complexity, goals and objectives of installation and operation will affect the overall implementation time line. Obviously, simple solutions will require less time than more complicated, integrated solutions. Testing is a key issue in implementation. Testing the system prior to actual go-live is a necessary step in ensuring success of the IT implementation process.

Vendors can be helpful in providing faster implementation time lines, but their assistance increases the cost of the product. However, for those facilities with fewer IT staff members, utilizing vendors and consultants will speed the implementation process.

Automation Issues

"As defined in the Institute of Medicine patient record study report (The Computerized-based Patient Record: An Essential Technology for Health care) the computer-based patient record is 'an electronic patient record that resides in a system specifically designed to support users through availability of complete and accurate data, practitioner reminders and alerts, clinical decision support systems, links to bodies of medical knowledge and other aides. . . . As the nation's vision moves toward a computer-based patient record, one must not lose sight of the individual's constitutional right to privacy. A computer-based patient record is electronically maintained information about an individual's lifetime health status and health care. It replaces the paper medical record as the primary record of care, meeting all clinical, legal and administrative requirements. It also serves the providers and patients better than a paper medical record. A computer-based patient record system also provides reminders and alerts, linkages with knowledge sources for decision support, and data for outcome research and improved management of the health care delivery. . . . In order to achieve the electronic medical record, health data must be gathered and stored. Standard terminology and data content is necessary to capture data in a more structured manner which enables location of information and enhances the ability to perform analyses on data" (CPRI 2003).

To accomplish this, common data sets have to be identified and common terminology defined. HIPAA has begun to establish standards. Nursing taxonomy has been developed to provide a standardized language for nurses but is not fully functional. The following issues must be examined and resolved in order to achieve the EHR:

- Application functionality

- Sources of data (input validation)

- Data entry devices

- Data input (interfaces)

- Data capture (storage, process, communication, security)

- Permanence

- Maintenance

- Backup and recovery

- Durability

Reengineering of Clinical Processes

"Much like the physical sciences with their system of weights and measures, health care must be able to communicate information in a manner which permits creation of comparable data across health providers in the natural course of care delivery, enabling risk adjusted benchmarking, clinical guideline development, aggregate outcomes analysis, and shared decision support rules development. Additional guidelines are being developed to address:

- Information security items

- Implementation of electronic signatures

- Methods for identifying and authenticating users of computer-based records

- Development of confidentiality statements and agreements
- System application security features
- Security audit functions and processes" (CPRI 2003)

Clinical processes must be reengineered to best capture data for the computerized systems. Redesign of forms, practice, and processes must be accomplished to use the system to its maximum capacity. Keystrokes, log-ons, and password management all hinder documentation. There are times when clinical staff, particularly physicians, will not accept seconds of delay if an individual's life is on the line. "In fact, the quality is quite variable and in some cases software purchasers wind up with systems that fall short of their expectations" (Austin and Boxerman 1998, p. 101).

Differences among Software Applications

Computerized systems are not readily accepted because of the time, expense, effort, and education required to implement them. The paper record and charting systems are familiar, comfortable, and consistent across most healthcare providers. As clinicians change jobs, the charting process remains consistent and customary. However, software applications can differ considerably. Each computerized system is adapted to the setting and the institution. Software applications do not have the same look and feel as the paper charting process. They do not interface with each other, leaving much to be desired as a true EHR.

As mentioned earlier, software application vendors are often purchased by other companies and their software application eliminated by the new owner. That could mean another major purchase of a software application that will be supported by the new vendor. As each vendor's product is eliminated, more money is required to purchase new software, which translates to more time, effort, and training requirements for clinical staff.

Technology is limited in certain situations. Many more products are available for the acute care setting than for the long-term care setting. Clinical EHR packages differ greatly among vendors. Finding the correct package for the institution is time-consuming and can be cost prohibitive. And, as discussed earlier, there are many problems with user acceptance, education, and expectation. There are no guarantees that the package chosen is the best solution, will provide the results expected, or will be a viable product in the long run.

Creation of a Standardized Language

If lifetime resident records are to become a reality, there needs to be a standardized language, or taxonomy. Each clinician, system, entity, and country must use the same standard nursing language to identify the collective observations of each resident. Systems cannot share information that is not standardized. Blood pressure must be captured the same way in each system, office, and facility in order for it to be used across a resident's lifetime. A blood pressure captured as B/P 140/70 will not match BP 140/70 or blood pressure 140/70. Blood pressure is a simple example to demonstrate the different ways in which the same data elements are captured using different styles. Electronic transfer of the B/P, BP, or blood pressure may not be accepted across all systems.

HIPAA has begun to set U.S. standards for the EDI of resident data for billing. Code sets, EDI standards of ASC X 12 N and HL 7, are now mandated nationwide. These allow data to be shared instantly and transmitted in a standardized format. Healthcare plans, clearinghouses, and healthcare providers have the same definitions and requirements for the EDI because of this federal legislation.

However, HIPAA covers only the EDI of resident identifiable information for billing and healthcare coverage. It does not mandate standards for nursing language.

Having standards for nursing language will ensure that a particular diagnosis or intervention will be identified and interpreted in the same manner across the entire continuum of care. Thus, diagnoses or interventions can be transmitted, carried, charted, read, shared, and understood uniformly within every clinical contact.

> In order to provide the legal record of care, the system must capture the clinician's expression of [resident] assessment, diagnosis, goals, the plan of care, the care actually delivered, the [resident's] responses to care, and the actual [resident] outcomes. A nomenclature that captures all of the enormous richness of this data set across the spectrum of [resident] care settings must have what is known as *domain completeness*. Existing nursing nomenclatures cover various aspects of the nursing process in varying depths in one setting or another, but none can claim domain completeness (Zielstorff 1998, p. 1).

The process to electronically capture nursing language must fit naturally into the clinician's work flow. Clinicians have to see a benefit in the system that outweighs the burden of changing their documenting methods. Careful integration of the work flow into an institution's work flow processes is extremely important. "If you cannot name it, you cannot teach it, research it, practice it, finance it, or put it into public policy. And—most certainly—you cannot implement it in a computer-based system" (Henry, Warren, and Zielstorff, 1998, p. 1).

The translation of existing nursing taxonomy into other languages is not easy. "Translation must transfer the concepts behind the words, and concepts which are well recognized in one culture may not be recognized in another" (Clark 1998, p. 2).

"Today's health care environment demands that automated [resident] record systems deliver the following functions:

1. Provide the legal record of care

2. Support clinical decision making

3. Capture costs for billing, costing and/or accounting purposes

4. Accumulate a structured, retrievable data base for

    a. administrative queries

    b. quality assurance

    c. research

5. Support data exchange with internal and external systems

All of these functions depend on data. Each function places requirements on the nomenclature that is used to capture and store that data. As we will see, sometimes these requirements conflict with one another, which further confounds the effort to develop a single, comprehensive nomenclature for use in automated systems" (Zielztorff 1998, p. 5).

Summary

Aligning the information technology goals and objectives with facility goals and objectives is of importance from a quality outcome perspective. If the goals and objectives do not match, the end product will not provide the required results and expectations.

Understanding system requirements, infrastructure demands, and facility needs is an important step in the computerized environment. Following each step of the implementation process and testing rigorously are important to quality outcomes. Well-thought-out, effective information solution implementation allows the organization to provide better services and programs for each resident and enhances staff productivity, which reflects on the facility's competitive edge. The key steps in selection and implementation must be achieved to produce a high-quality outcome.

The ultimate goal of implementing clinical IT solutions should be to ensure that the resident receives the highest-quality care. The outcome of any clinical installation of IT software should be to ensure that the resident maintains or improves functional ability and that the facility is able to "provide the necessary care and services to attain or maintain the highest practicable physical, mental, and psychosocial well-being" (CMS 2001, PP-83).

References

Austin, Charles J., and Stuart B. Boxerman. 1998. *Information Systems for Health Services Administration,* 5th ed. Chicago: Health Administration Press.

Henry, Suzanne Bakken, Judith J. Warren, and Rita D. Zielstorff. 1998. Nursing data, classification systems, and quality indicators: what every HIM professional needs to know. *Journal of AHIMA* 69(5): 48–54. Available at http://www.ahima.org/journal.

Centers for Medicare and Medicaid Services. 2001 (October 31). Guidance to Surveyors—Long-Term Care Facilities, appendix PP in *State Operations Manual.* Available at www.cms.gov.

Clark, June. Year. 1998. The International Classification for Nursing Practice Project. Available at http://www.ana.org.

Computerized Patient Record Institute. 2003. Available at www.himss.org.

Haag, Stephen, Maeve Cummings, and James Dawkins. 2000. *Management Information Systems,* 2nd ed. Boston: Irwin McGraw-Hill.

Health Information Management Systems Society. Available at http://www2.himss.org.

Health Insurance Portability and Accountability Act of 1996. Available at http://aspe.os.dhhs.gov/admnsimp.

Nursing Informatics. Available at http://www.cpmc.columbia.edu/homepages/joz9001/NL.html.

Priest, Stephen. 2000. *HSA Management Information Systems.* Standish, Me.: St. Joseph's College.

Zielstorff, Rita D. 1998. Part one: characteristics of a good nursing nomenclature from an informatics perspective. Available at http://www.ana.org.

Chapter 22

Confidentiality, Security, and Privacy

Privacy is a resident's fundamental right. Healthcare providers have always dealt with the detailed, sensitive information of a resident's health history and current medical and physical condition. The health information management (HIM) professional has a long-standing dedication to protecting the **confidentiality, security,** and **privacy** of any health record maintained by the healthcare provider. Confidentiality, security, and privacy are not new topics for discussion because of the Health Insurance Portability and Accountability Act (HIPAA) of 1996 but, rather, old acquaintances to be constantly and diligently protected.

Even the Hippocratic oath contains language to ensure the protection of **individually identifiable health information.**

> Whatever, in connection with my professional practice, or not in connection with it, I see or hear, in the life of men, which ought not to be spoken of abroad, I will not divulge, as reckoning that all such should be kept secret.

The reason for confidentiality is to ensure that the resident's fundamental right to privacy is maintained. HIPAA developed standards to ensure that a resident's right to privacy is better achieved.

However, HIPAA does not fully cover confidentiality, security, and privacy. Rather, it only provides a foundation for privacy and security from which healthcare facilities must constantly monitor compliance and policy. Many states have comprehensive legislation in place that will not be affected by the HIPAA mandates. Indeed, state laws that are more stringent supersede specific HIPAA regulations.

Long-term care facilities must monitor changes in the HIPAA regulations and also closely watch state requirements and regulations. As the laws and regulations change, facilities must adapt their policies, procedures, and programs defining confidentiality, security, and privacy accordingly.

Security and Privacy Program

Compliance with HIPAA, state laws, and regulations governing the confidentiality, security, and privacy of patient information is mandatory and enforced by civil and criminal penalties promulgated by HIPAA. Facilities must provide policies and procedures for the confidentiality, security, and privacy of individually identifiable health information. These policies and procedures should be part of a comprehensive privacy and security program that includes compliance records and reports defining practice parameters and expectations. Under each specific standard discussed in this chapter are listings of suggested policies and procedures.

In addition, facilities should require every employee, whether new or established, to sign a confidentiality statement to be kept in the employee's human resources file. This agreement is the foundation of the facility's security and privacy program. Facility policy should determine the need to review and renew this statement, but generally it is a good idea to update it annually.

In addition to having policies, procedures, and practices in place to demonstrate compliance, the facility must ensure that its staff is educated on the importance of confidentiality.

Examples of educational opportunities include:

- Accessing only the information required to do the job
- Discussing the resident's private information with the correct people in the correct areas
- Disclosing private information as per policy
- Protecting passwords
- Keeping the resident's private information out of public access areas
- Protecting computer screens and medical records from easy access
- Locking file cabinets, doors, and desk drawers when no one is available in the area
- Asking for identification of unknown individuals
- Wearing name badges at all times
- Copying policies and procedures
- Faxing protected information per policy
- Reminding each other of the importance of confidentiality
- Talking to only those who need to know
- Keeping conversations down at nursing stations and treatment areas to help protect confidentiality
- Questioning: How would I feel if this were my information?

Importance of Confidentiality

The importance of the confidentiality and privacy of resident information cannot be understated. Understanding regulations at the state and federal levels is crucial, and applying that knowledge to everyday working patterns in the long-term care setting is key to ensuring that the resident's right to privacy is upheld. Knowing the policies and thinking before acting will help each staff member protect the resident's information.

Staff members must only have access to the information they need to know to perform their job functions. The HIPAA privacy rule applies to resident health information in every type of format—electronic, written, and oral; thus, knowing and understanding the implications of a breach of confidentiality is vital. Confidentiality, security, and privacy rules and regulations are not meant to burden the facility or the staff but, rather, are intended to protect and ensure each resident's fundamental right to be left alone.

Patient information concerning drug and alcohol abuse, psychology and psychiatry, and HIV/AIDS treatment information was restricted from disclosure prior to the regulations contained in HIPAA. The federal restrictions governing these confidentiality areas have not changed under HIPAA.

It is important to be familiar with "more stringent" as defined in the privacy regulations. "The Privacy Rule provides a floor of privacy protection. State laws that are more stringent remain in force" (DHHS 2002). There are six defining categories contained in the more stringent definition in the *Federal Register.*

Monitoring Change in HIPAA and State Privacy Requirements

HIPAA privacy standards were implemented on April 14, 2003. Being ever diligent and proactive will ensure that the facility will keep abreast of the changing healthcare environment and the promised changes to HIPAA and implementation of state-specific privacy and security legislation.

Confidentiality, security, and privacy do not go away, but HIPAA will change. Protecting the resident's right to privacy will never be fully completed because rules and regulations change. There will be tests of the regulations and facility programs through the legal system that may drive even more change.

For example, electronic systems and electronic health records will require improvements in security techniques. Technology will advance to meet the rising needs of society and with those changes will come new transaction standards, new privacy rules, and greater security measures. Facilities cannot afford to be complacent. Complacency is a driving force behind failure and noncompliance.

Existing facility policies and procedures on confidentiality, security, and privacy must be reviewed and rewritten as required. The state hospital association, facility legal counsel, or skilled nursing home associations may provide valuable ongoing support as HIPAA regulations are reviewed and revised. The notice of privacy practice that the facility will develop and provide for its residents will provide a good source document for listing all facility policies and practices, and can be referred to in the future if the regulations are indeed revised.

Health Insurance Portability and Accountability Act of 1996

The **Health Insurance Portability and Accountability Act (HIPAA) of 1996** was created "To amend the Internal Revenue Code of 1986 to improve portability and continuity of health insurance coverage in the group and individual markets, to combat waste, fraud, and abuse in health insurance and health care delivery, to promote the use of medical savings accounts, to improve access to long-term care services and coverage, to simplify the administration of health insurance, and for other purposes" (HIPAA 1996, p. 1).

HIPAA was signed into law on August 21, 1996, by President Clinton. The delegation of authority set in the HIPAA regulations falls under the Department of Health and Human Services (DHHS), Office for Civil Rights. The law, Public Act 104-191, contains the following five provisions:

- Title I. Insurance Portability

- Title II. Administrative Simplification

- Title III. Medical Savings/Tax Deduction
- Title IV. Group Health Plan Provisions
- Title V. Revenue Offset Provisions

The focus of this chapter is administration simplification. "It is the purpose of this subtitle to improve the Medicare program under title XVIII of the Social Security Act, the Medicaid program under title XIX of such Act, and the efficiency and effectiveness of the healthcare system by encouraging the development of a health information system through the establishment of standards and requirements for the electronic transmission of certain health information" (HIPAA 1996, section 2612).

HIPAA provides three distinct, yet interconnected, standards for managing electronic data interchange (EDI): transaction standards, security standards, and privacy standards. These are outlined as follows:

- Transaction standards

  —Published on August 17, 2000

  —Final October 16, 2000

  —Must comply by October 16, 2002

  —March 2002 provided a means to file an extension to the transaction standards. The extension allowed facilities to extend the compliance date with the transaction standards to October 16, 2003, and required testing of transaction sets by April 16, 2003.

- Security standards

  —Originally published August 12, 1998

  —Proposed as of October 31, 2002

  —Republished Feburary 20, 2003

  —Final April 20, 2003

  —Must comply by April 20, 2005

  —The security standards contain the following requirements:

    –Administrative safeguards

    –Physical safeguards

    –Technical safeguards

- Privacy standards

  —Published December 28, 2000

  —Comment period extended in February 2001

  —Initial Final Rule April 14, 2001

  —Privacy guidelines published July 6, 2001

  —Revised privacy standard published March 2002

  —Finalized in August 2002 with new guidelines

  —Compliance required by April 14, 2003

These three sets of standards are discussed in detail in this chapter.

The purpose of HIPAA is to reduce administrative overhead. HIPAA provides standards to replace hundreds of forms and formats for claims and other administrative and financial transactions. In providing standards for EDI, the legislators were compelled to provide privacy and security standards to protect the privacy and safeguard individually identifiable health information contained in the resident's designated record set.

Compliance

All those payers, healthcare providers, and clearinghouses that submit health claim information electronically must comply with HIPAA. This means that any providers, including hospitals, nursing homes, physician offices and clinics, home and ambulatory services, must comply with the final regulations when they submit claims electronically.

Penalties

HIPAA sets civil penalties for failure to use all three sets of adopted standards. There are criminal penalties for wrongfully disclosing confidential information, which include:

- $100 for each violation of a standard

- Maximum of $25,000 per year per identical requirement

In addition, there are wrongful disclosure penalties for each offense of the standards.

- Wrongful disclosure

    —Fined not more than $50,000

    —Imprisoned not more than one year

- False pretenses

    —Fined not more than $100,000

    —Imprisoned not more than five years

- Intent to sell, transfer, or use

    —Fined not more than $250,000

    —Imprisoned not more than ten years

Deliberately selling patient identifiable information is illegal. Providing individually identifiable information to the media is illegal as well.

Discussing resident care with other healthcare workers involved in the resident's specific care is acceptable practice. However, discussing resident-specific information in the nonclinical setting (elevators, lunchroom, courtyard, home, and other places) with individuals who do not need to know about the resident is not appropriate.

Intent of Electronic Data Interchange

"Electronic Data Interchange (EDI) is the electronic transfer of information, such as electronic medical health claims in a standard format between trading partners. EDI allows entities within the health care system to exchange medical, billing, and other information, and to process transactions in a manner that is fast and cost effective. With EDI, there is a substantial reduction in handling and processing time compared to paper and the risk of lost paper documents is eliminated. EDI can eliminate the inefficiencies of handling paper documents, which will significantly reduce administrative burden, lower operating costs, and improve overall data quality" (DHHS 2000a).

The *Federal Register* reports that "currently, there are about 400 formats" for electronic submission of healthcare claims in the United States. Healthcare providers have always had to submit claims to payers in these different formats, which makes software maintenance more difficult because each format for each payer has to be created and updated.

The intent of EDI is to allow providers and payers to exchange information faster and more cost-effectively. It is meant to reduce the resource-intensive claims process. Each standard contained in the current HIPAA legislation, and those that will be reviewed and revised in the future, must fit the following objectives:

- Improve the efficiency and effectiveness of the healthcare system

- Meet the needs of the health data standards

- Be consistent and uniform with other HIPAA standards

- Have low development and implementation costs relative to using the standards

- Be supported by ANSI-accredited standards

- Have timely development, testing, implementation, and updating procedures to quickly realize administrative simplification benefits

- Be technologically independent of any computer platforms and transmission protocols unless the standards are obviously part of the standard

- Be precise and unambiguous

- Keep data collection and paperwork to a minimum

- Incorporate flexibility

Security and Privacy Program Development

Facilities should develop a security and privacy program that details compliance with the HIPAA regulations. The program may contain the following components:

- Philosophy for the organization

- Purpose

- Policy

- Statement of commitment

- Definitions

- Objectives

- Accountability and responsibility

- Classification of information

- Collection of information

- Risk factors

- Access to information

- Retention and destruction

- Physical security

- Resident and employee rights inherent in the program

- Caregiver information

- Privileges and obligations of research

- Requirements for release

- User authentication

- Disaster recovery/business resumption plan

- Security and privacy administration

- Information security awareness training

- Monitoring and auditing

- References

- Attachments as appropriate to the program

Policies and Procedures

The facility should review and revise its policies and procedures to ensure compliance with the HIPAA regulations. As mentioned earlier, suggested policies and procedures are contained in the following specific HIPAA standards sections of this chapter.

HIPAA does not include telephone voice messaging or voice response nor does it discuss facsimile use. However, this does not mean that the facility should not consider policies and procedures to incorporate security and privacy mechanisms for these technologies.

Transaction Standards

The transaction standards were established to set the "standard" for sending and obtaining information electronically. These standards were designed to cut the cost of administrative overhead by creating an environment whereby the daily activity of claims processing, from admission to discharge and final billing, can be accomplished with fewer personnel, online, and in one format. Using this philosophy, the cost of providing claims-processing services would be reduced. However, to achieve compliance, many institutions are required to spend money to purchase improved system support, architecture, and new software products or update existing software capability.

According to the DHHS (2000a), "Standard means a prescribed set of rules, conditions, or requirements describing the following information for products, systems, services or practices:

1. Classification of components.

2. Specification of materials, performance, or operations.

3. Delineation of procedures."

HIPAA also defines transaction as the "the exchange of information between two parties to carry out financial or administrative activities related to health care."

The standards set by HIPAA regulation include ASC X 12 developed by the ANSI Accredited Standards Committee and National Council for Prescription Drug Programs (NCPDP) for pharmacy claims.

Benefits of Transaction Standards

HIPAA's transaction standards set technical specifications for the way healthcare data or individually identifiable health information is electronically communicated to healthcare payers, providers, and clearinghouses. They are the standards for the eleven specified types of information listed later in this chapter in the section on other pertinent information. When providers and payers can have set standards to receive all of this information electronically, it will provide faster, higher-quality healthcare with lower cost benefits for everyone involved.

> The use of these standard transactions and code sets will improve the Medicare and Medicaid programs and other Federal health programs and private health programs, and the effectiveness and efficiency of the health care industry in general, by simplifying the administration of the system and enabling the efficient electronic transmission of certain health information (DHHS 2000a).

Those healthcare facilities that send any health information in electronic form must comply with the transaction standards as well as the other standard sets in the final regulations. The reason behind the development and implementation of HIPAA is to provide facilities with a mechanism to receive faster reimbursement with less manual processing through a uniform method of EDI while implementing security mechanisms to ensure the protection of the privacy of all patients and residents.

The transaction standards provide the uniform method of EDI. Those designated ASC X 12 and NCPDP standards as well as the designated code sets provide the defined field requirements for data to be exchanged—sent and received—by provider and payer through a clearinghouse, if the facility so chooses.

Using the transaction standards offers the following benefits:

- Cleaner claims
- Electronic payment
- One format for EDI
- Decreased staff hours for manual claims processing
- Decreased paper use and storage
- Fewer pending or denied claims because of the standard claims forms
- Standardized clinical and resource databases
- Consistent information to determine fee schedules, cost analysis, and patient-mix data
- Verification of eligibility and benefits prior to billing
- Improvement of cash-flow management
- Automated precertification or preauthorization for service
- Decreased phone usage

- Improved data quality (EDI only works when data are accurate)

- Lower cost of software development and maintenance (one format decreases cost)

Moreover, the software will work with all providers, payers, plans, and clearinghouse submissions.

Compliance with Transaction Standards

All facilities, payers, and clearinghouses must comply with the transaction standards when—and only when—there is an electronic data interchange of healthcare claims. Compliance dates were effective by October 16, 2002, unless the facility submitted an extension as outlined by the Centers for Medicare and Medicaid Services (CMS). Any facility that filed an extension would have to be compliant by October 16, 2003. Under the extension, testing of claims must have begun by April 16, 2003.

Under the CMS compliance plan, a facility must abide by the transaction standards in order to reach full compliance with regulatory standards and mandates. Proper use of code sets and proper bill submissions reflect on the organization's compliance program against fraud and abuse. Under HIPAA, coding, proper billing, and claims submission are extremely important functions within the facility. Qualified coders and updated references are mandated by HIPAA as well as fraud-and-abuse provisions under CMS guidelines. Compliance and HIPAA are closely related, although they were developed for different purposes and through different methods.

Importance of the Transaction Standards

The importance of using the transaction standards through the use of EDI is self-evident. Administration simplification provides a faster, more efficient method for reimbursement and, simply put, reduces the burden on the organization by simplifying and improving the efficiency of the administration of healthcare claims and processing through EDI methods. The speed and accuracy of online data exchange makes way for improved services, customer satisfaction, and real-time data transfer through a secure and private methodology.

Documentation

Every healthcare facility must develop policies for compliance with the transaction standards. However, the policies should be kept to a minimum. For example, some facilities combine the policy and procedures into one to make the process easier to follow. Also, staff members must understand the facility's policies to ensure compliance with HIPAA. These policies may be reflected in the notice of privacy practice, if applicable. Testing plans and all steps taken in the facility's compliance process for the transaction standards should be documented and retained for reference.

Quality Considerations

The data fields required by HIPAA transaction requirements must be accurate. If the data fields change, the facility should contact its vendors and test the changes prior to implementation of the new requirements.

EDI will not function properly unless the transaction standards and code sets as outlined within HIPAA are met. Failure to have transaction standards correct could result in delayed reimbursement for the facility.

Assessment criteria for monitoring compliance with transaction standards may include the following:

- Data fields are correctly designed.

- Data in the fields are correct.

- Code sets (that is, references) are up-to-date and include all required digits.

- Code sets reflect Official Coding Guidelines.

- Quality checks on ICD-9-CM and CPT are completed as outlined by the facility.

- Billers have complied with submission policy.

- Data fields are complete.

- Coding and billing staff are updated on HIPAA requirements as policy changes occur.

- Denial of claims is monitored.

For the facility to submit claims in a timely manner, code assignment and claims processing must be completed according to policy. The policy for coding practice should stipulate the timeliness of code assignment at admission, during interim billing, and at discharge. Claims processing should be outlined in facility policy so that coding staff understand the time frames for claims submission and provide coding assignment as expected.

Other Pertinent Information

The facility must continue to monitor changes for requirements of transaction standards because the transaction could change and the code sets could evolve. The standards do stipulate that ICD-10-CM will replace ICD-9-CM in the future.

The facility should develop standards for a testing procedure and practice with their vendors to help facilitate the processing of transaction standard changes. This process will ensure that data transaction has been tested prior to actual submission and will determine problems prior to actual claims processing. The testing environment allows the facility to ensure that claims processing will continue to be fast and effective and allow reimbursement to flow into the facility without unnecessary delays.

The claims-processing policies and procedures must consider the following types of information exchanges:

"1. Healthcare claims or equivalent encounter information

2. Healthcare payment and remittance advice

3. Coordination of benefits

4. Healthcare claim status

5. Enrollment and disenrollment in a health plan

6. Eligibility for a health plan

7. Health plan premium payments

8. Referral certification and authorization

9. First report of injury

10. Health claims attachments

11. Other transactions that the Secretary may prescribe by regulation" (DHHS 2000a)

Transaction standards also define code sets to be used in EDI as follows:

- Volumes 1 and 2 of *International Classification of Diseases, Ninth Edition, Clinical Modification* (ICD-9-CM) and Official Guidelines for Coding and Reporting

- Volume 3 of *International Classification of Diseases, Ninth Edition, Clinical Modification* (ICD-9-CM) and Official Guidelines for Coding and Reporting

- **National Drug Codes** (NDC)

- Code on Dental Procedures and Nomenclature

- **Health Care Procedural Coding System** (HCPCS)

- *Current Procedural Terminology, Fourth Edition* (CPT-4)

The transaction standards require that these code sets be valid and that up-to-date references be used in the facility.

Reevaluation of the Transaction Standards

The facility must reevaluate its EDI processing as implementation of HIPAA progresses. It must keep abreast of changes and look at ways to improve EDI to minimize costs and improve services and reimbursement. Overall, the facility should be mindful of the purpose of the implementation of HIPAA transaction standards and continually evaluate its systems and processes to ensure full compliance with current and changing transaction requirements.

Other issues concern the use of unique health identifiers for individuals, employers, health plans, and healthcare providers. The facility must keep abreast of developments or changes in these specifications as well.

Policies and Procedures

Types of policies that the facility may develop as it complies with HIPAA transaction standards include:

- Access to electronic systems and processing requirements

- Admission processing

- Auditing process for quality and accuracy in each area as needed

- Charge entry procedures

- Chargemaster monitoring

- Claims processing and submission

- Code set accuracy

- Coding assignment processing

- Coding time frames
- Complaint management
- Compliance plan
- Data submission criteria
- Denial processing and monitoring
- Documentation required to code accurately
- EDI processes detailed for each payer
- Managing resident request for claims-processing information
- Oversight of claims-processing function
- Oversight of coding function
- Partnership with health information management for code assignment
- Reference material required for code assignment
- Security and privacy mechanisms used
- Testing criteria
- Vendor listing for healthcare claims processing for tracking purposes

Privacy Standards

Privacy is a resident's fundamental right. HIPAA's privacy rule provides the first national standards to protect individuals' identifiable health information by:

- Providing patients and residents with more control over their health information
- Setting boundaries on the use and disclosure of **protected health information**
- Establishing safeguards that protect privacy
- Establishing accountability by implementing civil and criminal penalties
- Protecting public health through required disclosures
- Providing the ability for the patient or resident to make informed choices
- Enabling patients and residents to know the privacy practice of the facility
- Limiting disclosure to a minimum
- Giving patients or residents the right to review and receive their records

The standards established by the privacy rule distinguish *use* from *disclosure* to help facilities understand the two distinct terms as they relate to HIPAA and implementation. Privacy standards also call for business associate contracts. The "'business associate' is generally any independent party that performs activities on behalf of a covered entity using [protected health information] PHI, or provides any of a wide range of services relating to a covered entity involving the use or disclosure of PHI" (DHHS 2002).

This rule includes standards to protect the privacy of individually identifiable health information . . . which apply to health plans, health care clearinghouses, and certain health care providers, present standards with respect to the rights of individuals who are the subjects of this information, procedures for the exercise of those rights, and the authorized and required uses and disclosures of this information (DHHS 2002b, p. 82462).

The terms *disclosure* and *use* are defined as follows (DHHS 2002b):

Disclosure means the release, transfer, provision of access to, or divulging in any other manner of information outside the entity holding the information. . . . Use means, with respect to individually identifiable health information, the sharing, employment, application, utilization, examination, or analysis of such information within an entity that maintains such information.

Purpose of the Privacy Standards

The privacy standards were established to help improve the efficiency and effectiveness of public and private health programs and healthcare services by furnishing improved protections for individually identifiable health information. They indicate that there has been "growing public concerns" about the progress made in electronic technology and the use of technology in the healthcare industry. The standards also were developed to protect the public's perception that there is "a substantial erosion of the privacy surrounding individually identifiable health information maintained by health care providers, health plans and their administrative contractors" (DHHS 2002b, p. 82462).

These national standards were designed to permit greater control, set boundaries, and establish safeguards for residents' health information. They establish accountability within the healthcare industry while enabling the government to protect the public's health.

In addition, the privacy standards provide a means for residents to find out how their information may be used and disclosed, provide mechanisms to establish minimum necessary guidelines and controls, and provide a federal requirement to give residents the right to inspect and obtain copies of their health information. Many states already allow residents to access their records, but the privacy standards now create a federal mandate to ensure national rights to privacy and access for each individual who uses the healthcare industry.

Specific Components of the Privacy Rule

HIPAA clearly provides direction on compliance with its privacy standards.

The privacy rule requires facilities to share a general notice of privacy policy with their residents. This notice summarizes the facility's practices as they relate to privacy of individually identifiable health information.

The privacy rule also requires that authorizations be obtained prior to release of individually identifiable health information in specific cases.

In addition, the privacy rule's standards provide specific requirements for fundraising, marketing, restrictions on uses and disclosures, confidential communication, access to information, amendments to health information, and the ability to receive an accounting of disclosures. Facilities must assign responsibility for oversight of the privacy standards as well.

The regulations of August 2002 clarify the term *minimum necessary*. Facilities need to understand the minimum necessary requirements of the privacy standards and to make reasonable efforts to limit the use and disclosure of protected health information to the minimum necessary to address the need.

Importance of Privacy in Healthcare

The resident's right to privacy is no different from any other right inherent in the long-term care environment. The concept of preserving the resident's health goes hand in hand with ensuring the resident's right to privacy with regard to his or her health information. In the *Federal Register,* concern has been identified among the general public that the advent of new technology such as electronic health records will result in invasions of privacy. In the long-term care environment, MDS data collection and submission is a vital component of the facility's quality of care structure. These data are required to be submitted electronically to the specific state for monitoring and quality reporting. The privacy standards enhance the privacy and security of this data submission.

The privacy standards provide each facility with the tools to build a strong and secure health information management process complete with transaction standards, security mechanisms, and privacy policy, procedures, and techniques. Ensuring that each staff member, resident, volunteer, vendor, visitor, and student understands the facility's commitment to privacy is essential and further defines and clarifies the facility's responsibility to protect resident's health information.

Documentation for the Privacy Standards

A number of required components must be documented within specific privacy standards. Documentation may consist of form development and review of existing documentation to ensure its compliance with the privacy standards. Documentation should include the notice of privacy practice, uses and disclosures, authorizations, amendments and resident access to health records, and an accounting of releases of information. Designation of a privacy officer also must be documented in some manner, whether through the security and privacy program or a job description, and communicated to staff, residents, volunteers, vendors, visitors, and students within the facility.

Documentation must be implemented by the compliance dates and reviewed as needed or as regulations change and new laws at the federal and state level are implemented.

Quality Considerations

Authorizations to disclose or use health information have specific requirements that must be met and must comply with existing state laws. The notice of privacy practice must include every aspect of privacy policy and practice. This document is provided to the resident, so it must be easy to understand and read. State and federal law must be examined in conjunction with each other to ensure that all components of the facility's program reflect accurate practice. Legal review is required for this process.

Assessment criteria for monitoring compliance with the privacy regulations may include the following elements:

- Authorization contains the proper components.

- Authorization is signed as appropriate.

- Authorization is complete prior to release of information.

- Notice is accurately reflective of privacy practice.

- Notice was changed appropriately as policy was changed.

- Pertinent auditing programs are implemented and reevaluated as deemed necessary.

- A confidentiality statement has been signed as per facility policy.

Other Pertinent Information

Modification and changes to the privacy rule can and will be proposed and implemented. The process is defined in the regulations and can occur on an annual basis. Facilities should be mindful of when changes occur with any regulation or standard contained within the HIPAA requirements.

As mentioned earlier, state law may preempt the privacy standards. There is a formal complaint process defined within the privacy standards. Refer to the federal regulations for specifications and implementation provisions. (See figure 22.1.)

The facility must implement policies and procedures related to the privacy standard requirements. The policies must be reasonably developed in accordance with the facility's size and type of programs and services. In addition, they must be in language that is easily understood so that they can be implemented successfully. Policies must be updated, as indicated, to comply with changes in the regulations. If the policy changes, the notice of privacy practice must be reviewed and revised, as necessary, to be consistent with the standards.

Policies and Procedures

The following may be included in the list of policies that a facility may need under HIPAA privacy standards:

- Assigning and disabling access to systems and facilities
- Business associate contracts
- Chart order
- Computer tracking
- Computer usage
- Confidentiality statement
- Corrections, errors, omissions, and other documentation standards
- Crisis communication
- Data ownership (establish who owns the data for training and monitoring)
- Designated record set
- Documentation on discharge
- Documentation (general health record)
- E-mail
- Faxing
- Institutional review board
- Maintenance of resident records
- Media release
- Medical staff rules and regulations
- Minimally necessary

Figure 22.1.   General listing of privacy standard requirements

Uses and disclosures discuss the following components:
General rule
Minimum necessary
Restrictions
De-identified information
Business associate contracts
Deceased residents
Personal representatives
Confidential communications
Consistency of "notice"
Whistle-blowers

Organizational requirements:
Hybrid entities
Affiliated covered entities
Group health plans

Consent clarification (August 2002 rule):
Permitted uses and disclosures
Consent (not a requirement but may be used)
Treatment, payment, and healthcare operations

Authorizations:
Uses and disclosures
Psychotherapy notes
Core elements

Opportunity to agree or object:
Directory
Disclosure to family

Authorization not required:
Required by law
Public health activities
Victims of abuse, neglect, or domestic violence
Healthcare oversight activities
Judicial or administrative activities
Law enforcement activities
Coroners and medical examiners
Cadaver or eye and tissues donation
Research
Board approval of a waiver of authorization
Avert a serious threat to health or safety
Specialized government functions
Worker's compensation

Other:
De-identified information
Reidentification
Minimum necessary
Limited data set
Fundraising
Underwriting
Verification requirement

Notice:
Content (if used)
Provision of notice
Joint notice
Documentation

Restrictions:
Right to restrict
Terminating a restriction
Confidential communications

Access:
Right to access
Request for access and timely action
Provision of access
Denial of access
Documentation

Amendment:
Right to amend
Request for amendment and timely action
Accepting amendment
Denying amendment
Action on notice of amendment
Documentation

Accounting:
Right to accounting
Content of accounting
Provision of accounting
Documentation

Personnel designation:
Designation and documentation
Training
Safeguards
Complaints
Sanctions
Mitigation
Refraining from intimidating or retaliatory acts
Waiver of rights
Policies and procedures
Documentation

Transition provisions:
Effect of prior authorizations
Other than research
Research
Business associates
Deemed compliant qualification

Compliance dates:
Privacy rule was effective April 14, 2003.

- Password privacy
- Patient's right to amend individually identifiable health information
- Release of individually identifiable health information
- Resident to restrict individually identifiable health information
- Resident's access to individually identifiable health information
- Retention of records
- Security and privacy committee
- Security and privacy oversight
- Security and privacy program
- Telephone voice messaging

Security Standards

The HIPAA security standards provide protection for the transaction and privacy standards. They provide a mechanism to ensure that data are protected when shared electronically, and certain security mechanisms can ensure the privacy of oral and written health information as well. The security standards help safeguard data integrity and protect the confidentiality and availability of data when implemented correctly and used according to established policy. Each standard is either required or addressable as indicated in the regulation, giving the security standards a more flexible approach to compliance. Those areas that are identified as required must be instituted by the facility to ensure that implementation of the standards is completed.

Security refers to the technical measures taken to safeguard the confidentiality of health information. It supports data integrity, which is the property of accuracy and completeness of data—data quality. Proper security ensures that health information is available when needed for use or disclosure.

Purpose of the Security Standards

The purpose of the security standards is to provide those protective devices or methodologies that the facility will need to ensure that privacy is maintained as defined in policy. Under the security standards,

Covered entities must do the following:

- Ensure the confidentiality, integrity, and availability of all electronic protected health information, the covered entity creates, receives, maintains, or transmits.
- Protect against any reasonably anticipated threats or hazards to the security or integrity of such information.
- Protect against reasonably anticipated uses or disclosures of such information that are not permitted or required (DHHS 2003).

The security standards provide the infrastructure for secure EDI and protect elements contained within an electronic system that captures protected health information. These include such things as firewalls, virtual private networks, secure e-mail, and encryption capabilities as defined by facility need.

For consideration to meet the requirements of the security standards, the facility may choose to use other less-sophisticated technological computer techniques such as locks, employee ID badges, facility structure and access, padlocks, keyed or keyless entry systems, and safe combinations. Each of these, plus other security mechanisms, protects the privacy of resident information.

The security standards are comprehensive and coincide well with the privacy requirements; indeed, each supplements the other. The final security standards call for a "flexibility of approach" (DHHS 2003).

General Requirements

The security standards call for a risk assessment and gap analysis to be completed. Figure 22.2 provides the security matrix from the *Federal Register* to help facilities quickly see each required or addressable component of the security standards.

Importance of the Security Standards

Security mechanisms are those areas that are established to protect the electronic flow of information as well as methods to manage paper processes and oral communication more securely. Posting signs that remind individuals to be confidential is a security mechanism and thus one way to become compliant with the security standards. Of course, much more is needed, but this example provides a down-to-earth, less-expensive option to implement quickly and easily.

Security mechanisms exist today in all facilities. Locks on doors, visiting-hour requirements, health record processing, and job function delineation are all security mechanisms. Even in the paper world, job function protects the resident's right to privacy. The policy that defines who can document in the resident's record establishes security mechanisms for paper records. That is defined in job roles or job functions, so the written job description is a security mechanism, if used correctly. It is simply an access control.

The importance of security measures to protect resident privacy cannot be understated. The best devices and the best policies cannot always protect resident privacy when used inconsistently or followed improperly. For example, employee passwords should never be shared. The password is an access control that enables employees to complete their job functions and provide high-quality care or ancillary services to the resident. Sharing passwords is a breach of security and a breach of the resident's privacy.

One of the most important security mechanisms is the staff member, resident, volunteer, vendor, visitor, and student him- or herself. Following policies established to keep information private is key. Shouting resident names, talking over people to discuss resident conditions or problems, or open discussions about the resident are all breaches of compliance that can be eliminated through education.

Shift-to-shift reports must be done privately. The resident's mealtime in the community dining room is not the appropriate time or location to openly discuss his or her conditions. One of the most important security mechanisms is to think before sharing information in inappropriate areas or with individuals who do not have a need to know it. Staff, volunteers, and students must be made aware that information learned in the course of their work must remain in the facility; it does not go home to family and friends.

Security mechanisms do not have to involve expensive toys and tools; rather, they begin with the individual and progress to more sophisticated measures. It is important to keep in mind that about 80 percent of HIPAA addresses behavioral changes, not the acquisition of expensive devices or the development of lengthy policy.

Figure 22.2.   HIPAA matrix components

<table>
<tr><td colspan="3" align="center">**Appendix A to Subpart C of Part 164—Security Standards: Matrix**</td></tr>
<tr><td>**Standards**</td><td>**Sections**</td><td>**Implementation Specifications**
(R) = Required, (A) = Addressable</td></tr>
<tr><td colspan="3" align="center">**Administrative Safeguards**</td></tr>
<tr><td>Security Management Process</td><td>164.308(a)(1)</td><td>Risk Analysis (R)
Risk Management (R)
Sanction Policy (R)
Information System Activity
Review (R)</td></tr>
<tr><td>Assigned Security Responsibility</td><td>164.308(a)(2)</td><td>(R)</td></tr>
<tr><td>Workforce Security</td><td>164.308(a)(3)</td><td>Authorization and/or Supervision (A)
Workforce Clearance Procedure
Termination Procedures (A)</td></tr>
<tr><td>Information Access Management</td><td>164.308(a)(4)</td><td>Isolating Health Care Clearinghouse Function (R)
Access Authorization (A)
Access Establishment/Modification (A)</td></tr>
<tr><td>Security Awareness and Training</td><td>164.308(a)(5)</td><td>Security Reminders (A)
Protection from Malicious Software (A)
Log-in Monitoring (A)
Password Management (A)</td></tr>
<tr><td>Security Incident Procedures</td><td>164.308(a)(6)</td><td>Response and Reporting (R)</td></tr>
<tr><td>Contingency Plan</td><td>164.308(a)(7)</td><td>Data Backup Plan (R)
Disaster Recovery Plan (R)
Emergency Mode Operation Plan (R)
Testing and Revision Procedure (A)
Applications and Data Criticality Analysis (A)</td></tr>
<tr><td>Evaluation</td><td>164.308(a)(8)</td><td>(R)</td></tr>
<tr><td>Business Associate Contracts and
Other Arrangement</td><td>164.308(b)(1)</td><td>Written Contract or Other Arrangement (R)</td></tr>
<tr><td colspan="3" align="center">**Physical Safeguards**</td></tr>
<tr><td>Facility Access Controls</td><td>164.310(a)(1)</td><td>Contingency Operations (A)
Facility Security Plan (A)
Access Control and Validation Procedures (A)
Maintenance Records (A)</td></tr>
<tr><td>Workstation Use</td><td>164.310(b)</td><td>(R)</td></tr>
<tr><td>Workstation Security</td><td>164.310(c)</td><td>(R)</td></tr>
<tr><td>Device and Media Controls</td><td>164.310(d)(1)</td><td>Disposal (R)
Media Re-use (R)
Accountability (A)
Data Backup and Storage (A)</td></tr>
<tr><td colspan="3" align="center">**Technical Safeguards (see §164.312)**</td></tr>
<tr><td>Access Control</td><td>164.312(a)(1)</td><td>Unique User Identification (R)
Emergency Access Procedure (R)
Automatic Logoff (A)
Encryption and Decryption (A)</td></tr>
<tr><td>Audit Controls</td><td>164.312(b)</td><td>(R)</td></tr>
<tr><td>Integrity</td><td>164.312(c)(1)</td><td>Mechanism to Authenticate Electronic Protected
Health Information (A)</td></tr>
<tr><td>Person or Entity Authentication</td><td>164.312(d)</td><td>(R)</td></tr>
<tr><td>Transmission Security</td><td>164.312(e)(1)</td><td>Integrity Controls (A)
Encryption (A)</td></tr>
</table>

Source: DHHS 2003.

Documentation for Security Standards

Documentation is a key component of the security standards. The risk assessment and gap analysis must be documented and updated as appropriate. In addition, required business associate contracts must be maintained. The facility's contingency plan and disaster recovery plan are documents to follow as conditions arise.

Security standards call for policies concerning access controls to be in place. The facility must have a formal process for record management or processing. Moreover, an internal audit control must be done and documented, as must a security configuration.

Security breaches or incidents must be maintained and decisions documented. The security management process must be documented, maintained, and updated as necessary. Termination procedures must be in place, and training should always be documented to show proof of compliance.

At a minimum, designation of the person responsible for security should be contained in the job description and security and privacy program documentation. A listing of policies and procedures later in the chapter further defined documentation requirements of the security standards.

Quality Considerations

Privacy and security standard documentation should reflect the crossover requirements that exist in both sets of standards. Assess control and records processing should contain requirements from both sets of standards. Care should be taken to ensure that business associate contracts contain the appropriate language.

Auditing of access is a key quality concern. Facilities should consider developing a manageable auditing program. However, the program should not be so complicated that the auditing is too time-consuming. Development of this aspect of the security standards also is tied to the privacy standards auditing requirements.

Several areas in the security standards should be included in the auditing process. The facility must determine, based on its risk assessment, which areas to monitor for the most effective approach to compliance.

Assessment criteria may contain the following:

- Access control is accomplished according to policy.

- Disabling access occurs as required and is timely.

- Workstations are secure.

- Required controls are in place and are effective.

- Auditing program is continually monitored for effectiveness.

Information Technology Disaster Recovery/ Business Resumption Plan

The facility must have an information technology disaster recovery/business resumption plan in place. This plan may include the following components:

- Definitions of mission critical systems and inventory of business critical forms

- Up-to-date hard copy of all business critical documents

- Business critical procedures

- Defined minimum acceptable levels of service and minimum acceptable levels of system availability

- Prevention measures

- Backup procedures (hard-copy and local backup strategies; hardware, software, and network strategies)

- Recovery mechanisms and procedures ("hot site")

- Resources needed to support the recovery mode

- Human elements/team composition required to support the business critical functions

- Contingency plans, including responsibilities, authorities, and accountabilities

- Methods for quantifying degradation of service

- Media rotation schedules

- Physical and logical layout of the "hot site"

- Location of all critical reference manuals (on-site and off-site)

- Contact information (personnel, hardware/software vendors, utilities, and others)

- Work around procedures (referenced manual procedures of business critical functions, needed equipment, personnel required, services required, communications required to support the business critical functions)

- Emergency notification process and responsibilities

- Alternative work procedures, including a prioritized list of critical business interface

- Business continuity plan distribution, maintenance, testing, responsibility, and authority policies and procedures

- Security policy and procedure for transfer of media to an alternate facility

- Periodic testing of the plan

- Roles and responsibilities involved in executing the plan

- Hardware restoration and replacement procedures, including service requests, purchase orders, and supply chain

- Procedures for returning from alternate site, parallel processing, cut-over processing, and alternate site shutdown

- Asset management inventory

- Procedures for returning to normal operations

- Procedure for managing identified risks

Security Standards Matrix

The security standards matrix published in the *Federal Register* is a very good summary of the requirements contained in the regulation. (See figure 22.2.) It provides a quick reference or checklist for facilities to follow to ensure compliance with security standards.

Additional Considerations

Security and privacy have components that will overlap at times. If separate policies are developed to reflect the standards, both must be reviewed and revised when the regulations change. It is recommended that both sets of regulations be reflected in policy to make review more accurate and complete and to ensure compliance is achieved.

It is important to remember that security does not just address the electronic environment. Security mechanisms must be implemented and documented for the management of paper records as well as electronic records.

Policies and Procedures

The following types of policies may be considered when implementing the security standards:

- Access control, contingency plans, and disaster recovery programs (paper and electronic)
- Damaged record recovery
- Downtime for electronic systems
- Downtime procedures for specific departments, fiscal, health records admitting, and others
- Incident and termination process
- Internal audit process
- Media controls
- Personnel security
- Physical access controls
- Records processing
- Security configuration details and management plan
- Security management plan
- Facility security plan
- Training guidelines
- Workstation use and location

Summary

HIPAA contains three sets of standards: transaction standards, privacy standards, and security standards. The regulation contains language on resident rights and was developed to protect the privacy of each resident's individually identifiable health information.

HIPAA transaction standards are required for electronic data interchange used in healthcare claims processing. They provide one set of standards to manage healthcare claims to help lower healthcare cost, be more efficient, and ensure quicker reimbursement for the facility.

HIPAA privacy standards are required to protect the privacy of resident identifiable health information. They must be used for electronic as well as paper and oral information. The privacy standards require facilities to develop policies and procedures to ensure that the standards are met and assign someone responsibility for privacy oversight.

HIPAA security standards provide technical mechanisms to ensure privacy and to protect the EDI of claims submission. Security measures must consider electronic systems as well as paper records.

Every healthcare facility is required by HIPAA to provide training for all staff members, residents, volunteers, vendors, visitors, and students on the confidentiality and privacy of resident information. Moreover, the training should be documented.

HIPAA regulations are new additions to confidentiality and privacy issues that health information management professionals have experienced in the past. Most facilities will find that they already have several policies and procedures in place to help manage the HIPAA regulations. These facilities must review their policies and procedures and revise them to incorporate HIPAA language.

References

Administration Simplification. Available at http://aspe.hhs.gov/admnsimp.

American Health Information Management Association. Web site: www.ahima.org.

CPRI Toolkit. Available at www.himss.org.

Department of Health and Human Services. 1998. *Federal Register* 63, no. 155, August 12. Available at http://aspe.os.dhhs.gov/admnsimp/nprm/secnprm.pdf.

Department of Health and Human Services. 2000a. CFR Parts 160 and 162, *Federal Register* 45, August 17. Available at http://aspe.os.dhhs.gov/admnsimp.

Department of Health and Human Services. 2000b. *Federal Register* 65, no. 250, December 28.

Department of Health and Human Services. 2002. *Federal Register* 67, no. 157, August 14. Available at http://aspe.os.dhhs.gov/admnsimp.

Department of Health and Human Services. 2003. *Federal Register* 68, no. 34, February 20. Available at http://aspe.os.dhhs.gov/admnsimp.

Health Insurance Portability and Accountability Act of 1996. Available at http://aspe.os.dhhs.gov/admnsimp.

Glossary

Abnormal Involuntary Movement Scale (AIMS): A standardized form that can be used in facilities to document involuntary movements

Accidents/incidents: Those mishaps, misfortunes, mistakes, events, or occurrences that can happen during the normal daily routines and activities in the long-term care setting

Acknowledgment: A form that provides a mechanism for the resident to acknowledge receipt of important information

Activities of daily living (ADL): The basic activities of self-care, including grooming, bathing, ambulating, toileting, and eating

Admission agreement: A legal contract signed by the resident that specifies the long-term care facility's responsibilities and fees for providing healthcare and other services

Admissions and readmissions processing policy: A policy that provides the guidelines that are required when a resident is admitted or readmitted to the facility

Advance directive: A legal, written document that specifies patient preferences regarding future healthcare or the person who is authorized to make medical decisions in the event the patient is incapable of communicating his or her preferences

Advanced practice registered nurse (APRN): The term being increasingly used by legislative and governing bodies to describe the collection of registered nurses that practice in the extended role beyond the normal role of basic registered nursing.

Against medical advice (AMA): The discharge status of patients who leave the hospital after signing a form that releases the hospital from any responsibility or who leave the hospital premises without notifying hospital personnel

Alias policy: A policy that is implemented when resident confidentiality is required by the resident, family, or responsible party

American Health Information Management Association (AHIMA): Professional membership organization for managers of health record services and healthcare information

American Occupational Therapy Association (AOTA): The nationally recognized professional association of more than 40,000 occupational therapists, occupational therapy assistants, and students of occupational therapy

American Physical Therapy Association (APTA): The national professional organization whose goal is to foster advancements in physical therapy practice, research, and education

Analysis of discharged health records policy: A policy that outlines steps to be taken to process discharged resident records

Antipsychotic Dyskinesia Identification System: One of several standardized forms for assessing and documenting abnormal movements (of face, eyes, mouth/tongue, or body) that may occur in the course of treatment with some psychotropic medications; also called the Discus monitoring form

Antipsychotic medications: Drugs that are used in the management of psychotic conditions, bipolar disorders, or major depression with psychotic features

Assessment: A process used to obtain information about an individual who wants to receive healthcare services or enter a healthcare setting

Assessment reference date (ARD): The date (MDS data item A3a) that sets the designated end point of resident observation for all staff participating in the assessment

Authenticated: Confirmed by signing

Authentication: Proof of authorship

Authorization: The resident's formal, written permission to use or disclose his or her protected health information for purposes other than treatment, payment, or healthcare operations

Care plan: The primary source for ongoing documentation of the resident's care, condition, and needs

Census-reporting policy: A policy that outlines the process for census reporting and tracking

Centers for Disease Control (CDC): A federal agency that oversees health promotion and disease control and prevention activities in the United States

Centers for Medicare and Medicaid Services (CMS): A division of the Department of Health and Human Services that is responsible for developing healthcare policy in the United States and for administering the Medicare program and the federal portion of the Medicaid program; formerly called the Health Care Financing Administration (HCFA)

Certification/recertification: Medicare requirement for the physician's official recognition of skilled nursing care needs for the resident

Chargemaster: A financial management form that provides information about the facility's charges for the healthcare services it provides to its residents

Chart depletion policy: A policy that outlines the documents that can be removed, or depleted, from resident records over time

Chart order policy: A policy that provides a detailed listing of all documents and defines their order and section location within the health record

Chart-tracking/requests policy: A policy that outlines the way in which charts are signed out of the permanent files and how requests for records are handled

Commission on Accreditation of Rehabilitation Facilities (CARF): A private, not-for-profit organization that develops customer-focused standards for behavioral healthcare and medical rehabilitation programs and accredits such programs on the basis of its standards

Confidentiality: The controlled release of patient-identifiable health information to a care provider or information custodian under an agreement that limits the extent and conditions under which the information may be used or released further

Confidentiality policy: A policy that outlines the steps to take organizationwide to protect information about residents and the facility from unwanted disclosure

Consent: A means for residents to convey to healthcare providers their implied or expressed permission to administer care or treatment or to perform surgery or other medical procedures

Consent to restrain: A consent that is used in instances when the resident must be restrained to ensure quality of life

Correction, addendum, and appending health records policy: A policy that outlines how corrections, addenda, or appendages are made in the resident's health record

Current Procedural Terminology (CPT-4): A comprehensive list of descriptive terms and codes published annually by the American Medical Association and used to report diagnostic and therapeutic procedures and other medical services performed by physicians

Damaged record recovery policy: A policy that outlines the steps the facility should take to recover paper and/or electronic records in the event of a disaster

Discharge summary: A summary of the resident's stay at the long-term care facility that is used along with the postdischarge plan of care to provide continuity of care for the resident upon discharge from the facility

Do-not-resuscitate (DNR) order: An order written by the treating physician stating that in the event the patient suffers cardiac or pulmonary arrest, cardiopulmonary resuscitation should not be attempted

Downtime procedures for health records policy: A policy that outlines the steps the department should take when computerized equipment fails or systems are down

Durable Power of Attorney for Health Care (DPAHC): A third party designated by a competent individual to make healthcare decisions for that individual should he or she become incompetent

Electronic data interchange (EDI): A standard transmission format using strings of data for business information communicated among the computer systems of independent organizations

Electronic health record (EHR): A computerized record of health information and associated processes; also referred to as a computer-based health record in an ambulatory setting

Face sheet: Usually the first page of the health record that contains resident identification, demographics, original date of admission, insurance coverage or payment source, referral information, hospital stay dates, physician information, and discharge information, as well as the name of the responsible party, emergency and additional contacts, and the resident's diagnoses

Faxing policy: A policy that outlines the steps to take for faxing individually identifiable health information and business records and usually limits what information may be faxed

Focus: An organized form of charting narrative notes in which nursing terminology is used to explain the resident's health status and resulting nursing action.

Forms management policy: A policy that outlines the process for the creation of new forms

General consent to treatment: A consent signed upon admission to the facility that allows the clinical staff to provide care and treatment for the resident and that usually includes the resident's agreement to pay for the services provided by the facility, to assign insurance benefits to the facility, and to allow the facility to obtain or release health records for payment purposes; also called general consent

General health record documentation policy: A policy that outlines documentation practices within the facility

Health Care Procedural Coding System (HCPCS): A coding system designed to promote uniform reporting and statistical data collection of medical procedures, supplies, products, and services

Health Insurance Portability and Accountability Act (HIPAA) of 1996: The act that limits exclusions for preexisting medical conditions, prohibits discrimination against employees and dependents based on health status, guarantees availability of health insurance to small employers, and guarantees renewability of insurance to all employees regardless of size

Health record: A paper- or computer-based tool for collecting and storing information about the healthcare services provided by a healthcare facility to an individual patient

Health record committee policy: A policy that outlines the goals of the committee, the audit tools used, the number of audits required and specific time frames for their completion, and the results-reporting mechanisms

Health record department access policy: A policy that outlines employee access to the health record department and the chart-tracking mechanism for signing out records

History and physical (H&P): The pertinent information about the patient, including chief complaint, past and present illnesses, family history, social history, and review of body systems

History and physical documentation requirements policy: A policy that specifies the detail required in the history and physical examination done by the physician or physician extender

Incomplete records policy: A policy that outlines how physicians are notified of records needing signatures

Individually identifiable health information: The term used in the HIPAA privacy rule to indicate any patient-identifiable health information, including demographic and/or payment information, that relates to the past, present, or future condition or treatment of an individual and that can be used to identify the individual

Informed consent: A legal term referring to a patient's right to make his or her own treatment decisions based on the knowledge of the treatment to be administered or the procedure to be performed

Interagency transfer form (W-10): A form that contains sufficient information about a resident to provide continuity of care during transfer or discharge

***International Classification of Diseases, Ninth Revision, Clinical Modification* (ICD-9-CM):** A classification system used in the United States to report morbidity and mortality information

Joint Commission on Accreditation of Healthcare Organizations (JCAHO): A not-for-profit organization that offers an accreditation program for hospitals and other healthcare organizations on the basis of predefined performance standards

Liability files policy: A policy that outlines procedures for limiting access to, and maintaining the security of, information related to liability cases

Living will: A directive that allows an individual to describe in writing the type of healthcare that he or she would or would not wish to receive

Master resident index: A listing or database that a long-term care facility keeps to record all the residents who have ever been admitted or treated there

Master resident index maintenance policy: A policy that outlines procedures on the maintenance of the master resident index and the steps to take to verify and cross-check all entries

MDS processing policy: A policy that applies when health record personnel are included in the MDS data entry or submission of the MDS data

Medication administration records (MARs): Tools used to capture the delivery of drugs to residents

Minimum Data Set (MDS): The instrument specified by the Centers for Medicare and Medicaid Services that requires nursing facilities (both Medicare certified and/or Medicaid certified) to conduct a comprehensive, accurate, standardized, reproducible assessment of each resident's functional capacity

Minimum Data Set for Long-term Care (MDS 2.0): A federally mandated standard assessment form used to collect demographic and clinical data on nursing home residents

National Drug Codes (NDC): Codes that serve as product identifiers for human drugs, currently limited to prescription drugs and a few selected over-the-counter products

No carbon required (NCR): A designation indicating that a copy is unnecessary

Nurse practitioner (NP): A healthcare professional authorized to provide basic primary healthcare, diagnosing and treating common acute illnesses and injuries

Nursing assessment record (NAR): A form used to track residents' functional status and support the Minimum Data Set (MDS) process; also referred to as an activities of daily living (ADL) flow sheet

Nursing facility (NF): A comprehensive term for a long-term care facility that provides nursing care and related services on a 24-hour basis for residents requiring medical, nursing, or rehabilitative care

Nursing Home Quality Initiative: A six-state pilot project performed in 2002 by the Centers for Medicare and Medicaid Services (CMS) that identifies quality measures that reflect the quality of care in nursing homes

Nursing Home Reform Act: A part of the Omnibus Budget Reconciliation Act of 1987 whose purpose is to guarantee the quality of nursing home care and to ensure that the care that residents receive helps them to achieve or maintain the "highest practicable" level of physical, mental, and psychosocial well-being

Occupational therapy (OT): A treatment that uses constructive activities to help restore the resident's ability to carry out needed activities of daily living and improves or maintains functional ability

Off-site storage policy: A policy that details how and when records are processed for shipment off-site

Omnibus Budget Reconciliation Act (OBRA) of 1987:   Federal legislation that required the Health Care Financing Administration (now renamed the Centers for Medicare and Medicaid Services) to develop an assessment instrument (called the resident assessment instrument) to standardize the collection of patient data from skilled nursing facilities

Patient Self-Determination Act (PSDA):   Federal legislation that requires healthcare facilities to provide written information on the patient's right to be given advance directives and to accept or refuse medical treatment

Physical restraint: Any manual or mechanical device, material, or equipment attached or adjacent to a resident's body that restricts freedom of movement and prevents the resident's normal access to his or her body

Physical therapy (PT):   The field of study that focuses on physical functioning of the resident on a physician-prescribed basis

Physician assistant (PA):   A health care professional licensed to practice medicine with physician supervision

Physician extender (PE):   A professional such as a physician assistant or nurse practitioner who "extends" the services of the physician to ensure continuity of care as issues or concerns arise in the long-term care setting and the physician cannot be present

Physician query process: A communication tool and educational mechanism that provides a clearer picture of specific resident diagnoses when in question

Physician query process policy: A policy that addresses requests from physicians for additional information as part of the coding and reimbursement process

Physician's certification: A statement from a physician confirming a Medicare-eligible resident's need for long-term care services

Policy: A governing principle that authorizes or limits actions

Postdischarge plan of care: A care plan used to help a resident discharged from the long-term care facility to adapt to his or her new living arrangement

Preadmission Screening Assessment and Annual Resident Review (PASARR):   A screening process for mental illness and mental retardation that must be completed prior to a prospective resident's admission to the long-term care facility

Privacy: The quality or state of being hidden from, or undisturbed by, the observation or activities of other persons; freedom from unauthorized intrusion

Procedures: The steps taken to implement a policy

Progress note: The means to capture the physician's documentation, continuing care needs, and involvement in the resident's medical health status

Prospective payment system (PPS):   A Medicare payment for medical care that is based on predetermined payment rates or periods and linked to the anticipated intensity of services delivered and beneficiary condition

Protected health information (PHI):   Under HIPAA, individually identifiable information that is transmitted by electronic media, maintained in any medium (paper or electronic), or is transmitted or maintained in any other form or medium

Quality assurance (QA): A set of activities designed to measure the quality of a service, product, or process with remedial action, as needed, to maintain a desired standard

Quality improvement (QI): A set of activities that measures the quality of a service or product through systems or process evaluation and then implements revised processes that result in better healthcare outcomes for patients, based on standards of care

Quality indicator (QI): A standard against which actual care can be measured to identify a level of performance for that standard

Records disaster recovery policy: A policy that establishes how records should be handled in a disaster such as a fire

Records purging policy: A policy that is used in conjunction with the off-site storage policy

Records removal policy: A policy that outlines how and when records may be removed from the health record department

Records retention policy: A policy that specifies the length of time that health records are kept as required by law

Registered nurse (RN): A graduate nurse who has passed examinations for registration

Release of protected health information policy: A policy that outlines how residents and others may obtain copies of their health records

Resident assessment instrument (RAI): A uniform assessment instrument developed by the Centers for Medicare and Medicaid Services to standardize the collection of skilled nursing facility patient data; includes the Minimum Data Set 2.0, triggers, and resident assessment protocols

Resident assessment protocol (RAP): A summary of resident problems and care needs in long-term care settings

Resident record: A term frequently used in long-term care in lieu of health record

Resident's right to access: A term encompassing the mechanisms in place to allow residents to review their own health information

Resource utilization groups, version III (RUG-III): The proposed prospective payment system for long-term care

Respiratory therapy (RT): The practice involved in enhancing respiratory function for the resident

Restorative nursing care: Care that incorporates resident-specific programs that restore and preserve function to assist the resident in maximizing functional independence and achieving a satisfactory quality of life

Security: The physical safety of facilities and equipment protected from theft, damage, or unauthorized access; also includes protection of data, information, and information networks from loss and damage, as well as unauthorized access and alteration

Sentinel health event: A term used by the Joint Commission on Accreditation of Healthcare Organizations to describe an unexpected occurrence involving death or serious physical or psychological injury, or the risk thereof; usually stated simply as sentinel event

Signing out of health records internally to other facility departments: A collection of mechanisms to ensure that charts are tracked when taken out of the HIM department

Skilled nursing facility (SNF): A long-term care facility with an organized professional staff and permanent facilities (including inpatient beds) that provides continuous nursing and other health-related, psychosocial, and personal services to patients who are not in an acute phase of illness, but who primarily require continued care on an inpatient basis

SOAP: An acronym for a component of the problem-oriented medical record that refers to how each progress note contains documentation relative to subjective observations, objective observations, assessments, and plans

SOAPIER: A form of charting narrative notes that requires subjective, objective, assessment, plan, intervention, evaluation, and revision in the note structure

Specific consent to treatment: A type of consent that explains the potential risks and benefits of a particular treatment or procedure and constitutes the resident's permission to the healthcare provider to perform the treatment or procedure

Speech–language therapy (SLP): A treatment intended to improve or enhance the resident's ability to communicate and/or swallow

Subpoena policy: A policy that outlines the steps required to handle the subpoena processing for protected health information

Terminal-digit filing system: A health record filing system in which the last digit or the group of last digits is used, followed by the middle and last groups of numbers

Unapproved abbreviations policy: A policy that defines the abbreviations that are unacceptable for use in the health record

Unit numbering system: A filing system in which the same health record number is applied to the record for a resident each time he or she is admitted or readmitted to the facility

Index

(Continued on next page)

(Continued on next page)

(Continued on next page)

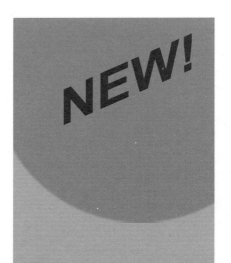
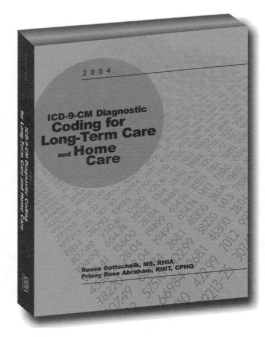
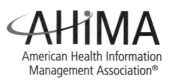

AHIMA Certification:
Your Valuable Career Asset

AHIMA offers a variety of credentials whether you're just starting out in the health information management (HIM) field, are an advanced coding professional, or play an important privacy or security role at your facility. Employers are looking for your commitment to the field and a certain competency level. AHIMA credentials help you stand out from the crowd of resumés.

- ✔ Registered Health Information Administrator (RHIA)/Registered Health Information Technician (RHIT)
- ✔ Certified Coding Associate (CCA), entry-level
- ✔ Certified Coding Specialist (CCS), advanced
- ✔ Certified Coding Specialist—Physician-based (CCS-P), advanced
- ✔ Certified in Healthcare Privacy (CHP)
- ✔ Certified in Healthcare Security (CHS), offered by HIMSS through AHIMA
- ✔ Certified in Healthcare Privacy and Security (CHPS), AHIMA in conjunction with HIMSS

In recent AHIMA-sponsored research groups, healthcare executives and recruiters cited three reasons for preferring credentialed personnel:

1. Assurance of current knowledge through continued education
2. Possession of field-tested experience
3. Verification of base level competency

AHIMA is a premier organization for HIM professionals, with more than 46,000 members nationwide. AHIMA certification carries a strong reputation for quality—the requirements for our certification are rigorous.

AHIMA exams are computer-based and available throughout the year.

Make the right move...pair your degree and experience with AHIMA certification to maximize your career possibilities.

For more information on AHIMA credentials and how to sit for the exams, you can either visit our Web site at www.ahima.org/certification, send an e-mail to **certdept@ahima.org,** or call **(800) 335-5535.**

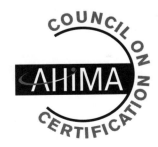